FRANK & JANET SHAW

KU-515-349

CHESHIRE

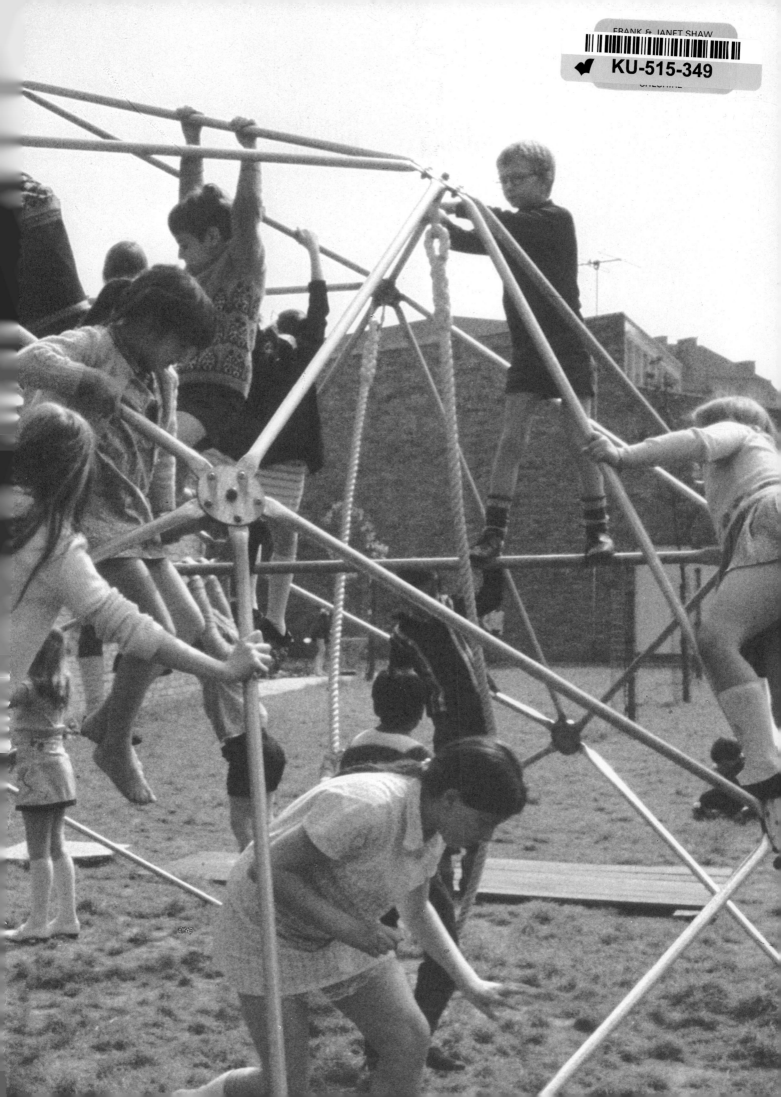

Family Health
An Illustrated Guide

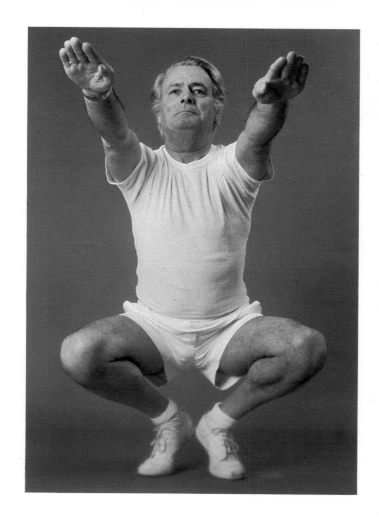

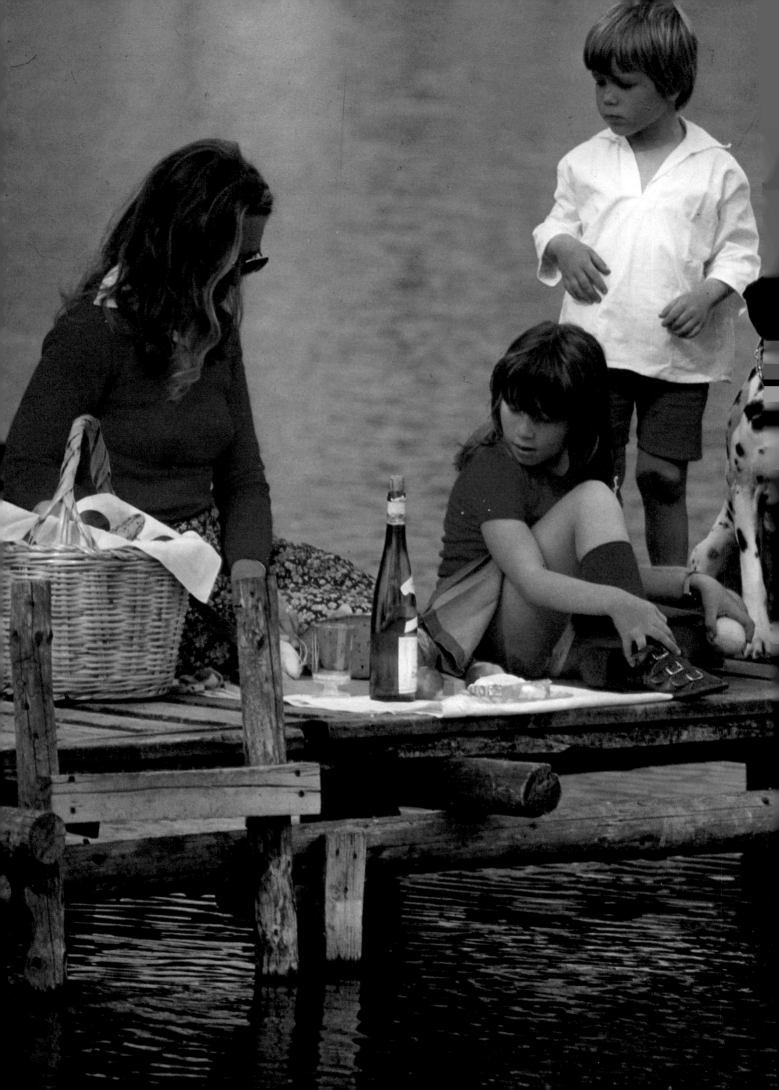

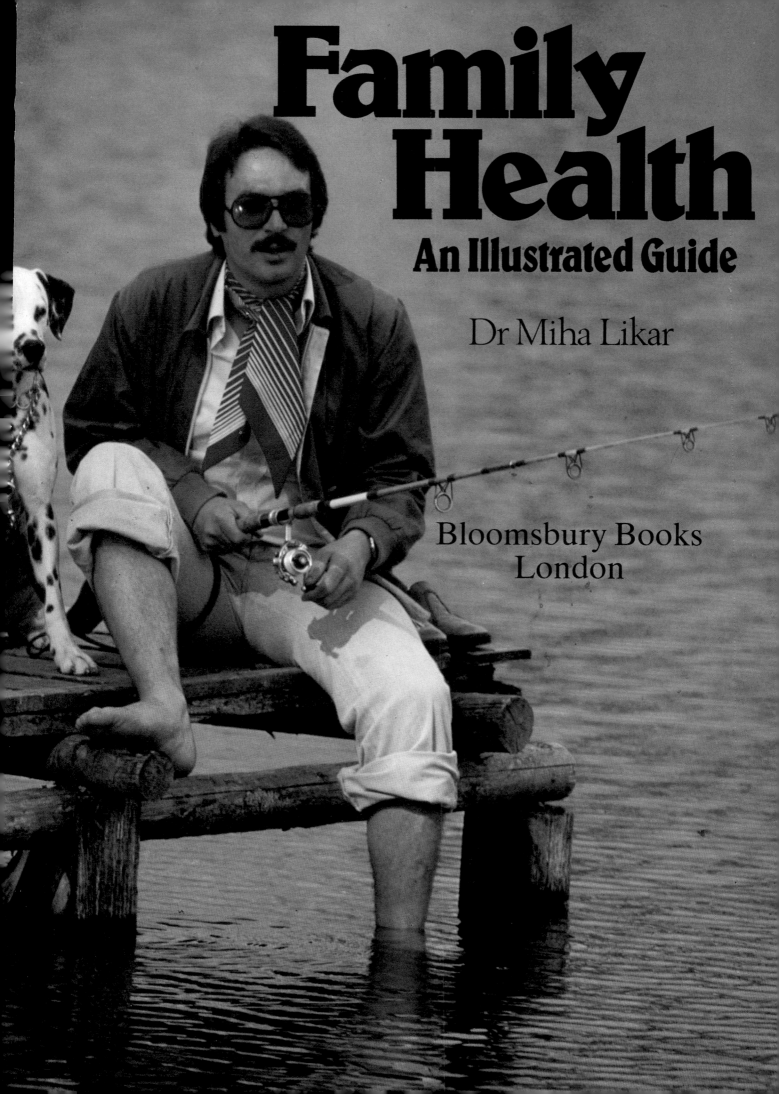

Family Health
An Illustrated Guide

Dr Miha Likar

Bloomsbury Books
London

© 1979 J. G. Ferguson Publishing Company USA

This edition published 1989 by
Bloomsbury Books an imprint of
Godfrey Cave Associates Limited
42 Bloomsbury Street, London, WC1B 3QJ
Printed in Hong Kong by Regent Publishing Services Ltd.
ISBN 1 870630 28 9

Introduction

Your family's health is precious and caring for it is a
major responsibility. The aim of this clearly written,
fully illustrated guide is to help you understand,
anticipate, and cope with a whole range of medical
problems. It covers general health and the particular
problems of each generation, from pregnancy and
childbirth, through the traumas of adolescence, to health
in the elderly. It discusses the major serious illnesses, how
they are treated, and the steps involved in undergoing
a surgical operation.
A sensible approach to health requires an understanding
of how the body functions. This is why a comprehensive,
but easily understood, section on human physiology
has been included. Prevention of illnesses is another
important factor, and the book also contains a program
for a healthier lifestyle. Finally, no guidebook to health
would be complete without a First-Aid section to enable
you to cope with the emergencies and accidents that
unfortunately occur so frequently.

Contents

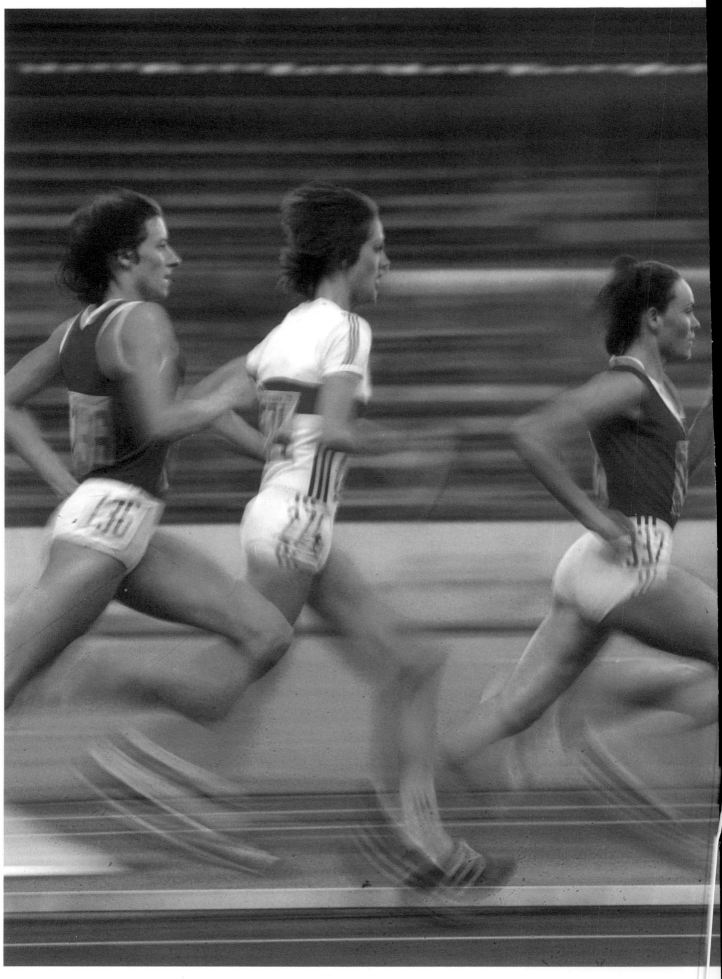

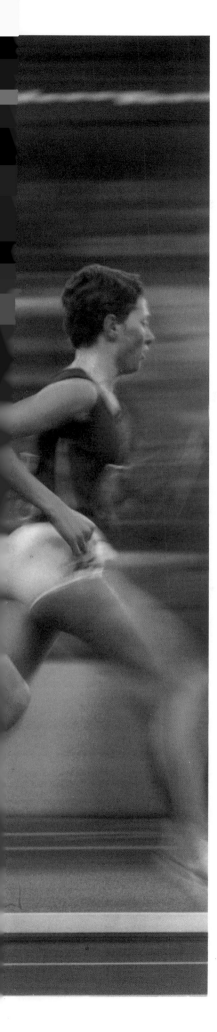

Chapter 1

Your Body as a Machine

When you take a car out on the road, as well as being able to control it safely, you should know a little of what goes on under the hood. This advice applies even more so when you are driving an infinitely more complicated piece of machinery – your own body. If we subjected our cars to the same abuse that we often inflict on our bodies we would be replacing them every month. The human body is very resilient but it does have one disadvantage over the car – it cannot be replaced. So, to keep your body in good working order, and to anticipate any breakdowns, you should have an understanding of each of its parts, and how they are combined to keep the whole organism running smoothly.

Opposite: stamina, endurance, and rigorous training have enabled the athlete to meet the physical demands of the track. It is the supreme example of a machine developed to operate at maximum efficiency.

Cells, the Units of Life

One of the miracles of human existence is that every person has developed from a single cell. And because our bodies consist of tissues made up of millions of cells, it is important to know something about these tiny compartments of living matter before we can understand how our bodies work, and before we can prevent diseases and keep ourselves healthy.

Nearly all cells have a nucleus which contains chains of deoxyribonucleic acid (DNA) molecules that form structures called *chromosomes*. Chromosomes contain the vital factors that play a basic role in determining our physical and mental characteristics; that is, they determine the ultimate specialized function of each kind of cell in the body.

In a healthy body, specialized cells are formed

Below: mitosis, the process by which a cell divides into two. Before the beginning of mitosis the chromosomes duplicate so that each daughter cell will have the correct complement of genes. The chromosome duplicates separate and move to opposite poles of the cell, a new membrane forms around each nucleus, and the cell constricts and splits in the center.

into groups that do the same kind of work. These groups are called *tissues*, which are also grouped into specialized organs or systems: respiratory tract, digestive system, heart and circulation, and many more. Muscle cells, for example, are fused into long fibers that make muscles move. Liver cells are shaped to do a different job: they convert foods into chemicals for the muscle cells to use.

The determining factors contained in every chromosome are called *genes* and the information they contain controls the formation of the proteins that are the foundation of all life processes. These proteins are built up from *amino acids* – often called the "building blocks of life."

The long molecule of DNA is made up of four kinds of units; or, described in another way, is a letter tapped out in Morse code in which there are two kinds of dots and two kinds of dashes. These dots and dashes always come in groups of three, and a group of three codes for a particular amino acid in the cell where it is then bound into a protein chain. In this way a string of protein is formed on tiny particles inside the cell called *ribosomes*, and a molecule of DNA types out, by a sequence of three (dots and/or dashes), the sequence of amino acids in a specific protein. It resembles a conveyor belt in an automobile assembly hall. If the DNA sequences are wrong, the wrong proteins will be formed and, since the genes are the basic units of heredity, diseases that may result can be passed on from

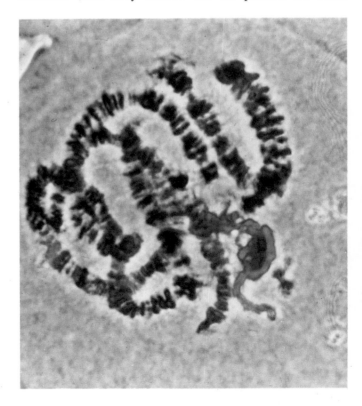

Above: giant chromosome from the salivary gland of the fruit fly *Drosophila*. The size of these chromosomes, due to repeated duplication along their length, makes them particularly useful for genetic research. The arrangement of genes along the length of the chromosome gives rise to the prominent pattern of transverse bands.

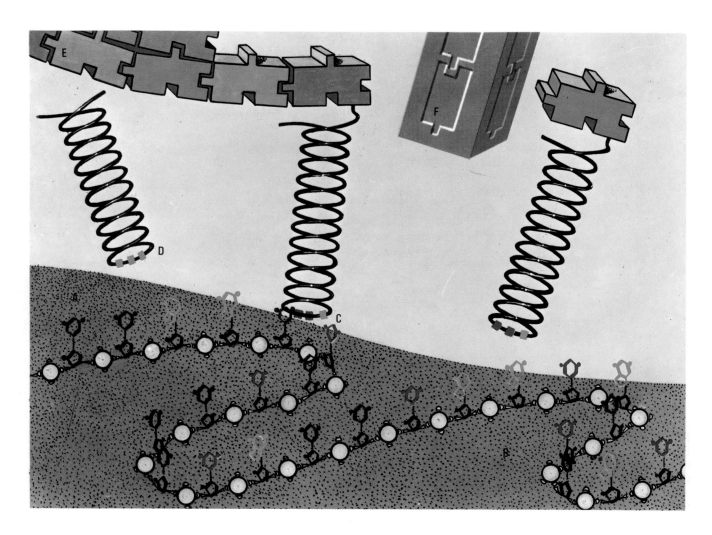

parents to their children. Sometimes the copying process itself goes wrong and a new DNA sequence results. Such a change is called a *mutation*. In the same way that changing a dot for a dash distorts a message in Morse code, most mutations are harmful.

Since the genetic code uses small molecules as its units, an enormous quantity of organized information is stored in the tiny chromosomes. This complexity is necessary because of our single-cell origin, and the information available must be enough to direct every step of the process of cell development into the varied and complex tissues and organs that make up the human body — and keep repeating the process for generation after generation.

Since the discovery of the genetic code scientists have been trying to modify it artificially. Some success with bacterial chromosomes has been achieved and similar success can be expected in the not too distant future in the fight against hereditary diseases. It would be wonderful, for example, if the gene which carries the information "you have hemophilia" could be artificially improved to become normal. Indeed geneticists have already succeeded in curing a small number of children suffering from a hereditary disease called *galactosemia* (increased quantities of galactose or "milk sugar" in the blood stream). They have done this by substituting a normal galactose metabolizing gene for a malformed one.

Above: A: ribosome, the site of protein synthesis. B: messenger RNA, a direct copy of the DNA 3-unit code. C: transfer RNA; it carries a specific amino acid to the site. D: 3-unit code on transfer RNA complements that on messenger RNA. E: amino acids combine aided by enzymes (F) to form proteins.

Below: a mutation in a cell during the early stages of development can result in striking differences in the same tissue, as for example, in this two-colored chrysanthemum. This type of organism is known as a chimera.

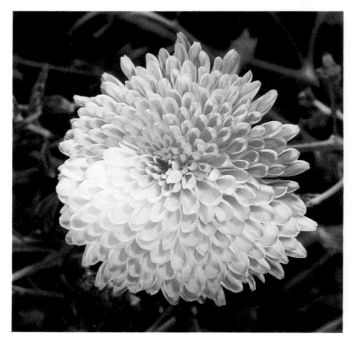

The Cycle of Life

The continuity of life depends on the transmission of living matter from parents to offspring. Man begets man in his own image, and the mechanism by which this occurs is remarkable. It was not until the middle of the 19th century that scientists discovered that when the male and female sex cells fuse they both contribute equally to the characteristics of the offspring.

Every cell in the human body contains a double set of 23 chromosomes and each set carries complete instructions for cell growth and development in specialized ways. One set comes from the sex cell of the father and another from the sex cell of the mother. It is the interplay between the two sets that determines the appearance and characteristics of the next generation. For instance, a sex cell with a chromosome carrying the gene for blue eyes may meet another carrying the gene for brown eyes. But as brown is dominant over blue, the child's eyes will most likely be brown. However, there is still a blue gene in every cell, and in some later generation it may find itself associated with another blue gene; in that case the new child will have blue eyes. Thus every generation carries the characteristics not only of its father and mother but also of all its ancestors.

Below: a spermatozoon in the process of penetrating the membrane of the ovum. The genetic material of both cells will fuse to produce a new individual with characteristics of both parents, a process known as fertilization. Among other things, fertilization initiates changes in the membrane of the ovum to prevent penetration by other sperm.

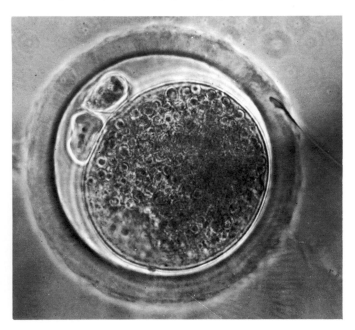

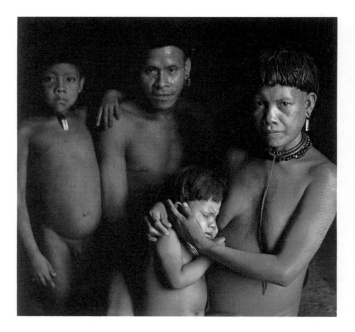

Above: during the early history of the human being, geographical isolation and adaptation to different climates resulted in the evolution of races with different genetic characteristics. Skin color, hair texture and facial structure are the most striking manifestations of this inheritance.

There are two different kinds of male sex cells, one containing a sex chromosome called X and the other containing one called Y. A woman has only one type of sex chromosome, called X. When a *spematozoon* (male cell) containing an X chromosome unites with an *ovum* (female cell), the offspring is female, but a sperm carrying a Y chromosome produces a boy. Sex determination is therefore determined by the man, and since the numbers of X and Y spermatozoa are roughly equal, this ensures that there will be roughly equal numbers of both sexes born.

An ovum is about the same size as a full stop on this page; a spermatozoon is about 20,000 times smaller. At birth, the *ovaries* of a girl contain their full complement of about 500,000 ova; no more are made subsequently. Between the ages of around 14 and 50 she releases about 500 ova; the rest degenerate. This is quite different from the way that male sex cells are formed. The production of spermatozoa starts at puberty, after the age of about 14, and goes on continuously up to the age of about 70, and often into extreme old age.

Once a month a single ovum (though occasionally two or more), escapes from an ovary and is conveyed down a duct called the *Fallopian tube*, which leads to the *uterus*, or womb. But it is only just after the ovum has escaped from the ovary that it can be fertilized by one of the spermatozoa that have swum in the opposite direction up the Fallopian tube after sexual intercourse. If this is achieved, the fertilized ovum, now called a *zygote* (but eventually to become a recognizable human *embryo* in the womb), travels down the Fallopian tube on its way to the uterus. But before it reaches its destination, it divides first into two cells, then into four and so on, so that by the time it reaches the uterus, about seven days later, it consists of a hollow sphere of many hundreds of cells known as a *blastocyst*. While the blastocyst is traveling down the Fallopian tube, the uterus prepares to receive it by thickening and developing a more concentrated network of blood vessels. The uterus knows what to do and when because it is affected by hormones from both the pituitary gland at the base of the brain and also from the ovary that sheds the ovum.

On arrival in the womb, the blastocyst literally attacks its wall, digesting its cells and burrowing in, until after four days it is finally embedded. During this period it feeds on the broken down cells and on the blood from ruptured blood vessels, but already it is converting this temporary source of material and energy into a completely new organ of contact between itself and the mother. This organ is a network of blood vessels, supported by connective tissue and coupled to the embryonic circulatory system that is by this time quite well developed. This network becomes intimately meshed with the blood vessels of the uterus, and provides a zone of exchange

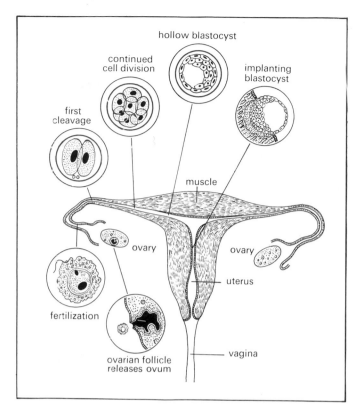

Above: the various stages of the fertilized egg as it passes through the oviduct to the uterus. During this stage of early pregnancy the cavity of the uterus is extremely small. Later it will stretch to accommodate the growing fetus and become more muscular in readiness for childbirth.

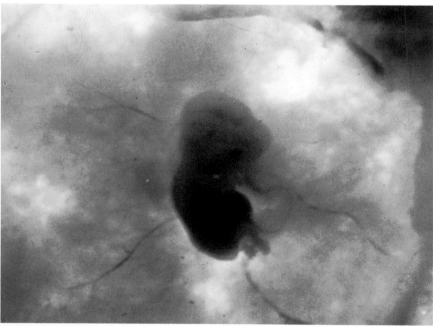

Left: a 6-week old fetus. By this stage the bulges of the heart and liver are discernible, and the brain, midbrain, and hindbrain have differentiated. The limb buds have elongated, and the ears and eyes have begun to develop. The fetus is enclosed and cushioned in a fluid-filled sac called the amnion.

between embryo and mother. However, the bloodstreams of embryo and mother must remain separate, because the mother's blood contains substances that would be harmful to the embryo and therefore must be held back. Carbon dioxide and nitrogenous waste are let out from the embryo into the mother's bloodstream, while food and oxygen travel in the opposite direction. The complete zone of exchange, with its blood vessels from both embryo and mother, is called the *placenta*. It is joined to the body of the embryo by the *umbilical cord*, and by this means the embryo lives a parasitic existence, making indirect use of the mother's organs of respiration, digestion and excretion, while its own

organs are shaping and growing in preparation for an independent life. At the same time the placenta also begins to produce hormones that, together with those of the pituitary gland and ovaries, prepare the mother for giving birth and suckling the newborn infant.

At the age of two months the embryo is clearly recognizable as a four-limbed human, and from then on until birth it is called a *fetus*. While it is growing and developing during the next seven months, the walls of the uterus become thicker and more muscular in preparation for the considerable effort that will be required to expel the fetus into the outside world.

Zones of Exchange

Throughout man's life, a number of chemical substances are in constant motion within the body. This process is essential, because most cells cannot wander about the body like single-celled animals in their environment. And if a cell is to stay alive and play its part as a member of one of the many body tissues, the incoming and outgoing of protein, sugar, water, salts and other dissolved substances vital to its well-being must be regulated to within very fine limits. The cell must obtain these substances from outside. It must also discharge into the tissue fluid either waste products or useful contributions to the body's welfare.

Therefore we have to think about what happens to these substances at the actual barrier between the cell and its surroundings, that is, at the thin cell membrane. Although their concentration is roughly adjusted before they reach the cells, the concentration of substances in the tissue fluid and in the cell itself is never the same. The cell membrane, therefore, is at one and the same time a selective barrier and an active agent of import and export that ceaselessly maintains a balance between the concentration of substances inside and outside the cell. It performs its tasks in several ways.

The simplest way that dissolved substances can pass through the cell membrane is by *diffusion*. This is the movement of a substance from a region of high concentration to one of low concentration, until the final concentration in the two regions is the same.

But only a few substances enter or leave cells by diffusion alone. Oxygen and carbon dioxide, for instance, cross the membranes by diffusion, and waste nitrogenous matter leaves the cells in the same way. But the cell membrane also works to "force" material into and out of the cell, just as an engine works to force an automobile up a hill against the

Below: representation of the cell-membrane sodium pump. This active transport mechanism has been postulated to explain how the cell maintains a low concentration (relative to the extracellular fluid) of sodium ions and a high one of potassium ions. The process obtains its energy from the high-energy molecules of adenine triphosphate (ATP).

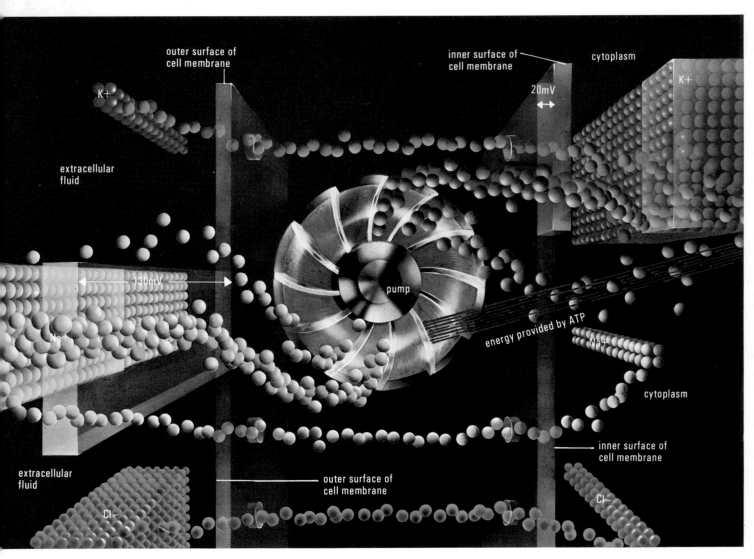

gradient. When this happens it is called *active transport*, or *active absorption*.

We can actually measure the energy consumed by cells in different parts of the body. Yet different tissues require different dissolved substances and in different quantities. Each gland has its special requirements. The needs of muscle cells differ greatly from those of nerve cells, and connective tissue lives at a very different tempo from that of the liver. Therefore each cell membrane not only pushes materials through "against the gradient," but also selects the correct weight of the particular dissolved substance that it needs at any one time. We often talk about energy being needed just to keep the body "ticking over," in contrast to the energy needed for muscular movement and body growth. We can be more precise about this and say that most of the energy used in keeping the body alive is spent on maintaining a critical balance of dissolved substances inside every cell.

The flow of water in and out of cells involves a different mechanism, called *osmosis*. The cell membrane is semipermeable, so called because it lets through the water but not the molecules of dissolved substances. The greater the concentration of dissolved substances inside the cell, the more the water will tend to enter it, and the force with which it does so is called the *osmotic pressure*. If too much water enters a cell it bursts. When water leaves a cell it collapses.

Certain cells of the complex human body have amazingly not altogether given up the type of feeding found in the simple amoeba. The membranes of these cells engulf fluids and fairly large particles, which then pass into the interior of the cell. This mechanism, called *pinocytosis*, when fluids are taken in, and *phagocytosis* in the case of solids, occurs in part of the alimentary canal and kidneys, and also in some white blood cells.

Thus we can see that although the cell membrane is extremely thin it is a complex and dynamic region, keeping the body's cells supplied with the correct balance of substances they need to function efficiently.

Right: electron micrograph of an animal cell. The double line corresponds to the protein layers of the membrane.

Below: amoeba engulfing a food particle by phagocytosis.

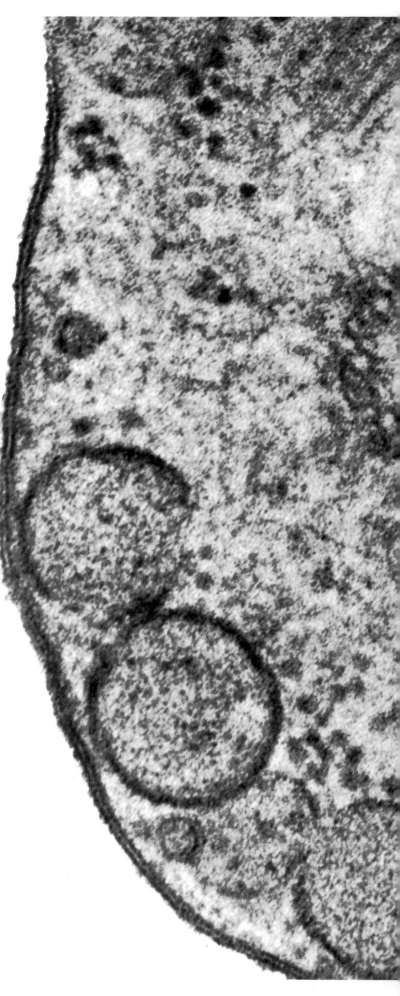

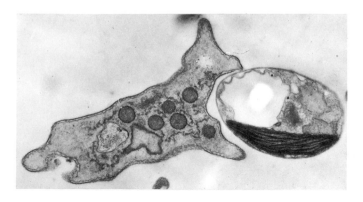

Tissue Specialization

Tissue consists of groups of similar cells that have been modified to perform specialized functions wherever they occur in the body. The degree of specialization depends on what the tissue is required to do. Tissues are classified into four major groups: conducting tissues, contractile tissues, supporting tissues, and lining and secreting tissues.

Excitability, the power to react to a stimulus, is a characteristic of all living tissues. A stimulus, such as that applied by an electric current at one site, may be transmitted to another part where it excites movement or other activity. A stimulus may also inhibit or diminish activity or movement. Although a property of all cells, excitability and its spread or transmission are especially developed in nerve and muscle cells. Conduction occurs not only from one part of the cell to another but also from one nerve cell to another, from nerve to muscle cells, from muscle cell to muscle cell in the case of some smooth muscle, and from nerve cell to secretory cell.

Nearly all motion in and of the body is the result of contraction of muscle cells. The finger movements of a pianist, the punch of a boxer, the beat of the heart, the expulsion of the fetus, and the constriction or dilatation of the pupil of the eye illustrate the variety of these movements. Muscular tissue must be capable of contractions which vary in speed, power, and extent. The different contractile func-

tions and methods of control are associated with differences in the structure of muscular tissues. In most mammals, including man, skeletal muscle makes up about half the body weight.

Connective tissues, such as bone, cartilage, fibrous tissue, elastic tissue, blood and lymph, make up a large part of the body. In spite of their variety, these tissue share the common property that their function is dependent on the quality of their *extracellular component* (the parts of the organ surrounding the cells). Supporting tissue consists of extracellular fluid, proteins and minerals which support the cells in their various organs, and by means of the bony skeleton support the whole body. Connective tissue contains cells which are responsible for manufacturing and maintaining extracellular material but they themselves play only a small part in its actual function.

Bile, urine, and intestinal contents are examples of fluids which are produced in the body, and they must be kept separate from each other and from the rest of the tissues. The cells whose function is to secrete and line are collectively called *epithelia*. In a

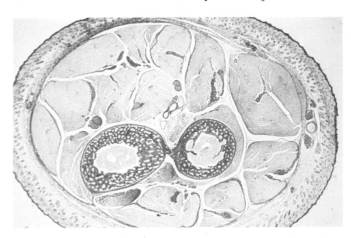

Above: developing bone in the leg of a young cat. Although bone is primarily a supporting tissue, the marrow contained in the center of limb bones has an entirely different function – producing blood cells.

connective tissue

muscle

blood

nerve

epithelium

bone

ligament

tendon

fat and areolar tissue

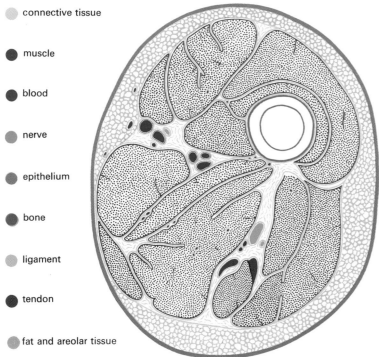

Left: cross section of a thigh, showing the arrangement of various tissues. Note the high proportion of muscle.

gland, the epithelium becomes specialized for a secretory rather than a lining purpose. The epithelia form both the internal and external surface of the body and they consist almost entirely of cells with little extracellular space and no contact with blood vessels. This uninterrupted layer cells is needed to control the passage of material across their surfaces, and they are separated from the underlying tissue by a layer called the *basement membrane.*

There is variation in the arrangement, shape, and number of cells which make up the various types of lining epithelium. This variety is due to functional requirements and the wide range of physical and chemical forces to which the surfaces are exposed. The external surface – the skin – is the most exposed, and is therefore covered with a strong *epidermis* (outer skin), the top of which consists of dry, dead, waterproof cells. Many of the moist internal surfaces of the body are lined with mucous membranes, for example the gastrointestinal tract. Mucous membranes usually contain glands of various kinds. The surface of the mucous membrane, sometimes called a *mucosa*, is kept moist by glandular secretions. The body cavities, housing the lungs, heart, and digestive organs, are lined by membranes that are kept moist by a thin film of fluid.

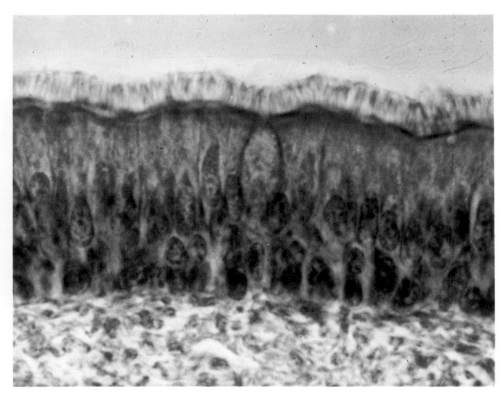

Photomicrograph of the trachea showing the mucous cells and ciliated epithelium. The cilia (fine, beating threads) move particles along while the mucus keeps the surface of the windpipe moist.

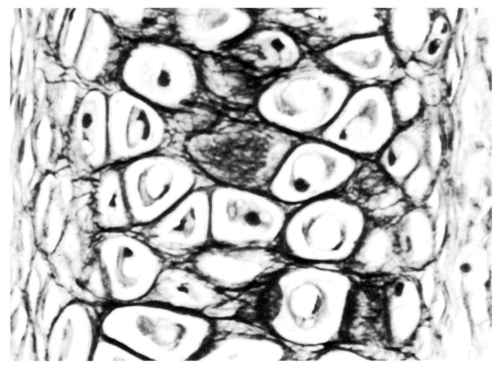

Cartilage, a connective tissue with a supporting function. This type, reinforced with yellow elastic fibers, is found in the ears.

Skin, our Outer Coat

Our bodies are encased in a tough, waterproof, elastic coat of skin. But skin does more than just protect us from the environment. It keeps us in contact with it by acting as a sense organ. It also enables us to adapt to the environment: a rich supply of blood vessels dilates or contracts depending on whether it is hot or cold, so that the temperature of our body remains constant.

Skin is a varied as well as a versatile organ. A baby's skin is dry, smooth, and clear, and cannot sweat very well. As the baby grows older marked changes occur. Blemishes appear and the sebaceous glands begins to secrete sebum. At puberty hair begins to grow more profusely and appears in previously hairless regions – the armpits, pubic region, and in men, on the face. As we get older our skin begins to show marks of use and abuse, and exposure to the elements. Hands become callused, wrinkles and lines become etched, and the skin loses its elasticity.

There are differences in skin between the sexes and between the races. Specialized cells in the skin produce a pigment called *melanin*. In darker skinned races more melanin is produced. This pigment protects the skin from harmful ultraviolet light, and in lighter skinned people can be seen to develop as part of the tanning process. It also collects in localized groups to form freckles and moles. The amount of melanin also determines the color of the hair and eyes. Some people, known as *albinos*, are born without the ability to produce melanin.

Skin consists of two layers: a thin upper layer or *epidermis*, and a thicker *dermis* which is richly supplied with blood vessels. The cells of the epidermis are continuously dividing and move up to the surface to replace the cells which are sloughed off or shed. They produce a protein called *keratin* which hardens the cells and is also the major components of hair and nails. The surface of the epidermis is thus covered with a protective horny layer of dead cells which waterproofs the skin and keeps out bacteria and harmful substances. The epidermis is particularly thick on the soles and palms – the areas subjected to the most friction.

Growing downward from the epidermis are tubular sweat glands, and follicles which produce hair. As the human being evolved, most of the body hair was lost and what remains has little function. The exceptions are the outcrops of hair in the armpits and around the genitals which reduce the friction around those sensitive areas.

In fur-covered animals hair serves to conserve heat. When the external temperature is low, erector muscles at the base of the hair follicles contract, raising the hair. This traps a layer of air which insulates the body. In humans the vestige of this system is the "gooseflesh" that appears when we suddenly get cold.

The dermis is bulkier than the epidermis and

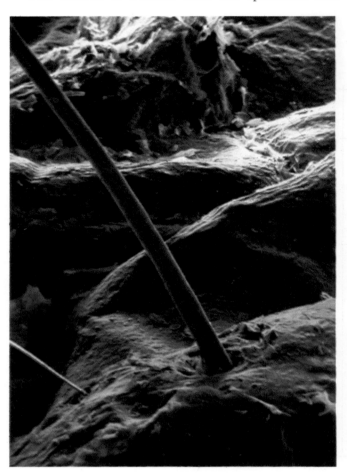

Highly magnified surface view of the human skin. The characteristic furrows and ridges become more pronounced with increasing age, use and weathering, and to the eye appear as a pattern of fine lines. This feature enables fingerprinting to serve as a means of personal identification. The other prominent features of the surface of the skin are hairs, pigmentation and pores.

contains nerves, sweat glands, and collagen fibers which give the skin its elastic properties. Below the dermis there lies the subcutaneous layer of fat, which further reinforces the skin's protective role. For that reason its thickness over the body is variable.

Because skin is visible its appearance and condition are of tremendous psychological importance. Not only has it generated a huge cosmetics industry, but any affliction, whether it is a symptom of an internal disorder or a disease of the skin itself, causes considerable distress. The effects of scars and disfiguring birthmarks illustrate this.

The skin harbors a large number of fungi, yeasts, bacteria, and numerous other creatures, most of which are harmless. In general unbroken skin pro-

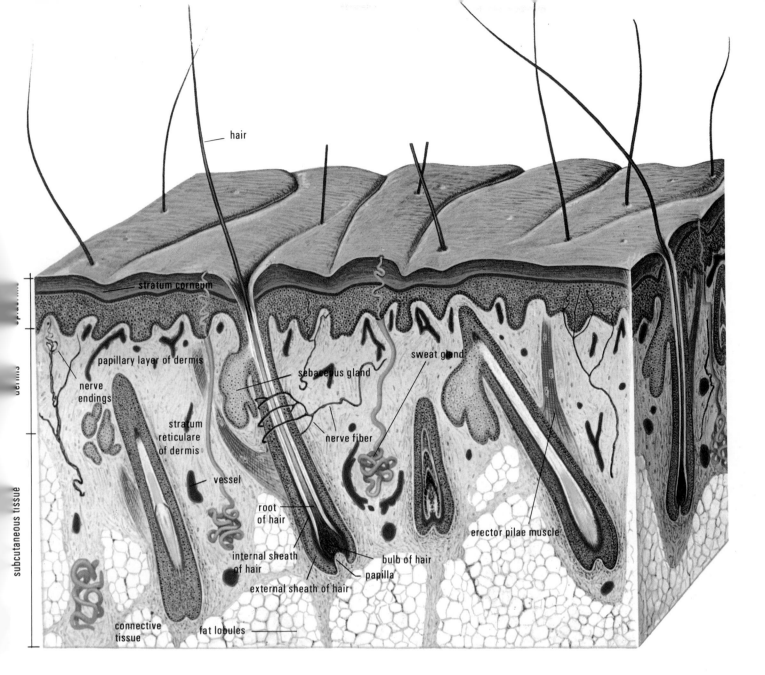

subcutaneous tissue

hair

stratum corneum

papillary layer of dermis

nerve endings

sebaceous gland

sweat gland

stratum reticulare of dermis

nerve fiber

vessel

root of hair

internal sheath of hair

erector pilae muscle

bulb of hair

papilla

external sheath of hair

connective tissue

fat lobules

vides a very effective barrier against infection; sebum and sweat are mildly antiseptic. Some parasites, however, burrow into the skin (scabies); or they puncture it to feed and can thus introduce dangerous viruses and bacteria into the body, as well as being highly irritating in themselves. These include fleas, ticks, and lice.

The majority of skin disorders come under the blanket term of *dermatitis*, literally an inflammation of the skin. This is often the response of the body to the presence of a substance to which it is allergic. The cure is usually to avoid the offending chemical, food, animal, plant, or whatever, but sometimes this is not possible. The body may become photosensitized by certain chemicals, in particular drugs, and every time the skin is exposed to sunlight a painful rash develops. Certain occupations carry with them the risk of *contact dermatitis*. Some people become sensitized to the chemicals that they have to come into daily contact with and develop highly irritating sores and rashes.

The constant renewal of the epidermal cells – on

Three-dimensional representation of the skin showing the epidermis, dermis and subcutaneous tissue, the sebaceous and sweat glands, the hairs, blood supply, nerve fibers, and nerve and nerve endings. Notice the angle of the hair follicles; contraction of the erector pilae muscles raises the individual hairs to a practically vertical position, so that they can trap an insulating layer of air.

average every month – can also produce problems. Most of the cells are shed, but they may collect in clusters on the scalp forming *dandruff*. They may multiply at an abnormally fast rate, resulting in the condition known as *psoriasis*. The epidermis may multiply faster than normal in response to physical pressure, producing calluses such as corns.

No skin disorder should ever be treated in isolation. The skin is an excellent monitor of the person's state of health and very often a disorder is the manifestation of an internal affliction. The cause may be a vitamin deficiency, an infection, an unsuitable diet, drug, or cosmetic, or an indication of a metabolic disturbance. The positive aspect of skin disorders is that at least there is no doubt of their presence.

19

Essential Materials

The cells and tissues of the body are not static structures. Tissue cells are continually being destroyed and replaced, and the substances within them replaced at varying rates. Many of the chemicals set free by the breakdown of substances within the cells are utilized again to manufacture new tissues. Some, however, cannot be used in this way and are lost in the *excreta* (urine and feces) and when the body perspires. These lost chemicals have to be replaced by a person's diet. In a healthy adult, who is neither gaining nor losing weight, the dietary intake of each of the elements must balance exactly the excretory losses. It is possible to know how much nitrogen, calcium, sodium, and potassium the body needs. It is also possible, but much more difficult, to determine the balance for other elements which form part of the structure of the body.

Carbohydrates provide the chief source of energy in most diets of a modern industrial community. They are found in such foods as cereals, vegetables and fruit, sugar, preserves and syrup, pulses and legumes. In a poor agricultural community, living mostly on cereals, the proportion of carbohydrates in the diet is higher and may be as high as 85 percent.

The chief carbohydrate is starch, which is present in all cereal grains, roots and tubers.

Some people may live on food entirely of animal origin, and have practically no carbohydrates in their diet. These include the Masai warriors of Africa, Eskimos, and South American gauchos. As these people are vigorous and healthy, carbohydrates are obviously not a dietary essential. The explanation is that the body can form glucose and derive energy from proteins and from fats.

Fats are the second largest source of energy in most diets. Fats are found in the tissue of animals and in plants, especially in the seeds. Fat supplies about 40 to 50 percent of the energy requirements of Western people. Many people living in underdeveloped countries get only a small amount of fat each day and their diets are almost always deficient in the fat-soluble vitamin A. Fat has an energy value more than twice that of carbohydrates and therefore provides a more concentrated form of energy. Polar explorers and others who need enormous amounts of energy may eat up to 10 ounces of fat a day, otherwise their diet would be impossibly bulky. Such large amounts of fat can be digested, absorbed, and used by the bodies of such active men.

Protein in the diet (contained in meat, fish, eggs, milk, and milk products) is essential to build up and replace body tissues. It is also used for the manufacture of many physiologically important chemicals. The protein requirements of children are relatively greater than those of adults. A newborn baby requires about five times as much protein as an adult per unit of body weight. This requirement falls as the rate of

	Essential Vitamins					
Vitamin	**A**	**B₁ (thiamine)**	**B₂ (riboflavin)**	**nicotinic acid**	**folic acid**	**B₁₂**
Source	Root vegetables and dark green vegetables; fish liver oils. Also in milk, cheese, eggs.	Bread, flour, potatoes, meat, vegetables.	Milk, eggs, cheese, and meat (especially liver)	Main sources are bread, flour, potatoes, fish, meat (especially liver).	Mainly green vegetables, liver. Also synthesized by intestinal bacteria.	Meat (especially liver), milk, eggs, fish. Very little in vegetables.
Function	Healthy respiratory surfaces. Needed for synthesis of visual purple; absence causes night blindness.	Energy reactions; absence causes depression and irritability, in severe cases, beri beri.	Energy reactions; lack causes sores and cracks near mouth, misting of cornea, etc.	Energy reactions; absence causes skin complaints, digestive upsets, mental confusion, pellagra.	Necessary for synthesis of nucleic acids.	Many enzyme systems. Necessary for healthy nerve cells; prevents certain types of anemia.
Vitamin	**B₆ (pyridoxine)**	**pantothenic acid**	**biotin**	**C (ascorbic acid)**	**D**	**E**	**K**
Source	Present in most foods, especially liver, cereals, peas, beans, yeast.	Liver, and in meat, cereals, milk and yeast.	Cows' milk, eggs, liver, yeast.	Fresh vegetables and fruits, especially citrus fruits; potatoes.	Liver, fish, margarine, butter, eggs.	Wheat germ, butter, cheese. Not very stable.	Green vegetables.
Functions	Present in several metabolic enzymes. Necessary for red cell formation, healthy skin and nervous system.	Present in enzymes concerned with carbohydrate metabolism. Health of skin.	Part of several enzyme systems.	Needed in large quantities, often deficient in the diet. Lack causes tiredness, and if severe, scurvy.	Essential for the absorption of calcium and phosphorus from gut. Absence causes rickets.	No evidence to suggest it affects fertility. Many other widespread effects.	Essential for normal clotting of blood.

growth declines, but young children need about two and a half times as much as adults and adolescents about one and a half times more.

Vitamins are organic compounds found in plant and animal tissue, some of which the body is unable to make itself and which must be supplied in the diet. Five major diseases – scurvy, beriberi, pellagra, keratomalcia, and rickets – are caused by a vitamin deficiency in the diet. In the past these diseases have been responsible for much ill health, and many deaths. Each can be prevented by the correct diet and they should no longer be a problem. However, although they rarely occur in the developed countries, they are still a major medical problem in many of the world's underdeveloped areas.

The body has three sources of *water*: the water present in food, the water drunk, and the water formed by the oxidation in the tissues of the hydrogen present in foodstuffs (called *metabolic water*). It is

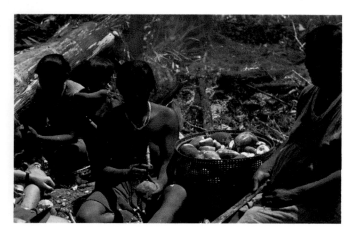

lost primarily in the urine, in the alimentary canal, and by evaporation from the skin (perspiration) and lungs. People cannot store water in the same way that some animals do. A normal adult man contains about 90 pounds of water in his body. If he is 4 pounds short, he is likely to be very thirsty. If he loses 8 pounds, he may well become very ill, and he will probably be dead before he has lost 18 pounds.

Certain minerals are essential to normal bodily function. The chief of these is common salt (sodium chloride). When the body is deprived of salt, the result is a reduction in the volume of the extracellular fluid and of the blood. Moderate salt loss can cause dizziness, fainting, weakness, and mental confusion. Severe deficiency leads to shock with a marked fall in blood pressure. A deficiency of potassium causes muscular weakness, dizziness, thirst, and mental confusion. It also interferes with the excitability of the tissues. Calcium is necessary for the formation and maintenance of bone, as is phosphorus. Iron is needed for the manufacture of the pigment hemoglobin, present in the red blood cells. Magnesium depletion is often present in people suffering from prolonged diarrhea, the chief features being depression, weakness, and increased irritability. In addition there are many elements that are present in minute quantities. These *trace elements* play a vital role in the body's wellbeing and must be replaced when they are used up.

The diet of the Makuna tribe, Columbia (left), is relatively high in carbohydrates. Meanwhile, that of the Eskimoes' (below), for whom whale meat is a staple food, is low in carbohydrate but extremely high in fat.

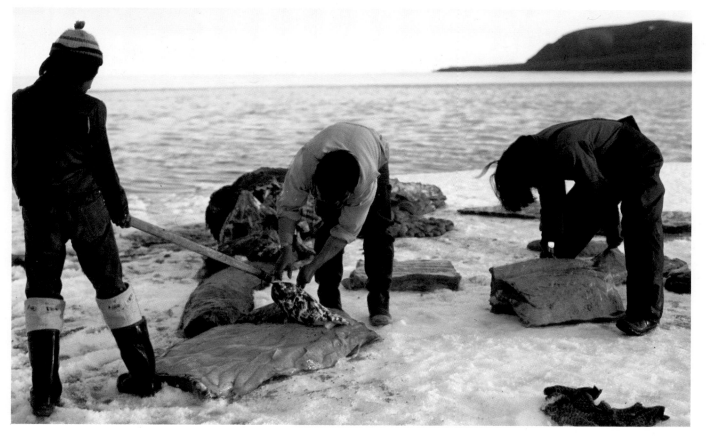

The Digestive Process

Digestion is the way in which the body breaks down food into the different chemicals it needs to re-generate cells and thus keep all the organs healthy. The breakdown of food in the stomach is only one of many processes by which its different parts are assimilated into the body from the *gastrointestinal tract* (stomach and intestines). The types of food in a diet vary greatly among individuals, depending on factors such as availability, economics, religious and social taboos, and personal taste. In general about 18

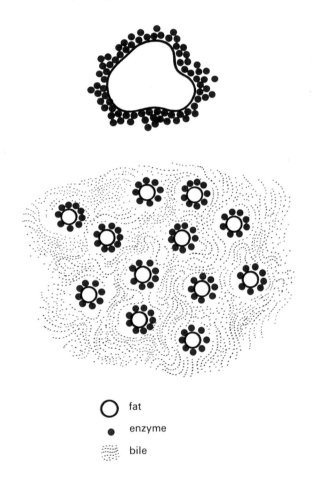

○ fat

● enzyme

⋯ bile

Large globules of fat are difficult to digest because the surface area : volume ratio is small (upper diagram). Bile (from the liver) aids fat digestion by emulsifying the fat into smaller droplets and presenting a greater surface area for attack by fat-digesting enzymes (lower diagram).

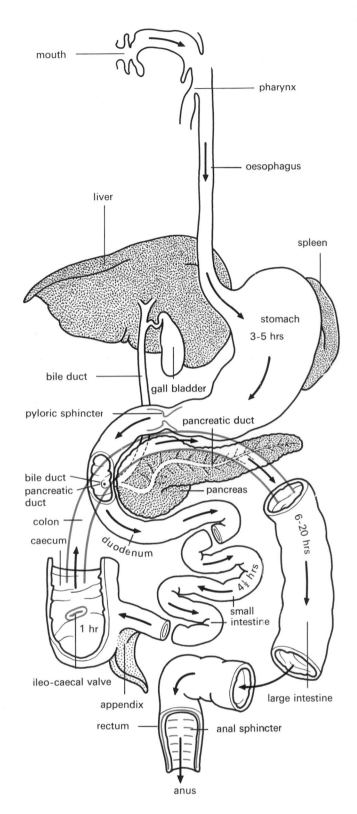

Passage of food through the alimentary canal. The primary motive force is peristalsis (circular muscle relaxes in front of the food and contracts behind it) starting in the esophagus. In the intestines it is coupled with a pendulum movement which mixes the contents.

ounces of solid matter and over half a gallon of water are taken in each day. This passes down the hollow muscular tube of the gastrointestinal tract and appears at its lower end, after an interval of 25 to 48 hours, as waste matter called *feces*.

The gastrointestinal tract forms part of the

alimentary canal, a long, muscular tube stretching from the mouth to the anus, lined with an epithelium which in some places is specialized for secretion of digestive juices and in others for absorption of food products into the body system. The main muscular coat of the canal is composed of layers of smooth

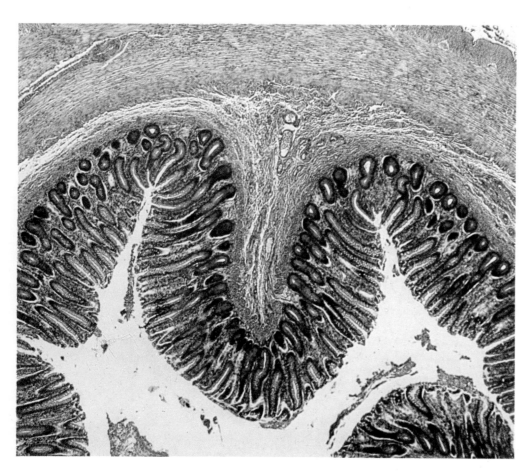

Left: transverse section of small intestine. Fingerlike projections called villi increase the surface area available for absorption.

Below: electron scanning micrograph of internal surface of small intestine, illustrating the villi. (Magnification ×200).

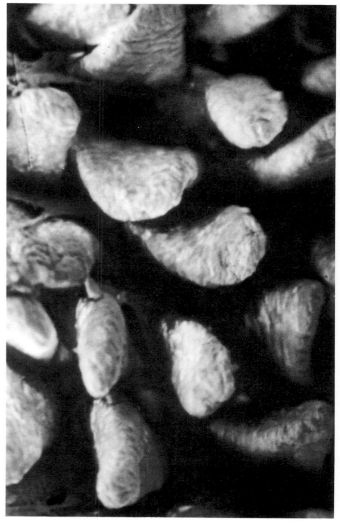

muscle which relax and contract to push food through the system. Much of the alimentary canal is covered with a *serosal* (thin, watery) layer. Blood vessels and nerves supplying the canal often travel in this layer before entering the muscle coat.

The alimentary canal has a large secretory capacity because in addition to many glands within its walls there is the group outside the tract consisting of the major salivary glands, liver and pancreas. Many pints of fluid are secreted daily into the interior cavities of the canal, most of the water being reabsorbed. Secretion occurs mainly in the upper part of the alimentary tract, from the mouth to the stomach; absorption occurs mostly in the middle zone, chiefly in the small intestine. The blood supply varies in different regions of the canal, but is very rich in segments that are busy secreting or absorbing, such as the stomach or small intestine.

A few minutes after a person has eaten a meal, food begins to leave the stomach, which is usually empty three hours later. On leaving the stomach the food passes fairly rapidly through the small intestine. Within about three to four hours the unabsorbed remnants of the meal begin to reach the *colon* (large intestine) and the residues of the various meals taken each day lie in the descending colon until they are expelled through the rectum. Defecation usually takes place once a day, but the variation is great and it is not abnormal for it to occur three times a day, or to be withheld for up to three days. The muscles of the alimentary canal regulate the passage of food to allow adequate time for digestion and absorption.

23

Transfer of Gases

The passing of gases into and out of the body – the taking in of oxygen and releasing of carbon dioxide and water vapor – is called breathing, or *respiration*. The lungs, the organs that perform this two-way exchange, are caged inside an ingenious atmospheric pump called the chest, or *thorax*. The thorax is walled in by the backbone, the breastbone and the ribs, along with the muscles that cover them. The *diaphragm* (a strong, dome-shaped muscle) separates the thorax from the abdomen.

In order to function properly the lungs need both a large surface area and an extensive blood supply. Both requirements are amply supplied. The lungs have altogether a surface area of 1000 square feet, and if spread out would cover a tennis court. This large area could not be achieved by simply having two hollow bags fed by numerous blood vessels. Instead each lung is infolded many times into about 300,000 round pockets called *alveoli*. These are the actual sites where gases are exchanged; they look like minute bubbles of air and give the lungs a foamy appearance. Large numbers of these alveoli are grouped together into sacs that lead into a tube called the *bronchiole*. The thousands of bronchioles join up

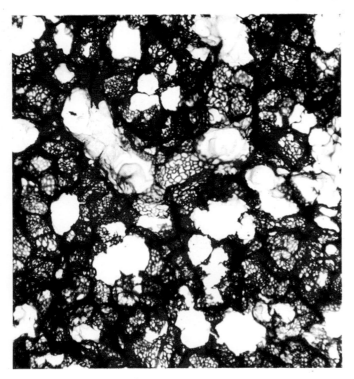

A section through a lung (×35). The spaces correspond to the bronchioles and air sacs. The granular appearance of the air sacs is due to their surface being convoluted into hundreds of compartments (alveoli).

repeatedly to form larger tubes. Finally, a single tube from each lung, called a *bronchus*, joins to form the windpipe, or *trachea*; this connects the lungs with the outer air.

The walls of the alveoli are extremely thin so that gases have the very minimum distance to travel between the alveoli and the blood. The alveoli are surrounded by a very dense net of blood capillaries that there is the maximum amount of blood available to collect and deliver gases from the lungs. The tubes and passages that connect the lungs with the outside also perform the vital service of air conditioning, by warming and moistening the incoming air. The *turbinates* (coiled tiny blood vessels) in the nose act like radiators on the walls of a room.

The trachea and the bronchi are lined with *cilia* (minute hairlike protrusions) and mucus. Small dust particles that have eluded the hairs in the nose become trapped in the mucus and, by the movements of the cilia, are swept up into the pharynx, where they are swallowed. Air reaching the lungs is thus practically dust-free, moist, and warm. The thorax is an airtight box. The lungs at all times occupy the available space within the box, and they are permanently connected to the outside air. The pressure of the atmosphere not only acts equally over the whole surface of the body, but also on the inside of the lungs. As the thorax expands, air flows into the lungs and distends them so that they fill the extra space.

This air enters the alveoli by diffusion, and oxygen from the air passes through the walls of the alveoli and enters the red blood cells. This oxygen-rich blood is transported to the heart and from here is pumped to all the body's cells. The cells use up the oxygen and give off carbon dioxide, which is returned to the lungs by the blood and enters the alveoli. When a person breathes out, the carbon dioxide is released and expelled from the body.

The amount of oxygen that the body needs depends on a person's activity. Muscle, for instance, requires over 40 times more oxygen when active than when at rest. The only way that the oxygen supply can be varied is by altering the depth and rate of breathing. Breathing at the normal rate of 15–20 times a minute, we pass in and out of the lungs the equivalent of 17 fluid ounces of air with each breath. During severe exercise, however, each breath may amount to as much as 140 fluid ounces, although with physical training this can be slightly increased. When we breath out the amount that remains in the lungs is quite large, about 100 fluid ounces. Thus the "fresh air" that we breath in is mixed with stale air already in the lungs.

During the course of a day hardly an hour goes by without some sharp break in our normal rhythm of breathing, because our emotions have a marked effect on the respiratory center of the brain. Laughter consists of repeated staccato expirations with a vocal accompaniment, alternating with deep inspirations.

Anxiety and fear give rise to rapid breathing, while mental concentration suppresses the breathing movements.

There is a very close interrelation between breathing and the voice. Sound is produced in the larynx, which is situated at the top of the windpipe. As soon as we wish to produce a sound, the vocal cords swivel so that they vibrate as air is forced past them. We vary the pitch and quality of the sound produced by pulling on the vocal cords with muscles and so altering the length and distance between them. In addition, the quality and loudness of the sound is modified by the resonance of the mouth, nose, sinuses, throat, and chest.

It is speech, though, and not mere sound, that is unique to humans. Although we are usually totally unaware of all the complex mechanisms involved, the continuous singing tone of the vocal cords is modulated, diverted and broken up by means of the epiglottis, teeth, tongue, and lips into an almost infinite variety of sounds out of which we build words and sentences.

A three-dimensional representation of the lungs showing their structural relationship with the trachea (windpipe). The left lung is divided into two lobes and the right into three. The tops extend as far upward as the neck, while the base of the lungs fits over the diaphragm. The lungs are separated from each other by the heart.

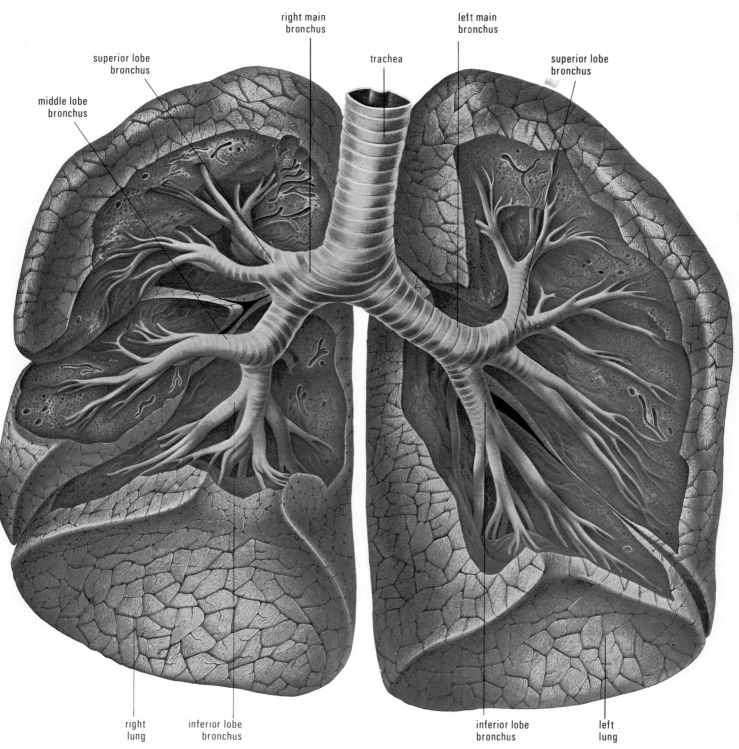

right main
bronchus

superior lobe
bronchus

trachea

left main
bronchus

superior lobe
bronchus

middle lobe
bronchus

right
lung

inferior lobe
bronchus

inferior lobe
bronchus

left
lung

Waste Disposal Units

The carbon dioxide and water that are produced in the body by the various chemical reactions do not present any great problems of excretion. They can accumulate without unduly harming the body. This is not the case with ammonia, produced from the breakdown of excess proteins. Ammonia is so poisonous that one part in 25,000 is fatal. Getting rid of this toxic substance is therefore restricted to one part of the body that is specialized to cope with this process. What happens is that proteins are broken down in the liver, first to amino acids, and then to ammonia. This is immediately converted into the relatively harmless substance urea, and is excreted by the kidneys, and also to a small extent by the skin during perspiration. But urea is soluble and must therefore be flushed out dissolved in water.

The excretion of water, salts, and urea through the skin, and of carbon dioxide through the lungs, is an uncontrolled process – that is, it goes on all the time regardless of how much water there is in the body. The only way of controlling excretion is by means of the highly organized kidneys.

The kidneys operate in two stages – a wholesale filtration process followed by a reabsorption of those substances that the body needs to retain. At each heartbeat, a quarter of the whole of the blood leaving the heart enters the kidneys through the *renal artery*. This vessel then divides into about a million *arterioles*; each of these goes to a funnel called the *Bowman's capsule*, which leads into a tubule, and the whole unit is called a *nephron*. Each arteriole divides into about 50 capillaries within the capsule to form the *glomerulus*. Blood enters the glomerulus at high pressure so that the smaller nonprotein components are forced through the capillaries into the cavity of the capsule. Every day about 50 gallons of filtrate are

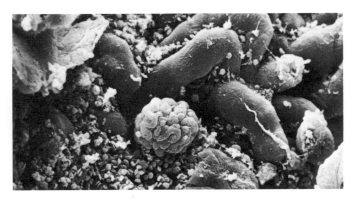

A surface view of the kidney glomerulus (center) and renal tubules. The platelike objects are red blood cells.

produced, equivalent to about two and a half times the weight of an average man.

The arteriole leaving the glomerulus winds around the kidney tubule, and it is from the tubule that reabsorption takes place. As much as 99 percent of the filtrate is reabsorbed. This is possible only because of the enormous total length of all the kidney tubules, amounting to over 34 miles. Amino acids, sugars, fatty acids, and glycerol are all useful and are totally reabsorbed. Salts are also reabsorbed but in varying degrees depending on their concentration in the body. Water is absorbed by osmosis (the process is called *osmoregulation*), again in varying amounts. Harmful substances such as urea are not reabsorbed at all.

The renal vein carries purified blood away from the kidneys for distribution around the body. The kidney tubules themselves unite to form a tube called the *ureter*. This transports what remains of the filtrate – now called *urine* – to the bladder and when the bladder is full, sense organs in its wall tell us it is time to empty it.

The osmoregulation performed by the kidneys is more important even than excretion, for although we can survive for several days without excreting urea, we cannot live for one hour if the osmotic pressure which depends on the amount of water and the concentration of dissolved substances, especially salts, deviates markedly. Our main supply of water is, of course, the watery component of what we drink. But the body loses a lot of water during the day. About 17 fluid ounces are lost by perspiration; 13 fluid ounces as vapor in expired air; 3 fluid ounces in the feces; and 50 fluid ounces as urine. The only conscious control that we have over this gain or loss is by drinking more or less. After a drink the kidneys serve as a fine adjustment, retaining or discarding water so that the correct amount remains in the blood and tissue fluids.

Just as important, the kidneys work continuously to maintain not only the total salt concentration but also a balance between the different salts, with an accuracy of 1 percent or even less. Some salts are needed for structural purposes, like bone building, and many processes work only in the presence of very exact salt concentrations. The heart, for example, stops if there is a small increase in the potassium concentration of the blood, and a small increase in magnesium puts us to sleep – an effect that is sometimes used in the anesthesia.

The normal way that kidneys function is by filtering a constant amount and by varying the reabsorption. The main influence on the kidneys, however, is hormonal. For example, a hormone called *antidiuretic hormone* (ADH) regulates water reabsorption and *aldesterone*, a hormone secreted by the adrenal glands, regulates salt reabsorption. The secretion of these two hormones is controlled from the brain's hypothalamus in which there are organs sensitive to the degree of dilution of the blood.

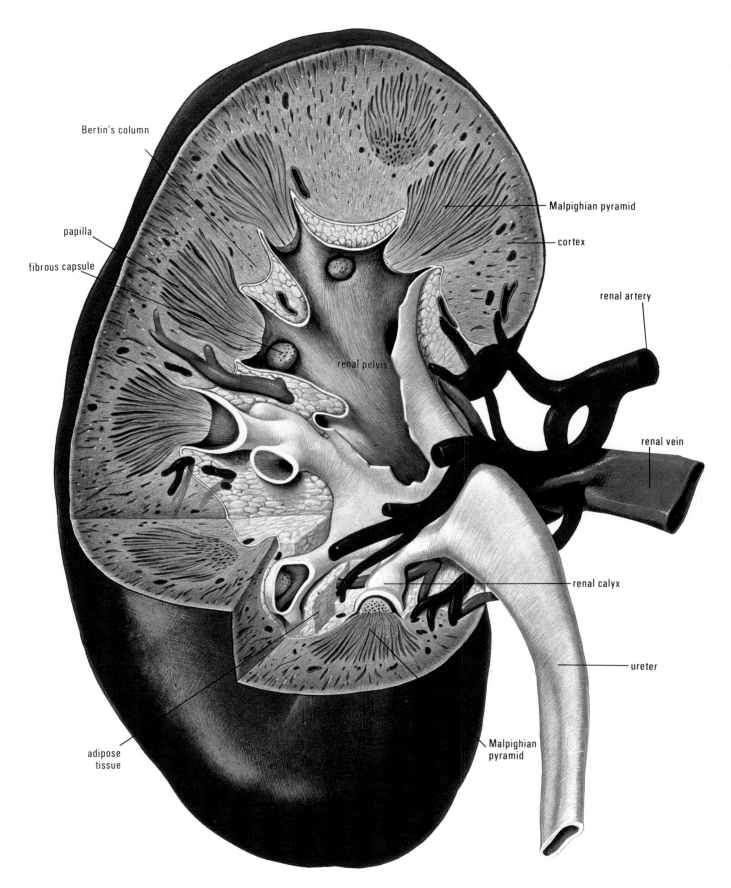

Bertin's column

papilla

fibrous capsule

Malpighian pyramid

cortex

renal artery

renal vein

renal pelvis

renal calyx

ureter

adipose
tissue

Malpighian
pyramid

Three-dimensional representation of the kidney. The outer
cortex contains the Bowman's capsules, and the distal and
convoluted tubules. The inner medulla contains many
Malpighian pyramids which consist of the loops of Henle
and the collecting ducts. The apexes of the pyramids project
into the renal pelvis, which is an extension of the ureter. The
entire kidney is enclosed in a fibrous capsule and embedded
in fat for protection.

Chemical Messengers

Organs or sets of cells that produce or secrete a useful substance such as saliva or bile, are called *glands*. But there are two kinds of glands. One kind, known as an *exocrine* gland, transports its secretions through a duct or tube to where they are needed. The other kind of gland has no duct; its cells secrete directly into the bloodstream. This second kind is called an *endocrine* gland and its secretion is a *hormone* (Greek *hormaein* – to stir up). These chemical messengers travel throughout the bloodstream to control the activities of other organs and such long-term activities as bodily growth and sexual development. They also maintain a constant balance between the activities of specialized organs to meet the needs of the body as a whole.

The endocrine system provides an alternative means of communication to the nervous system, and the two systems either act separately or supplement each other. The relationship between hormones and nerves is comparable to the communications system of an airport. Information and instructions destined for individual travelers are transmitted rapidly by telephone or teleprinter; these are equivalent to nerve messages. But certain kinds of information and instruction are broadcast to everyone over a public address system, and they are also flashed on closed circuit television screens, where they remain visible for some time; these messages thus reached a large number of people, though not all of them respond because they may not be concerned. These are the equivalent of the long-lasting hormone messages that are broadcast to every cell of the body.

Yet endocrine glands and the nervous system also work closely together, for endocrine activity is under the control of the hypothalamic region of the brain. Appropriate nerve impulses stimulate the hypothalamus to cause the release of hormones. This neuroendocrine cooperation is aptly demonstrated by the events that occur toward the end of pregnancy. When the *cervix* (the narrower outer end) of the uterus dilates, it initiates a nervous reflex. This excites hypothalamic neurones that terminate in the posterior lobe of the pituitary gland, often called the body's "conductor" because it regulates the whole "orchestra" of other endocrine glands. Its cells release among others the hormone *oxytocin* into the blood. Oxytocin causes the strong rhythmical contractions of the uterus which aid the birth of a baby. When the mother begins to feed the baby, a similar reflex stimulates another flow of oxytocin which causes milk to flow more readily from her breasts.

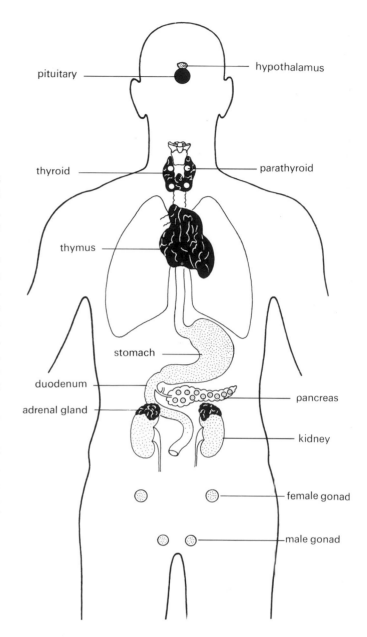

Location of the body's endocrine glands. The organs colored solid purple have a purely secretory function, while those stippled are tissues that secrete hormones in addition to their other functions.

When we feel frightened or angry, impulses from the hypothalamus travel down the spinal cord and excite other nerve cells – "sympathetic" neurones – which end in the *adrenal medulla*. The adrenals are a pair of small yellowish glands located just above the kidneys; the medulla is the central part of each adrenal. The adrenal medulla releases the hormone *adrenaline* into the bloodstream. It prepares the body for "fight or flight": the heart beats faster and more strongly, the air passages in the lungs and the blood vessels that supply muscles dilate, and the concentration of glucose (blood sugar) rises.

In a healthy person the neuroendocrine system is self-regulating. Excessively high concentrations of any particular hormone in the bloodstream suppress the activity of the gland that secretes it until the system is in balance again.

28

Hormones are needed only in very small quantities. However, they are quickly destroyed after completing their task. Some, such as ADH (antidiuretic hormone, which regulates the body's water balance), are excreted by the kidneys. This is just as well, for if hormones were not destroyed, their effects would go on for too long; it is easier to destroy them and replace them when needed. Some hormones are secreted in a daily rhythm; others, such as female sexual hormones, are produced in cycles of roughly 28 days, or in much longer periods when a woman is pregnant. Other hormones are produced at irregular intervals. For example, when we eat, the stomach, already stimulated by the prospect of food, secretes a hormone called *gastrin* that circulates through the bloodstream and back to the stomach, which is then stimulated to produce gastric juice. Here is an instance of an organ secreting a hormone to stimulate itself.

One of the most important side-effects of hormones is their effect on the central nervous system. *Cortisol*, for instance, strongly affects our mood and awareness of reality. Furthermore, many emotional disturbances activate the hypothalamus, which in turn disturbs the workings of the pituitary gland. If these disturbances go on for too long, the pituitary may be unable to resume normal activity, and the same applies to many other glands. The total behavior of man is thus controlled by the constant interplay of nerve impulses and hormones.

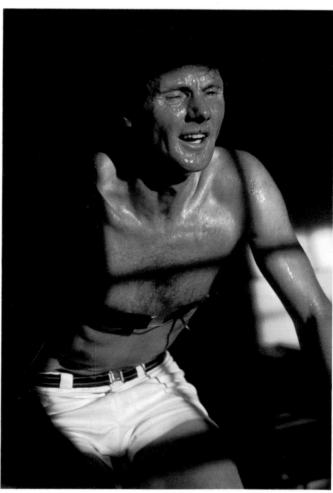

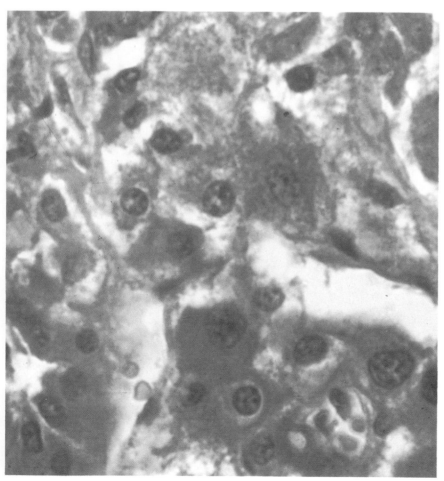

Above: in situations of stress the sympathetic nervous system stimulate the adrenal medulla to pour out large amounts of adrenaline. This hormone increases the heart beat, raises the metabolic rate and blood pressure, and stimulates breathing. The circulation of blood to the muscles is increased and the liver is stimulated to release more glucose. Adrenaline thus enables the body to cope with emergencies, and for this reason it is known as the "fight or flight" hormone.

Left: cells of the adrenal medulla, essentially a modified nerve ganglion. By secreting adrenaline it increases the body's efficiency and enables it to cope with short-term stress.

29

The Nervous System

These signals are small currents of electricity that travel along the nerve in a similar way to a current flowing through a telegraph cable. But unlike metal wires, nerves are not very good conductors of electricity. In order to keep signals large enough, nerve fibers have small "boosting" stations (called the *nodes of Ranvier*) at regular intervals. These nodes

If you have ever tried to make a doll stand up, you know how small a push it takes to make it lose its balance. In the living body, however, nervous control mechanisms make some muscles contract and others relax, so that the body retains its balance. In the muscles there are special cells, called *receptors*, that detect changes in the length of the muscle. When the body is pushed backward, some muscles are stretched and their receptors send nerve signals to the spinal cord. These signals then excite the nerves that control the muscles so that the stretched muscles now contract. The body is pulled forward and rights itself.

You can perform a simple experiment to demonstrate this mechanism. Sit with your knees crossed and tap your free leg just below the kneecap. If the tap is strong enough, it will pull on the tendon and slightly stretch the muscle above the knee. This stretch will excite the muscle receptors and the leg will kick forward automatically.

When you perform this experiment, you may be surprised by the speed with which it works. There is only a minute fraction of a second between the tap and the muscle contraction. In this time the nerve signals must travel to the spinal cord and then back to the muscle. Nerve fibers can do this because they are specially adapted to conduct signals at relatively high speeds of well over 300 feet a second.

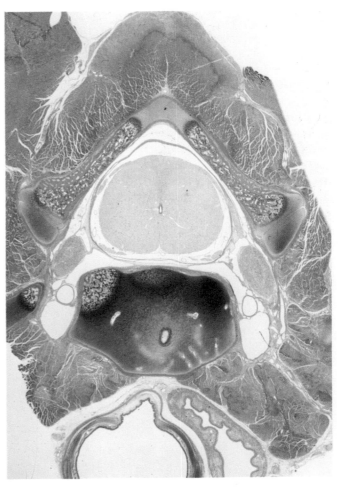

Above: a section through a vertebra. In humans, 33 vertebrae make up the vertebral column or backbone. In addition to acting as a support for muscles, the vertebral column protects the spinal cord, which runs as a continuation of the base of the brain. The spinal nerves emerge through gaps between the vertebrae.

Below: relaxed (left) and contracted (right) striped muscle filament. Voluntary muscle filaments consist of overlapping bands of the proteins actin and myosin. When a nerve impulse arrives at the terminal it releases a transmitter chemical which flows onto the muscle membrane and causes the bundle of actin and myosin to pull together.

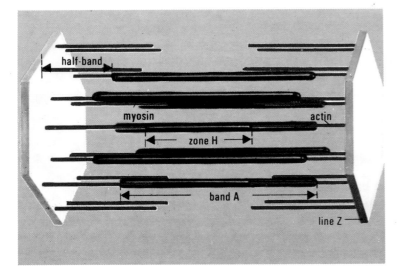

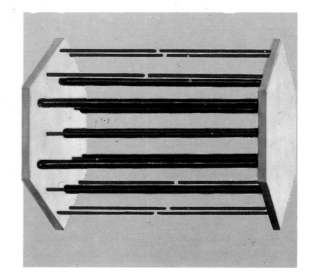

amplify the signal up to its original size before passing it on to the next node. When the signal reaches the end of the nerve fiber it causes the release of a chemical that excites the next nerve or muscle to which the fiber is attached. An electric charge takes place in the muscle and causes it to contract.

The brain and spinal cord consist of large numbers of nerve cells arranged in a complicated network about which scientists still know only a little. Some parts of the brain receive and analyze signals coming from the receptors. These are called the *sensory areas*. Other parts, the *motor areas*, send signals to the muscles and glands. There are, however, large areas of the brain that are neither sensory nor motor. It is assumed that these areas are concerned with learning, memory, and other higher activities.

Thus even when a person is performing a relatively simple activity, such as regaining his balance after stumbling, balance and stretch receptors are sending signals to the brain about the body's position in space and many different nervous mechanisms are brought into action.

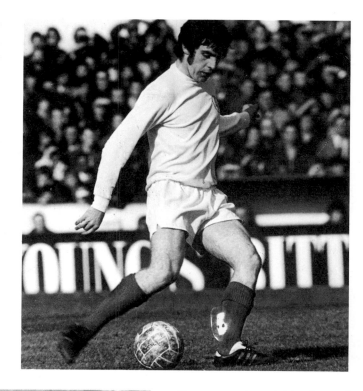

Above: certain activities demand an extremely high degree of nervous and muscular coordination. The brain perceives visual stimuli – the ball, or the position of the other players. Some of the footballer's resulting movements will be conscious – a result of his judgment – and part will be automatic (learned behavior). These activities are controlled by the central nervous system. Meanwhile the autonomic nervous system enables the body to cope efficiently.

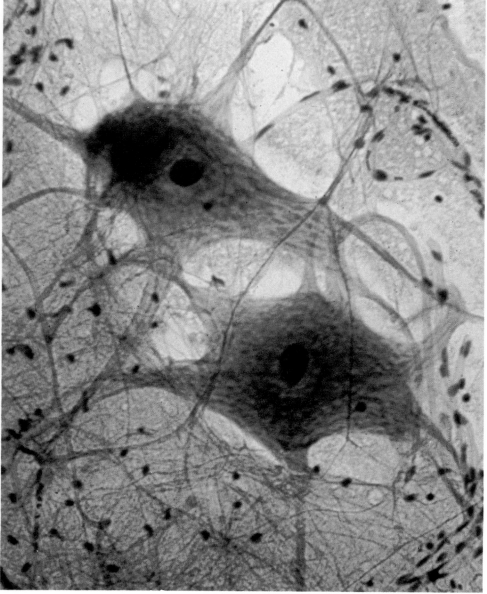

Left: two motor neurones (nerve cells) taken from the spinal cord. Radiating from the cell body are processes known as dendrites and a long fiber – the axon. The black knobs are synapses (connections) from afferent (sensory) fibers.

Muscles and Bones

Nearly everything we do depends on movement of one kind or another. Our way of life demands that we stand erect. We solve this problem, as well as that of moving the body about, by operating an elaborate system of passive structural members – the bones held together firmly by ligaments and

moved by active muscles. If we look at the bone-muscle complex with the eye of an engineer, we find that its design is almost perfect for its purpose. Each bone is the right shape and is strongest in compression, that is it can carry heavy loads imposed from either end. In this task it is eight times stronger than concrete. Protection against bending stresses is provided by muscles and ligaments that support the bone similar to the way struts and ties in a bridge absorb part of the load on the main beam at intervals along its length.

Bones are not dead and dry matter; the skeleton supports the body, protects the brain, heart, and lungs, manufactures red blood cells, and stores many essential minerals. Man's skeleton bears the hallmark of evolution which relates him to all other vertebrates, the animals with backbones. This feature is so familiar that it has become a part of everyday language. Someone who is weak and will collapse under pressure is often described as being "spineless" in many of the world's languages.

The skeleton can be divided into two distinct parts. The *axial* skeleton includes the skull, vertebral

tendon

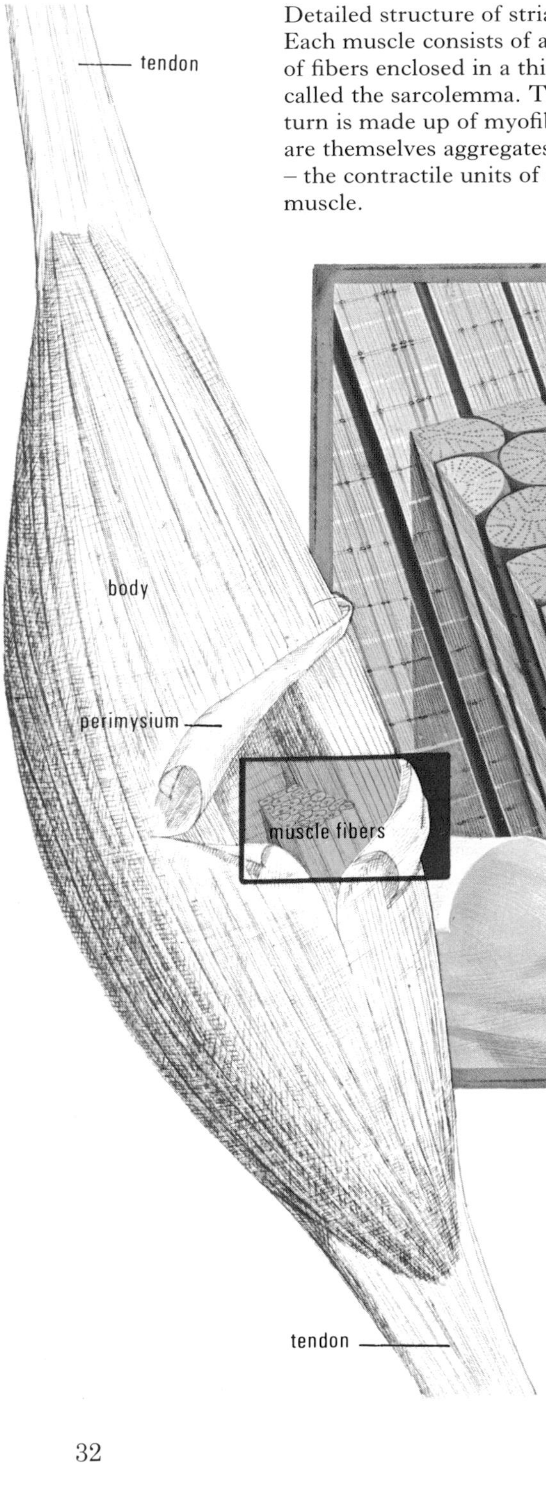

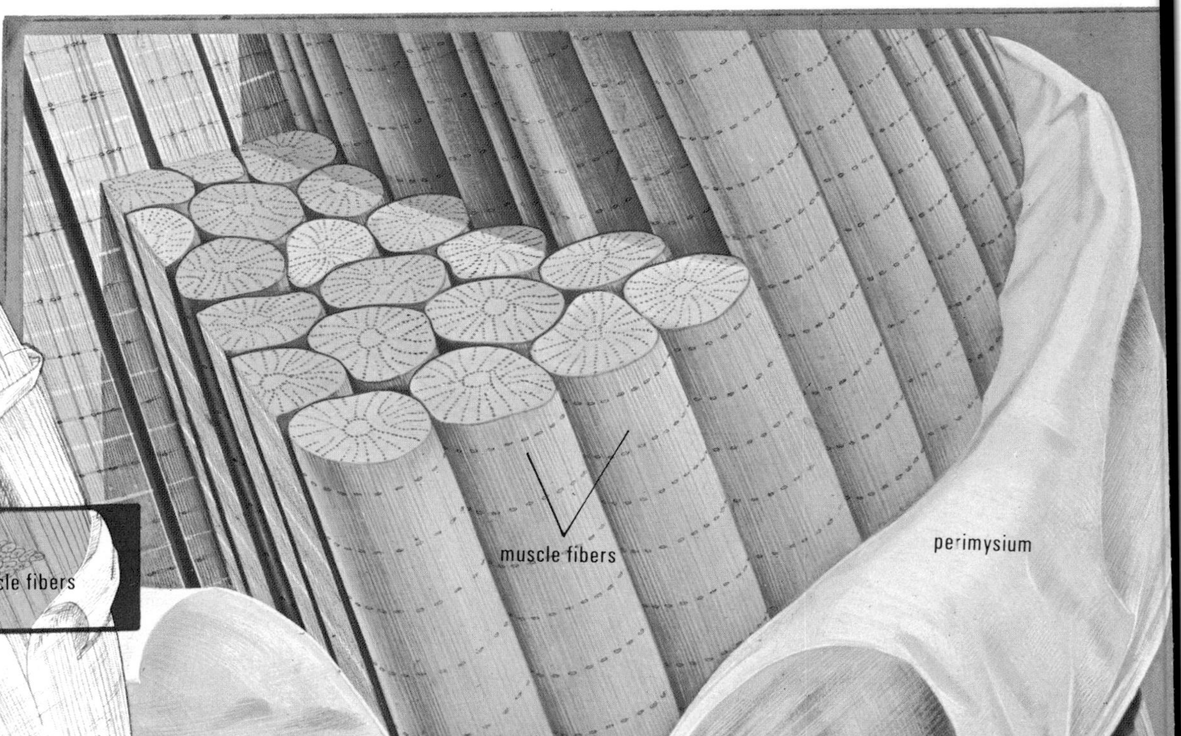

Detailed structure of striated muscle. Each muscle consists of a large number of fibers enclosed in a thin membrane called the sarcolemma. The fiber in its turn is made up of myofibrils which are themselves aggregates of myofilaments – the contractile units of striated muscle.

body

perimysium

muscle fibers

muscle fibers

perimysium

tendon

column and ribs; the *appendicular* skeleton is made up of the pectoral and pelvic girdles and the bones of the legs and the arms. Muscles are attached to the skeleton in pairs; while one contracts the other relaxes, and vice versa. In this way muscles can exert forces at opposite points, and thus move bones, and since bones articulate at joints the whole body becomes extremely mobile.

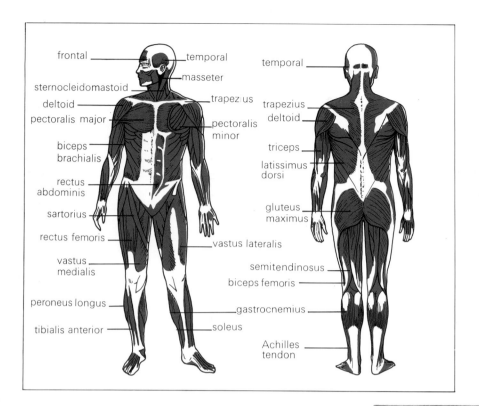

frontal
temporal
masseter
sternocleidomastoid
deltoid
trapezius
pectoralis major
pectoralis minor
biceps
brachialis
rectus
abdominis
sartorius
rectus femoris
vastus lateralis
vastus
medialis
peroneus longus
tibialis anterior
soleus

temporal
trapezius
deltoid
triceps
latissimus
dorsi
gluteus
maximus
semitendinosus
biceps femoris
gastrocnemius
Achilles
tendon

Left: illustration of a front (left) and back (right) view of a man, showing the main voluntary muscles. These skeletal muscles work in pairs; when one contracts the other relaxes. Flexors are the muscles responsible for bending large joints; extensors straighten them.

Below: striated muscle fibrils. The banding is due to the partial interlocking of actin and myosin filaments (see P. 30). As the fibrils contract the band pattern changes.

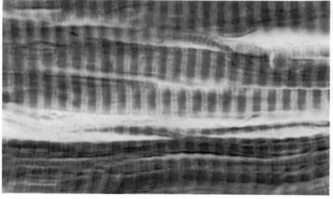

Each muscle is encased in a connective tissue membrane, which is continued at each end to form the tendons through which the pull of the muscle is transmitted to a bone. Because of their association with bones, the muscles that move the body are called *skeletal* muscles. Another way of distinguishing them from cardiac (heart) and smooth muscle is to call them *striated* muscles, because under the microscope such muscle tissue shows conspicuous transverse bands. Skeletal muscles are known as *voluntary* muscles and we have some degree of control over them. Cardiac and smooth muscle are *involuntary*, working entirely without our awareness.

Skeletal muscle works by contraction and consists of thousands of millions of long fibers, arranged in bundles, every fiber consisting of a great many tiny *fibrils*. These fibrils are composed of overlapping strands of the proteins actin and myosin. When stimulated, these strands slide against each other. This action repeated hundreds of times along the length of a single fibril results in a substantial shortening of its original length, and thus every time we make a movement thousands of parallel fibrils perform this shortening action.

The two ways in which muscles work are well illustrated in the effort of opposing tug-of-war teams. When the teams are perfectly matched, muscles contract without shortening. This is called *isometric* contraction. But when one side begins to win and pulls the other side along, the contraction of the winners' muscles produces movements by shortening, and this movement is called *isotonic*.

Nerves in the muscles branch over hundreds of muscle fibers: one nerve cell and its attached muscle fibers is called a *motor unit*, and it is the number of active motor units in a muscle that determines the force of contraction. But a muscle can contract with variable force, depending on how many motor units are employed at one time. There is another way in which the force of a contraction can be varied. A controlled muscular contraction is the response to a train of impulses that produces a sustained contraction called a *tetanus*. The serious disease called tetanus, or lockjaw, is caused by a type of bacteria entering the body and producing severe spasmodic muscle contractions.

The brain can vary the force of muscular contraction in two ways – by bringing a variable number of fibers into action, and by varying the frequencies of impulses in the motor fiber. One factor is obvious: a muscle cannot shorten if it is already fully contracted, nor does the brain try to tell it to do so. This means that the brain is well informed of the state of muscles, their position and degree of tension. The brain has up-to-the-second information on the position of the body in relation to its surroundings. So that the brain can be constantly supplied with this information, muscle receptors are at work ceaselessly day and night, all of our lives.

Temperature Control

Whether you play tennis on a warm summer day or ski on a day when the air temperature is below freezing point, your body maintains a temperature of about 98.4 °F. It has a "thermostat" that works a little like the mechanical thermostat that switches a heater off or on when the room temperature rises or falls from a predetermined level.

When blood flowing to the brain drops below normal temperature, receptors in the hypothalamus that serve as the body's thermostat go into action to restore the heat lost. But before this happens, an even quicker response is usually triggered off by receptors in the skin. They pass information to the hypothalamus that results in adjustments before appreciable changes in blood temperature can occur.

These adjustments affect both the source of all body heat – the burning of food in the body's cells – and the circulation of the blood which takes heat from the cells and carries it to the lungs and skin. If the body becomes too hot, temperature-regulating mechanisms cause the small vessels in the skin to expand; more blood flows through them and the air absorbs some of the excess heat.

Sweat glands throughout the skin are stimulated too. Sweat evaporation causes cooling and carries heat away from the skin – and therefore from the blood. If the air is hotter than normal body temperature, heat control depends entirely on evaporation. But if high humidity is coupled with high temperature, the sweat cannot evaporate into the air. In hot, moist climates ventilation with either moving air or dry air is essential. One can use either fans to set the

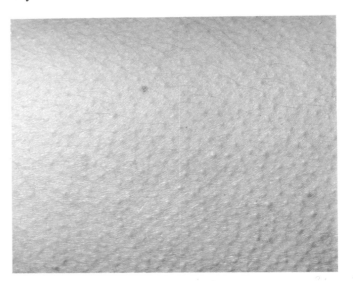

Above right: "gooseflesh" is all that remains in humans of the hair's role in temperature control. In furry animals the hair becomes erect in the cold, trapping a layer of air.

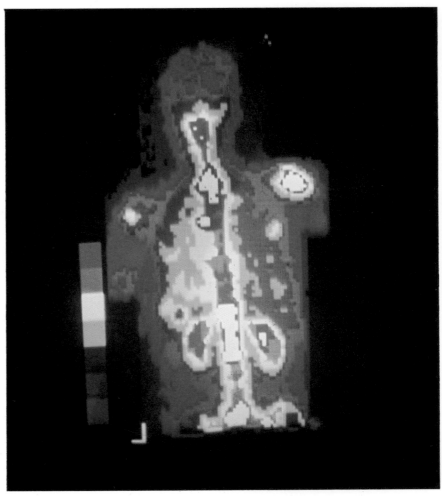

Right: thermographic infrared scan showing the distribution of heat throughout the body. White and yellow are the hottest areas, blue and green the coolest.

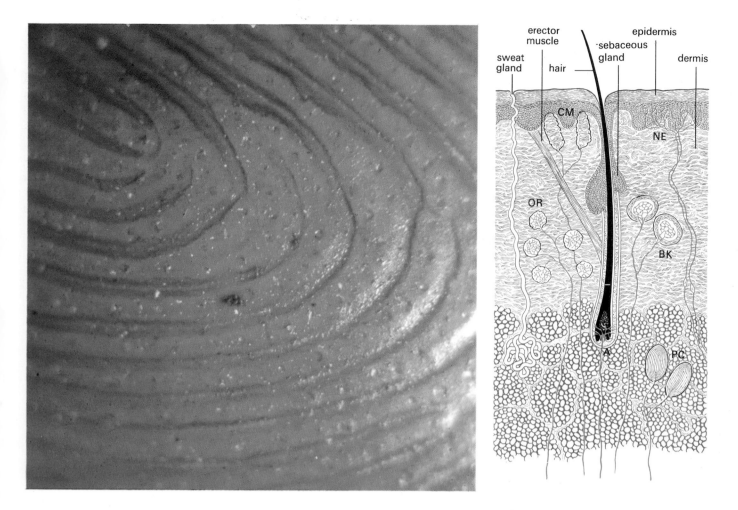

Above the diagram labels: erector muscle, sweat gland, hair, epidermis, sebaceous gland, dermis. Labels within diagram: CM, OR, A, NE, BK, PC.

Above: pores on the surface of the finger. **Above right:** skin receptors. NE: nerve endings (pain); CM: corpuscles of Meissner (touch); A: axons (touch); PC: Pacinian corpuscles (pressure); BK: bulbs of Krause (low temp); OR: Organs of Ruffini (high temp).

air in motion, or mechanical dehumidifiers and air conditioners to dry it.

When the weather is cold, the small vessels constrict and reduce blood flow to the skin, and more blood stays in the warm interior of the body. If the cold is intense, feet and hands unprotected by adequate clothing are especially vulnerable, since they depend for heat almost entirely on blood flow through the skin. Heat can be produced by exercise – since muscle contractions liberate heat – or by shivering – involuntary muscle contractions that are a kind of automatic "exercise."

When we exercise, many body cells need more of the oxygen and food supplied by the blood. Mechanisms located in the brain regulate blood pressure to insure an adequate blood supply. The heart beats faster and the selective enlargement (*vasodilation*) of small arteries called *arterioles* causes extra blood flow into the microscopically small capillary vessels that serve the muscles. Essential nourishment contained in the blood seeps through capillary walls in the form of *lymph*, the watery fluid that bathes all of our body's cells.

Without a control mechanism, local vasodilation would cause pressure to fall in the larger arteries,

endangering blood flows to the brain, heart, and other vital organs. What in fact happens is that arterioles elsewhere are constricted; those in the skin, for example, or in organs which, like the stomach, do not need an increased blood supply when the muscles contract and are active. The process depends on the elasticity of the blood vessels. "Hardening of the arteries," what are called *arteriosclerotic* changes of the artery walls, describes what happens when blood vessels lose this elasticity with age and cannot adjust to changes in blood pressure.

The control system's receptors are located in the large arteries that deliver blood to the brain. Without their constant vigilance, we would faint every time we got out of bed in the morning. Gravity, which influences circulation to a limited extent, would cause blood to rush from the brain as soon as we stood up.

Other receptors regulate breathing when there is either not enough oxygen or too much carbon dioxide in the blood on its way to the brain. They send impulses to the brain's respiratory center, which acts instantly to increase the size and frequency of the involuntary movements of the chest and diaphragm that make up normal breathing. More air is sucked into the lungs so that the blood flowing in capillaries can absorb oxygen through the thin walls. At the same time, the blood gives up carbon dioxide that is expelled when the lungs deflate.

35

The Body's Defenses

Mankind lives in an actively hostile environment. We have to face many dangers from the moment we are born. Some of our most vulnerable organs are protected by bone; the heart and lungs, for example, are caged within the ribs, and the central nervous system is heavily fortified. The kidneys, too, are embedded in a shock-absorbing mass of fat. The central nervous system, aided by receptors, helps us to avoid many hazards, while the experience and learning stored in the brain help us to choose whether or not we avoid danger or take a course of action that may lead us to it.

But our main defense is the normally unbroken shield of skin and the mucous membranes of the alimentary canal and throat. If the skin is pierced or burned, it creates a breach in the fortifications through which germs may enter. So the body closes the gap without delay; the blood provides its own plug by forming a clot, and later the surrounding tissues repair themselves. Mucous membranes, being delicate and moist, are more vulnerable than the skin, but they protect themselves by their own secretions; the surface of the eye is bathed in antiseptic tears; the salivary glands produce antibiotics; and the acid secretion of the stomach helps to sterilize our food intake.

However the defenses of the body's external surface are not completely effective. There still remains a variety of *pathogenic* (disease producing) bacteria and viruses that can penetrate the body. These cause illness either by disrupting the body's cells or by producing poisons called *toxins*. But defensive white blood cells are lying in wait. Some, called *phagocytes*, engulf bacteria and digest them. Other white cells, called *lymphocytes*, secrete special proteins called *antibodies*, which inactivate the germ or its poison.

These special proteins are worth looking at in some detail. Your body rejects a skin graft from another person (except from an identical twin) because it contains proteins called *antigens* different from your own. The body fights off foreign proteins by making special proteins called antibodies. Lymphocytes can manufacture antibodies that in some way match the foreign bodies, like a key fits its lock, so that a combination of the two renders the antigen harmless. And since most of the foreign proteins that invade the body are bacterial or viral, the ability to make antibodies is one of our main lines of defense against disease.

We can now follow what happens in the battle that takes place when pathogenic organisms attack the body in numbers sufficient to make us ill. In a local infection, such as a wound or a boil, we can feel and see more of what is happening. The first symptom is redness and heat, as local vasodilation brings more blood and hence more blood cells to the site of the infection. Then, as toxins begin to circulate, the bone marrow and lymph nodes are stimulated to produce extra reserves of white cells.

Because the germs multiply at a tremendous rate, the white cells and antibodies have to destroy them faster than they can reproduce. The mass of battling germs and white cells builds up to form a visible swelling, and the resulting pressure, together with the extra heat of cell activity, stimulates receptors to send messages to the brain; these are interpreted as sensations of pain, heat, and throbbing. The glands themselves often become swollen and tender; sometimes they become infected. The final outcome depends on many factors, the most important being on the one side the ability of the germs to multiply and produce an overwhelming number of dangerous

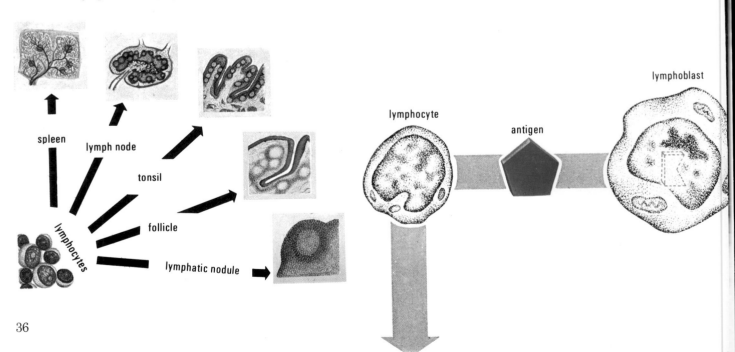

spleen

lymph node

tonsil

lymphocytes

follicle

lymphatic nodule

lymphocyte

antigen

lymphoblast

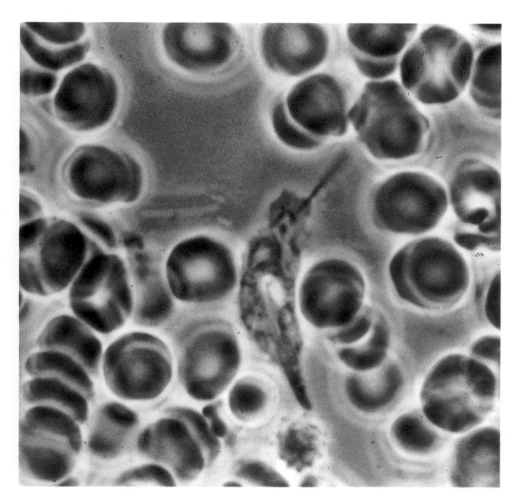

A phagocyte in a sample of human blood. These mobile cells engulf and digest bacteria and dead cells.

toxins, and on the other the ability of the body to muster its defenses quickly and in sufficient strength. Luckily for us, the body's defenses are extremely efficient, and are able to defeat most of the onslaughts upon it – provided we are reasonably healthy before the attack.

One of the greatest triumphs of medicine during the past century is the way in which the antibody mechanism has been harnessed to give us immunity to disease in advance of an infection. One way of doing this is to prepare weakened or dead strains of bacteria and viruses called *vaccines*, of such deadly diseases as typhoid, cholera, polio, and bubonic plague. These strains are too weak to produce dangerous symptoms when administered to a person, but they are strong enough to stimulate the production of antibodies, which persist in the body and can combat any subsequent infection. Another method is to inoculate with blood serum that contains ready-made antibodies; but this works only when it is performed immediately we are infected, and even then it does not provide immunity for very long.

Some lymphocytes remain in the lymphoid organs and never encounter an antigen. They do not multiply. Others circulate, and when they meet an antigen become active lymphoblasts. These may divide to form either antibody-producing plasma cells or alternatively long-lived lymphoblasts. The latter are "primed" to recognize that particular antigen and can deal with it rapidly when they encounter it elsewhere in the body or in a secondary infection.

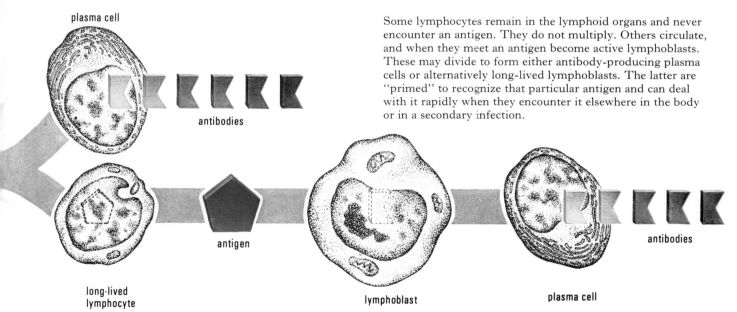

plasma cell

antibodies

long-lived lymphocyte

antigen

lymphoblast

plasma cell

antibodies

Biological Rhythms

All of us live in a world in which day and night follow one another in a fairly precise 24-hour cycle, even though the proportion of light and darkness varies with the seasons. Social life, work and leasure, sleep and meals, are geared to this cycle. So it is not surprising that many processes within the body oscillate with a 24-hour period. All biological measurements vary, and the statistician analyzes this variation into component parts: random variation in any individual, variations between one individual and another, and so on. One cause of variation which is very often ignored is the *circadian* (Latin *circa dies*, approximately a day) rhythm, or oscillation, with a period of around 24 hours.

At one time it was believed that urine flow is low at night because we neither eat nor drink at this time, because body temperature is low when we are at rest, and that blood plasma and urine become alkaline

after breakfast because the stomach secretes acid during the course of the meal. However, all these variations persist even if we break the rhythmic circadian habits which have been held responsible for them, for instance if we remain lying down for 24 hours, or indulge continuously in light work, or if we eat or take small identical meals regularly every hour. It appears that many rhythmic variations in bodily function result from an underlying process which continues to oscillate with an approximately 24-hour rhythm, independent of the alteration of light and darkness and the many other circadian rhythms which surround us. Other rhythms, often found in many animals, by contrast appear to be wholly dependent upon alternation of night and day, and are described as *nychthemeral* (Greek *nych-temeros*, night and day). For example most animals depend upon the alternation of light and darkness in their search for food or in their efforts to avoid being killed.

Many of our circadian rhythms are beneficial. We are wakeful during the day when we are attempting to work or use our mind to maximum efficiency. We are tired and sleepy at night when we most commonly sleep. The low urine flow at night gives us continuous uninterrupted sleep. The higher temperature during the day is an aid to muscular and

Diagram to show how circadian rhythms become established with increasing age, so that by the time it is 10 years old, a child has developed a 24-hour cycle. The colored sections represent sleep periods.

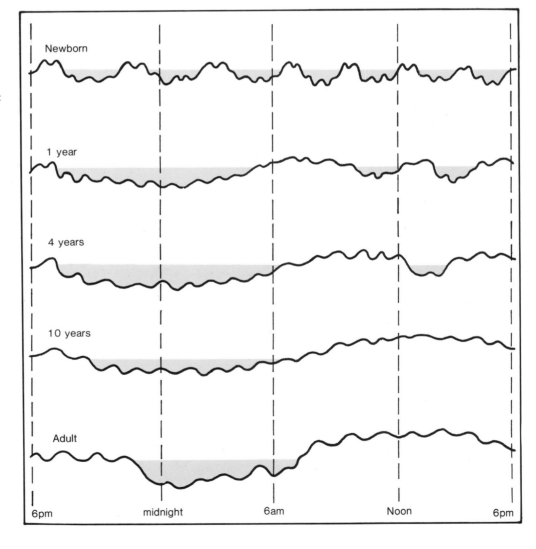

Newborn

1 year

4 years

10 years

Adult

| 6pm | midnight | 6am | Noon | 6pm |

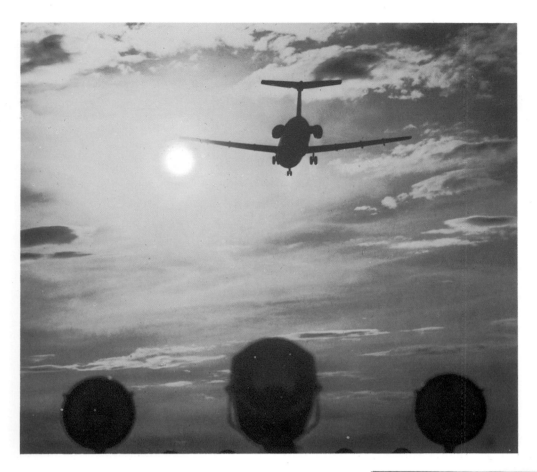

A session of travel involving
the crossing of several time
belts results in "jet syndrome," because the body
is still operating according to
the previous location's light
cycle.

The opening and closing of
the petals of certain flowers is
due to an internal mechanism.
Exposed to continuous light
or darkness the plants still
observe their natural circadian
rhythm.

perhaps mental efficiency. However, because of our ability to manipulate our environment and control, for example, temperature and lighting, we have no need to follow these rhythms. We can gather and store our food at virtually any time and in most civilized communities do not have to worry about predators. But this situation presents hidden dangers. Many of our inbuilt rhythms have a tendency to persist despite modification of habits or surrounding illumination, and they do not accord with our wish to depart from the circadian behaviour which nature or evolution intended for us.

Heavy capital investment in industrial plant demands that it shall operate continuously instead of merely in daylight hours. Road congestion may make night travel desirable for heavy commercial transport. Airplanes and submarines work round-the-clock schedules. Those who fly long distances around the world in short periods of time subject their rhythms to a large enforced shift which creates its own problems. Such travelers − businessmen, statesmen, sportsmen − are often anxious to perform at maximum efficiency soon after arrival at their destinations. Astronauts traveling to the Moon were entirely isolated from the usual circadian fluctuations in light, darkness, and other aspects of a normal environment. Those who have already orbited the Earth have subjected themselves to the remarkable rhythm of a day-night alternation taking only 90 minutes. All these different types of activity take their toll on human efficiency, and if carried on for too long may have a lasting effect on health.

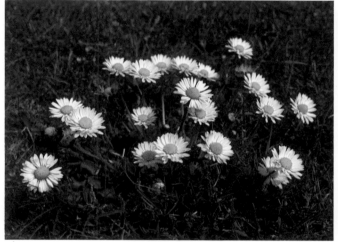

Even where they are least understood, the influences of circadian rhythms are widespread. The popular description of the small hours of the morning as a time of lowest ebb is borne out statistically by the fact that death is more common at this time than at any other. Little is understood of the mechanisms working these rhythms but it seems likely that they may reside in separate tissues and organs which under normal conditions are coordinated by some center in the brain, perhaps in the hypothalamus. Much more understanding is needed before we can manipulate these natural rhythms so that people can fly half way round the world and, instead of imagining it is time for bed and feeling only fatigued, accomodate themselves easily to the new time and be as alert as if they had just got up in the morning.

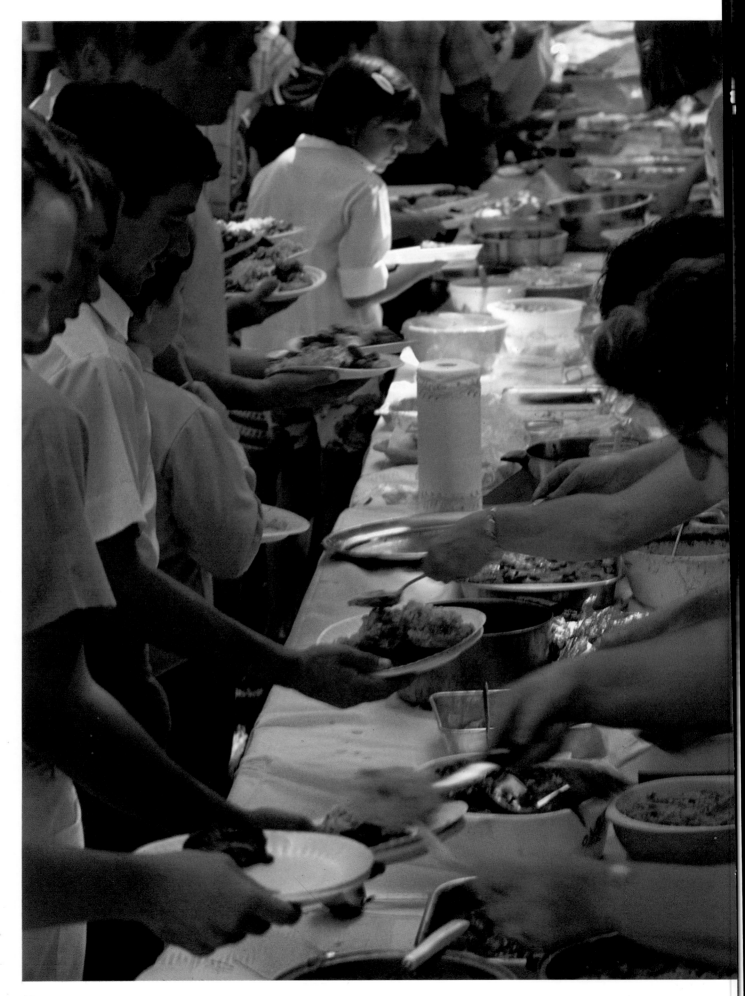

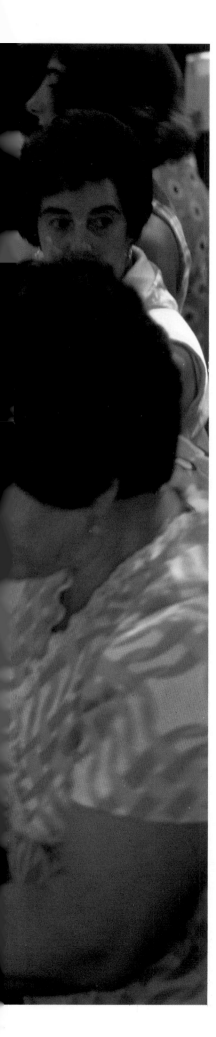

Chapter 2

The Digestive System

All the food and drink that we can take into our bodies needs a great deal of processing. Only then can its vital components be used for growth and energy to insure normal function while the unwanted, extraneous can be expelled as waste matter. This processing is carried out in the long digestive tract that starts at the mouth and finishes at the anus. The journey is not always smooth and uneventful. Breakdowns and malfunctions are liable to occur at any point, and if we can pinpoint the "troublespots," we will be better able to deal with them effectively.

Opposite: the essential process of eating has become ritualized to form the center of many social activities. Consequently, our eating habits are the result of culture and conditioning rather than health requirements.

Breaking down the Food

Until they discovered fire prehistoric men and women had to live on uncooked food. In fact raw food has one advantage over cooked food: more vitamins and salts are retained. By inventing and developing the art of cooking, human beings made three advances: they were able to make existing foods more tender, and hence more easily broken down for further processing; they were able to process food materials that they could not absorb at all in a raw state; and they found ways of mixing and heating a variety of raw materials that made their meals more enjoyable.

The kitchen is a kind of hit-or-miss biochemical laboratory in which the cook aims to achieve any or all of these three improvements. Biochemically speaking, very few cooks have any idea of what they are doing, even though they produce interesting and nourishing meals. But in fact they are making the molecules of food more vulnerable to attack by the body's chemical agents – and in this way help the processes of digestion. The effect of cooking is to soften the cell walls of the food, making it easier to masticate; this in turn increases the surface area that can be acted upon by the digestive juices. At the same time the starch grains within the cell swell; the cells may even burst, so making their contents more accessible. Potato, which contains lots of starch, is easily masticated after cooking, but vegetables such as celery and cabbage are more resistant, even after prolonged boiling.

The senses of smell and taste are closely linked. We often think we are tasting something, when really we are reacting to its odor as it enters the back of the nose from the mouth. The first stage of digestion works hand in hand with smell, taste, sight, and thought. Shakespeare's Macbeth sums up the situation in a nutshell: "Now good digestion wait on appetite, and health on both."

Even before we begin to eat, the sight, smell or thought of any food with pleasant associations starts the digestive juices flowing and causes waves of contraction in the muscles lining the stomach. These reflexes are conditioned – that is, we have learned to respond to bodily stimuli (an attractively presented dinner table, a restaurant menu) as well as merely physical or chemical stimuli. Saliva secretion, for example, can result from either the thought or smell of food (an acquired reflex) or from physical or chemical stimulation of nerve endings in the mouth by the food itself (an inborn reflex).

The process of digestion begins as soon as we put food into our mouths. As we chew, our food is mixed with saliva which breaks down large molecules (starches) into smaller ones (sugars) that can be absorbed by the intestines. Saliva can do this because it contains enzymes that help to break up these molecules.

As the stomach fills, gastric juices (composed of enzymes and hydrochloric acid secreted by gland cells in the stomach wall) take over chemical digestion. At the same time they excite reflexes that keep gastric juices flowing and stimulate the muscle contractions that move food and propel it through the long digestive tract. One such automatic mechanism secretes a hormone called *enterogastrone* that acts as a brake on the excessive secretion of hydrochloric acid. If this did not happen, acid would eat through the mucous membrane lining the stomach and duodenum and cause ulcers.

As food passes on through the intestines, physical and chemical stimuli continue to operate. Hydrochloric acid, for example, liberates a hormone that stimulates the pancreas and liver. Pancreatic juices pour into the duodenum where they break down fats, proteins and carbohydrates; bile (made in the liver and stored in the gall bladder) emulsifies fats into

Digestion is completed in the small intestine by various enzymes. The central chile duct collects part of the derivatives of fat breakdown and conveys them to the lymphatic system. The capillaries carry the other products to the liver via the portal vein.

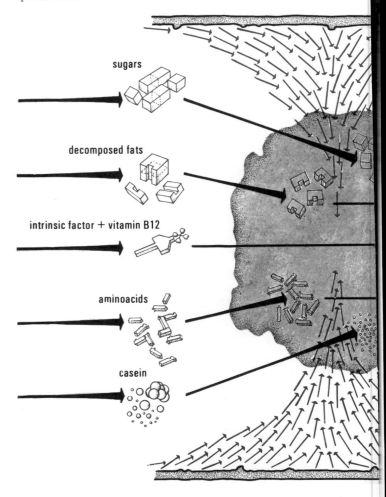

sugars

decomposed fats

intrinsic factor + vitamin B12

aminoacids

casein

tiny globules that are more accessible to the fat-digesting pancreatic enzymes. In a healthy system, this complex chain of self-regulating mechanisms, with others like them, makes sure that food is absorbed efficiently and that waste products are eliminated regularly. When one enzyme has finished its work, another takes over and then passes the product on to the next enzyme, and so on.

Eventually the food material is reduced to a state ready for absorption through the cell lining of the remaining 18 feet of the small intestine. The starch and sugars have now been changed into glucose, the proteins to amino acids and the fats to fatty acids and glycerol. Just as the large surface area of the alveoli of the lungs enables oxygen to be absorbed, so the huge surface of the small intestine, with its millions of minute projections called *microvilli*, enables nutrients to be absorbed in a similar manner.

Water recovery is the main function of the large intestine. About once every four hours the contents of the small intestine are discharged into the large intestine where *peristalsis* (a wavelike movement along the intestine) is very slow, providing the water enough time to be reabsorbed to the bloodstream. The residue that is left behind is known as the *feces*.

Finally the accumulated feces are passed to the rectum, which terminates at the anus, and are expelled by defecation. This transfer occurs by a remote-control reflex (the gastrocolic reflex) whenever food enters the stomach. It is thus normal to

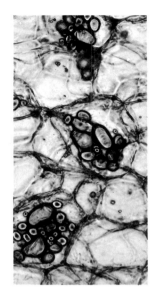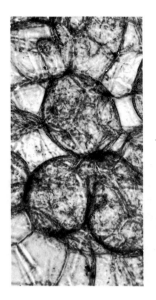

Photomicrographs of raw (left) and boiled (right) potato cells. In raw potatoes the starch grains are small and dense, and the cell walls tough. Cooking makes the starch grains absorb water and swell up, and it also softens the cell walls, thus making the vegetable more digestible.

want to defecate after breakfast. One special feature of digestion is its intermittent nature, even though we eat at more or less regular intervals during the day. The system that stores digested material and measures out a steady supply regardless of the nature of the food or the time of the day or night is situated in the liver.

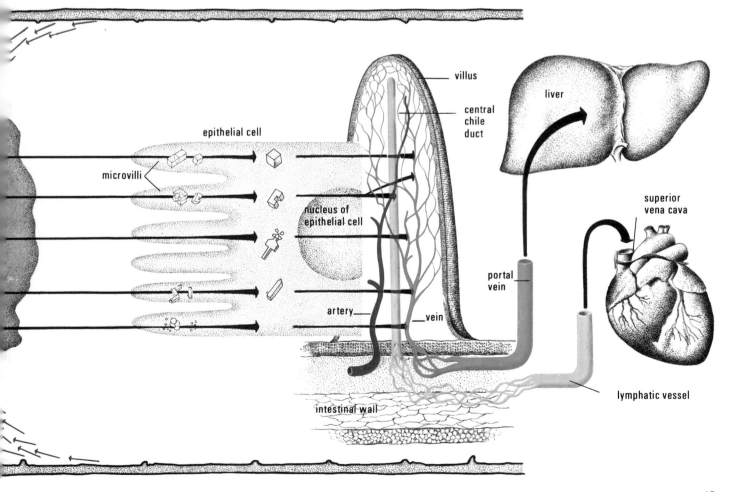

What is Indigestion?

"Indigestion" is a term frequently used by people to describe a multitude of symptoms generally experienced as some sort of pain or discomfort following a meal. To some people indigestion feels as if digestion has not taken its normal course. There is a sense of fullness in the tummy, a pressure or actual pain. Other people use the term "indigestion" to describe heartburn, belching, or flatulence. Nausea and vomiting are also often described as being due to indigestion. All of these symptoms can be associated with a great variety of ailments, not all of which are bound up with gastrointestinal disorders.

The abdominal pain experienced in indigestion is generally dull and aching, or felt as a fullness or pressure. Usually this type of pain is the result of distension or exaggerated muscular contraction of an organ or a part of the intestines. Pain under the chest bone is due to disorders in the gullet or upper half of the stomach. Sometimes this pain is difficult to distinguish from the pain caused by a heart condition. Pain in the middle part of the stomach is generally of gastric, duodenal, biliary or pancreatic origin. A pain in the region of the navel is mostly associated with diseases of the small bowel. Pain situated below the navel may arise because of trouble with the appendix or large bowel, or may be of pelvic origin.

The patterns of a person's complaints often provide clues as to the causes. With gastric cancer the symptoms are usually constant; in acute gastritis, following an excess of alcohol, they are intermittent. Symptoms are occasionaly seasonal; this can occur with peptic ulcer sufferers, the symptoms often being more prominent in the spring and autumn.

Another important factor is how soon after a meal the discomfort or pain occurs. Early symptoms after a meal may reflect a disease of the esophagus, cancer, or peptic ulcer in the stomach. Late symptoms, for instance those occurring several hours after eating, may be a symptom of duodenal ulcer, the pain occurring when the ulcerated mucosa is exposed to acid secretion of the stomach unprotected by the food. Conversely, the relief of pain following a meal is also common with people with a peptic ulcer and is presumably due to the neutralization of the acid by the ingested food.

In many cases, particular types of foods appear to be related to indigestion. For example, people with diseases of the esophagus might tolerate liquids well, but will experience discomfort from solid food. Certain foods are poorly tolerated because the intestinal tract cannot assimilate them adequately. This may happen when people suffering from pancreatic or bilary tract diseases eat fatty foods. In patients with ulcerative colitis after ingestion of milk, flatulence or diarrhea are common symptoms.

Certain circumstances, such as chronic anxiety, poor eating habits, or actual intestinal disease may produce an "indigestion" which would appear to be related to the presence of increased quantities of gas in the intestinal tract. Sufferers will often complain of flatulence. Also fatty meals delay gastric emptying and hence the passage of swallowed air down the intestine. This explains the prolonged sense of fullness after a fatty meal.

A number of diseases unconnected with the intestinal tract may result in indigestion symptoms by processes that doctors know little about. Symptoms of indigestion may occur, for example, after a heart attack, lung tuberculosis or a malignant

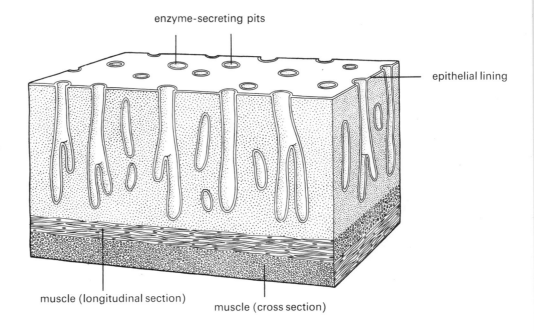

enzyme-secreting pits

epithelial lining

Diagram of the stomach wall, showing the pits opening on to the inner surface. The muscle layers of the stomach are thicker than in any other part of the digestive system, and their contraction churns up the food.

muscle (longitudinal section)

muscle (cross section)

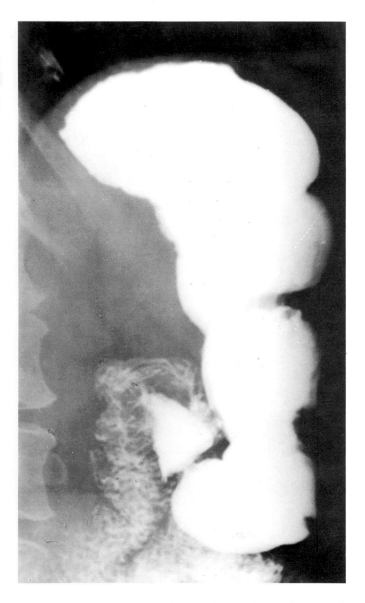

Above: an X-ray of a normal stomach after the swallowing of a barium meal. This procedure is used to investigate possible tumors, ulcers and hernias, and enables the movement of the stomach and its rate of emptying to be studied. The patient must fast for 12 hours beforehand.

acute infectious diseases, often accompanied by diarrhea. Severe nausea and vomiting may be prominent in viral hepatitis (inflammation of the liver), even before the appearance of jaundice. Migraine headaches and acute meningitis are examples of disorders of the nervous system that can lead to vomiting. Nausea and vomiting can also be side effects of some drugs and chemicals.

Because gastrointestinal disorders, especially stomach complaints, are among the most common of the body's malfunctions, it is not surprising that scientists are using many of their resources in an attempt to gain a better understanding of the mechanisms of digestion and how and why they go wrong. In one method a person swallows a small capsule containing a tiny radio transmitter. Once in the stomach the transmitter "broadcasts" back information about the concentration of acid in the gastric juices. Another method employs a gastroscope, a tiny lighted tube which is used by doctors to investigate directly different parts of the gastrointestinal system.

Mark had been suffering for some time from early-morning vomiting. As soon as he got up he vomited, but felt perfectly well after breakfast. He underwent all the clinical tests for gastrointestinal disorders. A duodenal ulcer was discovered, but the recommended treatment had no affect on his morning vomiting. It was later discovered that he was having difficulties at work and that he was a secret alcoholic. Now his doctor understood: the vomiting was a withdrawal symptom – his body demanded alcohol first thing in the morning! After being given additional treatment to cure his alcoholism, the morning vomiting stopped, and his peptic ulcer soon healed.

disease. Under these circumstances the symptoms of indigestion may be present with no unique features to suggest that they are in fact due to some other disease.

Anorexia, a loss of the desire to eat, is a prominent symptom in a wide variety of intestinal disorders. It may precede the appearance of jaundice in hepatitis, or it may be a prominent symptom in gastric cancer.

Nausea and vomiting are closely connected. Nausea is the feeling that you want to vomit and is usually associated with diminished activity of the stomach and alterations in the workings of the duodenum and small intestine. Nausea and vomiting commonly occur when there is inflammation, as in acute appendicitis (inflammation of the appendix), acute cholecystitis (inflammation of the gall bladder) or peritonitis (inflammation of the abdominal lining). But it is also a symptom of chronic indigestion, or

Below: photomicrograph of gastric glands in the stomach. There are three main types: mucoid cells which secrete mucus; zymogenic or chief cells responsible for the production of pepsinogen (from which the enzyme pepsin is formed; parietal or oxyntic cells, which secrete hydrochloric acid.

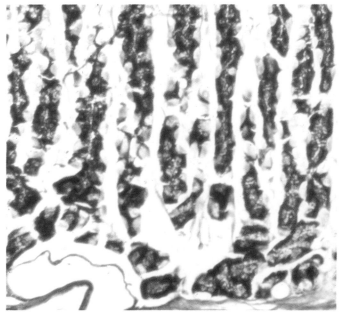

How the Mouth Works

Teeth and saliva are very important in the digestive process. Your teeth are highly refined tools for the breaking down of food, and their various shapes correspond to their special functions. The chisel-edged incisors in front cut the food. Next to them are the canines or eyeteeth. These are only moderately developed in man, but are powerful weapons for biting in the carnivorous animals. At the back of the mouth are the premolars and molars for grinding the food.

The other equipment in our mouth is ideally designed to help the teeth in the process of breaking down food. The muscles of the lips, cheeks, jaws, and tongue are coordinated and as a result of biting, chewing, and churning, the food is moistened, lubricated and chemically changed by saliva before it is swallowed.

Firstly the food is manipulated by the tongue, which pushes it sideways between the grinding surfaces of the molars. The broken food particles are well moistened with saliva and the masticatory muscles of the jaws work them back into the center of the mouth. This process continues until the food has been thoroughly broken up. Chewing promotes maintenance of the tissues in the mouth and gums, and can be compared to a healthy massage. As the mouthful of food becomes thoroughly mixed with saliva and reduced to a paste, the tongue squeezes it against the hard roof of the mouth into a mass called a *bolus* which can now be swallowed down into the stomach.

The adult human's 32 teeth are arranged in two rows. They bite together with a force that can support the whole weight of their owner. The upper and lower sets do not meet exactly. They fit neatly on

A general view of the mouth and teeth. There are 16 permanent teeth in the upper jaw and 16 in the lower.

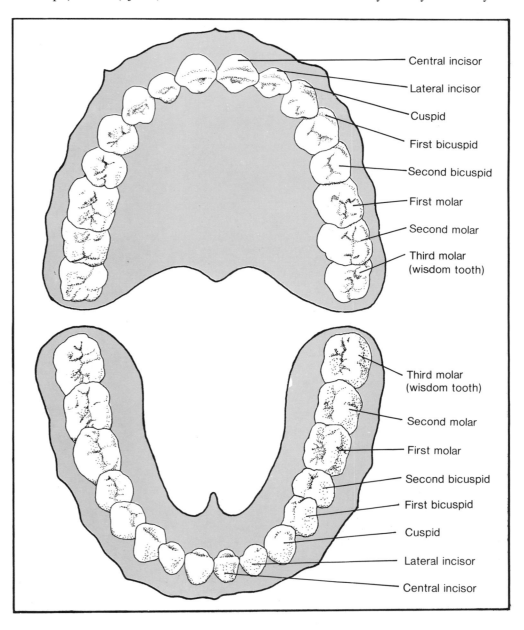

Central incisor

Lateral incisor

Cuspid

First bicuspid

Second bicuspid

First molar

Second molar

Third molar (wisdom tooth)

Third molar (wisdom tooth)

Second molar

First molar

Second bicuspid

First bicuspid

Cuspid

Lateral incisor

Central incisor

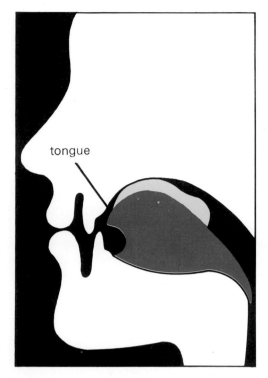

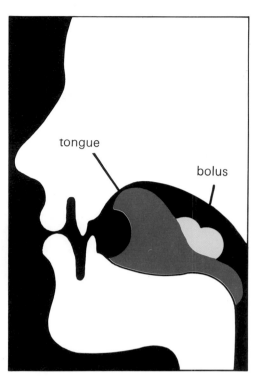

The tongue places the food in to the cavity of the mouth and manipulates its backward and forward into a bolus. This is then swallowed.

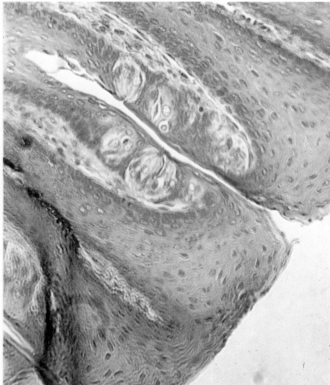

Section through the tongue showing the salivary glands and taste buds. There are four types of buds registering different tastes (sweet, bitter, salty and sour), and they appear to be concentrated in different areas of the tongue.

each other at the back of the mouth for grinding, but at the front, the upper teeth lie over the lower ones and act like a pair of scissors.

One of the yet unanswered mysteries is why modern man suffers more than his ancestors from the dental decay called *caries*. One theory is that the high incidence of caries today is related to the consistency of flour in the diet. The modern process of roller-milling removes all husks and fibrous debris; such a refined product needs no chewing and sticks to the teeth. It is well known that the rate of decay can be reduced by chewing a raw apple or carrot after eating a meal, and by cutting down on sweet, sugary foods. Another theory claims that germs, always present in large numbers on a thin layer covering the teeth's crown and gums, are the main culprit. It was proved in the 1940s that a concentration of about one part per million of the mineral fluoride in drinking water reduces dental caries in children. Since then, many countries have added fluoride as a regular constituent of their drinking water. Fluoride can also be applied directly to the teeth.

Salivary glands in the mouth produce the clear, slightly viscous fluid called saliva. It performs four functions: it lubricates the food and mouth as you eat or speak; it moistens the food and enables it to be swallowed; by dissolving food substances it enables them to be detected by the taste receptors on the surface of the tongue; and finally its enzyme, called *ptyalin*, transforms starch into sugars which can be assimilated. Ptyalin does not work in an acid medium and as soon as the bolus enters the stomach and becomes acidified by the gastric juices its action ceases. If you bolt your food in a hurry and do not chew it thoroughly, then the saliva is not being allowed to do its job properly – and you are wasting good food.

It should be obvious from what has been said about the role of different parts of the mouth that constant and adequate care is of the utmost importance. Both tooth decay and diseases of the gums can be prevented by scrupulous oral hygiene. Children should have regular dental checkups and be encouraged to continue this practice later in life.

The Facts about Ulcers

One of the common diseases of our age is peptic ulcer. About 80 percent of all peptic ulcers develop in the duodenum, and at some time during their lives approximately 10 percent or even more of the population will probably suffer from duodenal ulcer, many of which do not produce any symptoms and remain undetected. However, many lives are lost as a result of this disease – up to 2,000 yearly in West Germany alone – mainly because of hemorrhage or perforation. Duodenal ulcer is most common in men between the ages of 20 and 50.

Gastric and duodenal ulcers are often found in the same person, and it has been suggested that a chronic duodenal ulcer which causes delay in gastric emptying and consequent stagnation of food in the stomach (*gastric stasis*) stimulates the production of the hormone *gastrin* in the stomach, and thus the development of a gastric ulcer. But it is likely that a multiplicity of contributing factors are involved in the development of duodenal ulcers.

As duodenal ulcers never occur in the absence of acid, many doctors believe that they arise from abnormally high secretions. As already pointed out, emotional factors may alter gastric function. People with duodenal ulcers can often clearly point to an emotional upset which may have triggered off the

Stressful living has been implicated as a causative factor in the formation of peptic ulcers. The flow of gastric juices is under hormonal control. Chronic anxiety causes an increase in the flow and as a result the contents of the stomach become more acid.

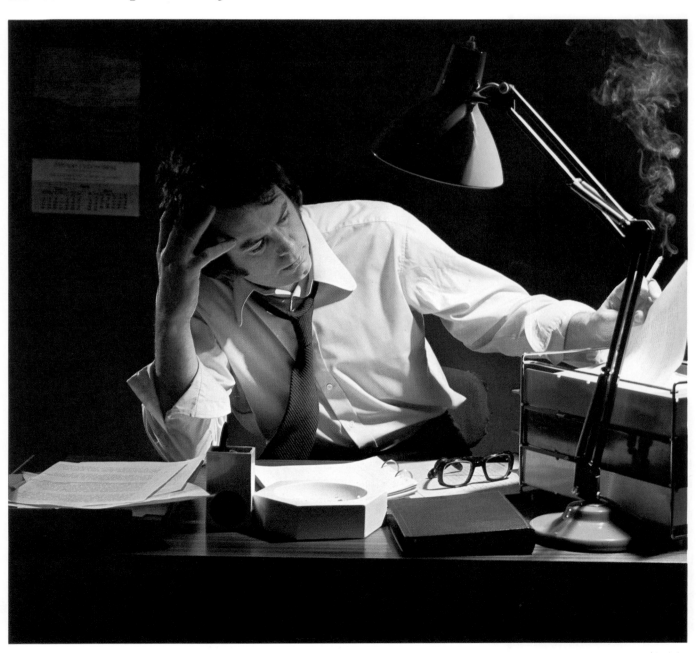

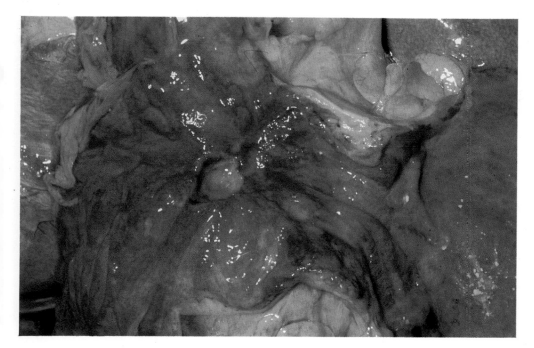

Left: a duodenal ulcer (center). The duodenum is particularly prone to ulceration because it has little protection against excess acid. The ulcers tend to heal up but the scars often open up again.

Below left: a barium meal X-ray of the stomach showing the formation of a gastric ulcer. These can sometimes become malignant.

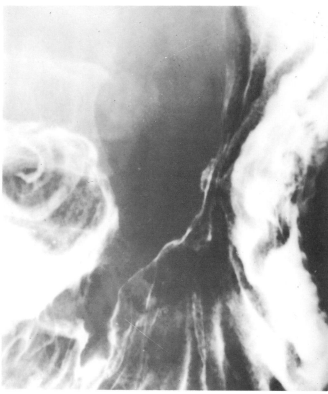

uniform: the development of pain followed by the relief of discomfort after a meal is such a common sequence that its absence usually indicates some other gastrointestinal disorder. The pain is a steady gnawing, burning, aching, or hungerlike discomfort over the upper part of the stomach.

Gastric ulcers are much less common than duodenal ulcers, predominating in men by a ratio of three to one – somewhat less than the predominance found in duodenal ulcer. Although gastric ulcers may appear at any time, they tend to occur between the ages of 45–50. They occur most often in the lower half of the stomach, usually singly. About 20 percent of gastric ulcers occur in people who have had past or present duodenal ulceration, but is very unusual for duodenal ulceration to follow the onset of pure gastric ulceration.

Several theories have been put forward to explain the development of peptic ulcers in the stomach. The majority of specialists support the idea that they are due to an oversecretion of gastric juice of hormonal origin, dependent upon prolonged or excessive liberation of the stomach's hormone gastrin. Unfortunately even this theory is by no means a satisfactory explanation for the vast majority of spontaneously occurring gastric ulcers.

Unfortunately, the familiar symptoms associated with duodenal ulcers do not always occur with other types of ulcer. Gastric ulcers are found without any symptoms, so that some are found by chance and others only by a severe complication such as perforation or bleeding. When symptoms occur they often take the form of a vague bloated feeling, or nausea after eating. Food often aggravates pain. The discomfort may include feelings of burning or cramp and is usually less localized than that found in those with duodenal ulcers. Weight loss is frequent, but pain at night is uncommon. All these symptoms of gastric ulcer tend to be chronic.

onset of their ulcer or made it worse. Many duodenal ulcer sufferers are hard-driving ambitious executives; but a great number of exceptions are found. Clearly, psychological factors may play a role in the development of duodenal ulceration, but are in all likelihood not the sole cause of the complaint. Because peptic ulceration is far more common in men, it has been suggested that estrogenic hormones, secreted mainly by women, may protect against the development of ulcer. But it is now thought that there is less gastric secretion in women because they have a smaller number of cells producing hydrochloric acid in the gastric mucous lining.

The symptoms of duodenal ulcer are remarkably

Treating Peptic Ulcers

Virtually every conceivable diet or drug has been advocated at one time or another for the treatment of peptic ulcers. Yet studies of various types of therapy show that few forms of treatment have any effect on the rate of healing. Certain recommendations, however, at least providing greater comfort and relief of symptoms, can be made. The aim is for each sufferer to be treated in a way in which suits his or her individual needs – and not to impose a strict set of rules.

Antacids are the mainstay of ulcer treatment. The reasoning behind this therapy is that if the acidity of the gastric juices is reduced, the pepsin loses its

The diet of the peptic ulcer sufferer is not restrictive. You can eat anything as long as it is not highly seasoned or fried. Small meals every two hours are preferred to fewer large ones. Alcohol and tobacco should be avoided.

capacity to digest proteins and the damaging effect due to acidity is cut to a minimum. Calcium carbonate is an extremely effective antacid, but absorbable antacids, such as the much-used sodium bicarbonate, should be avoided. They neutralize the acidity only temporarily; the stomach cells, in an attempt to restore the acidity, then overcompensate in their secretion of acid. Sodium bicarbonate is particularly dangerous when combined with the drinking of large amounts of milk. The milk washes out the alkaline bicarbonate and the stomach is left unprotected against the corrosive effects of the acid.

Observations have shown that special diets have no long-lasting healing benefit. However, the right kind of diet, consisting of small quantities of bland food taken frequently, will help to relieve the pain and discomfort. Six small meals a day, with plenty of high-protein foods and skimmed milk, is a good starting-point. Avoid highly seasoned foods, and roughage, and cut out fried or greasy foods altogether. As soon as the discomfort has disappeared, the diet can gradually be brought back to normal.

Relying solely on a good diet to act as a buffer against the excess acid is not advisable. This is because considerable amounts of acid are produced after the initial buffering effect of the meal has worn

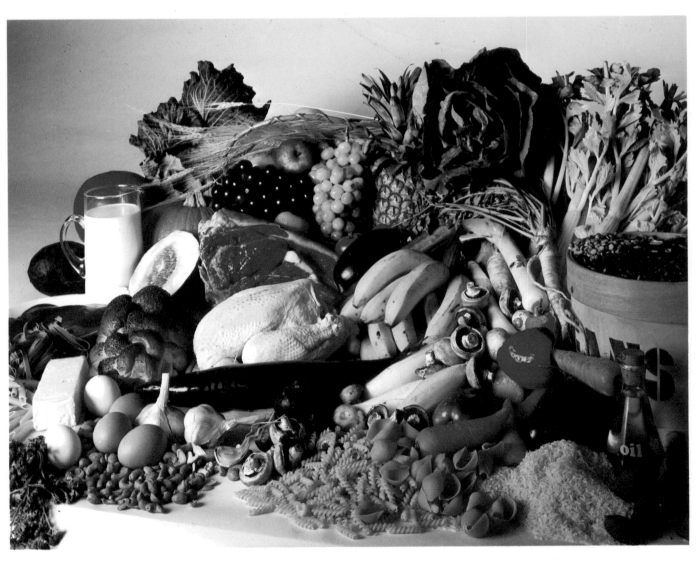

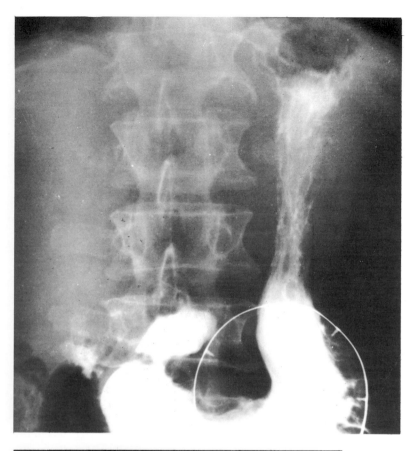

Left: barium X-ray of a stomach after a partial gastrectomy. If a gastric ulcer does not respond to therapy and there is a danger of bleeding or perforation, or if it recurs after healing, surgery is the next step. The region of the ulcer is excised and the remainder of the stomach is reconnected to the duodenum.

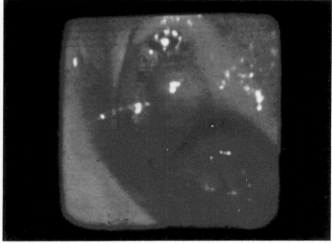

Below left: photograph of the interior of the stomach, taken with a gastrocamera.

off. So it is important that an antacid is taken one hour after eating.

Plenty of rest and sleep are strongly advised, and sufferers are urged to cut down on their business and social engagements. Resting in bed has proved beneficial for people with gastric ulcer. Care is an important part of treatment. A warm and sympathetic attitude, reassurance and support on the part of the family, are all helpful.

Alcohol should be strictly prohibited as it not only produces direct stimulation of the gastric juices, but may also induce the release of gastrin. In addition, it probably injures the gastric mucosal lining. Coffee, tea, and cola drinks stimulate gastric secretion because of their caffeine content and should also be avoided. It is sensible for the ulcer sufferer to give up cigarette smoking completely. It

has been found to cause delayed healing of gastric ulcers, although the reasons for this are not clear. However, total abstinence may produce adverse affects in heavy smokers, so it is best to consult your doctor on this point.

Many types of ulcer "cure" have been tried over the years, but none have proved to be of permanent value. Often the first results have seemed promising, but because ulcers have the remarkable tendency of suddenly reappearing without any warning or for no obvious reason, the true evaluation of any new form of therapy is very difficult.

In recent years, however, a drug has been developed which has revolutionized peptic-ulcer treatment. This drug – Cimetidine – selectively depresses the activity of the acid-secreting cells, without affecting the rest of the stomach's function. It is still not a permanent cure as the suppression lasts only as long as the drug is administered, but so far it is the most successful way of treating peptic ulcers.

Surgery is considered necessary for a minority of sufferers, and usually only when there are complications, such as perforation, obstruction of the passage, or persistent bleeding. But in nonemergency cases where other forms of treatment have proved completely ineffective, the risks of the disease must be balanced against those of an operation. On the one hand are the repeated discomfort, cost of frequent hospitalization, time lost from work, possible death, and the threat of complications. On the other hand are the operative and anesthetic risks, the possibility of recurrent ulcer, and postoperative symptoms.

The Large Intestine

One of the functions of the large intestine is to dispose of unabsorbed waste material through the anus in the form of feces (stools). The range of variations in bowel habits among apparently healthy people is extraordinarily wide, but there are two very common complaints – diarrhea and constipation.

Diarrhea is defined as the frequent passage of watery stools, and constipation as an undue delay in the evacuation of feces. The nature and the severity of such a functional disturbance is rarely easy to discover, because the gastrointestinal tract is a primitive organ which is affected by many different stimuli, from hunger to rage, from fever to fatigue, from infected or poisonous foods to the most subtle allergy contained in a highly refined food.

Acute disturbances of bowel function are relatively common and usually manifest themselves as diarrhea. The sudden onset of loose stools in a previously healthy person is due invariably to the toxins produced by an active infection and much less often to the taking in of poisoned foods, chemicals or drugs. If diarrhea has developed in a number of people within 28 to 72 hours after a common meal, then this may be due to a salmonella infection, a type of food poisoning. If diarrhea is accompanied by fever, muscle aching, severe abdominal discomfort, and complete lack of appetite (anorexia), then an inflammation of the small intestine is the possible cause. Inflammation of the small intestine due to a virus may cause diarrhea accompanied by bad

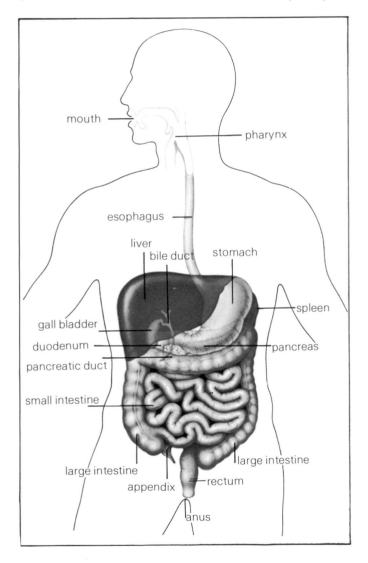

Above: the large intestine begins on the right side of the body as the ascending colon. It forms a T-junction with the lower part of the small intestine, the blind shorter part – the cecum – terminating in the appendix. The colon crosses the abdomen and descends along the left side into the pelvis, where it continues as the rectum.

Below: internal surface of the colon. Unlike the surface of the small intestine, there are no microvilli. Instead the surface contains a large number of tubular pits which increase in number toward the rectum. The outside of the colon is covered with bulges known as haustra.

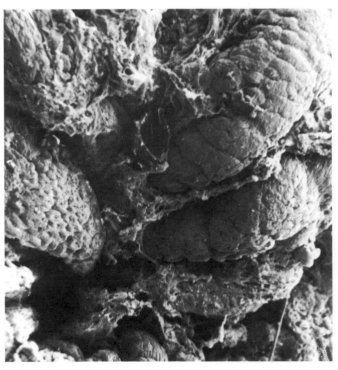

stomach pain and vomiting. Infections of the large intestine are usually accompanied by cramps and rectal urgency. If, in addition, blood is present in the stools, this may indicate dysentery or a parasitic infection.

A history of bouts of loose stools, extending over a period of months or years, calls for a careful investigation. The disturbance may have an emotional origin if it is not accompanied by fever, weight loss, blood in the stools, or a significant loss of zest for life. But when the diarrhea has been characterized by blood in the stools, or by fever and weight loss in addition, then a chronic inflammation of the intestine is a distinct possibility. Tuberculosis and cancer of the intestine can give similar symptoms.

Diarrhea in small babies should never be ignored. Unlike adults, an infant cannot compensate for the loss of water and salts by sweating or urinating less. Consequently, the baby will suffer severe dehydration and may even die as a result.

Whereas diarrhea may be a dangerous symptom, with its accompaniment of dehydration and loss of mineral salts, constipation in itself can do little harm. A long history of intermittent bouts of constipation accompanied by abdominal pain and distress relieved by the passing of small stools, is characteristic of what is called the "irritable colon syndrome," one of the most common reflections of anxiety met by doctors today. The overuse of laxatives over many years frequently adds to the underlying emotional disturbance, aggravating the symptoms, which are essentially an exaggeration of the normal workings of the large intestine and in mild degrees have probably been experienced by most healthy people, as for example the constipation associated with travel.

When a person believes that it is vital for bowel movements to be strictly regular, equating general health with "regularity," then this can lead to a dependence on laxatives to hasten what that person thinks is an overdue evacuation. Whatever the reason for this belief, often a result of childhood training, the overuse of laxatives over a long period can cause the large bowel to lose its sensitivity to stimuli.

Although both diarrhea and constipation occur usually as the result of relatively minor upsets, if the condition does not clear up, or if it gets progressively worse, then you should seek your doctor's help. Tumors of the gastrointestinal tract make up nearly half of all cancers, so early diagnosis is obviously of the utmost importance.

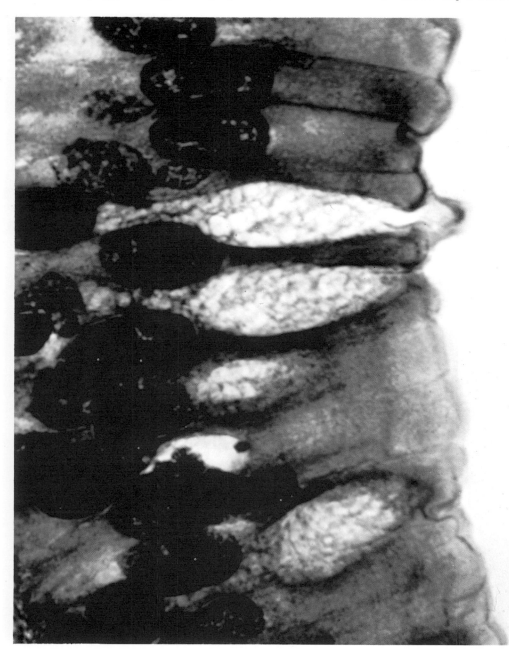

Section through the large intestine showing the goblet cells. These secrete mucin, the chief constituent of mucus. Other secretory cells in the large intestine include tubular intestinal glands and cells of Paneth.

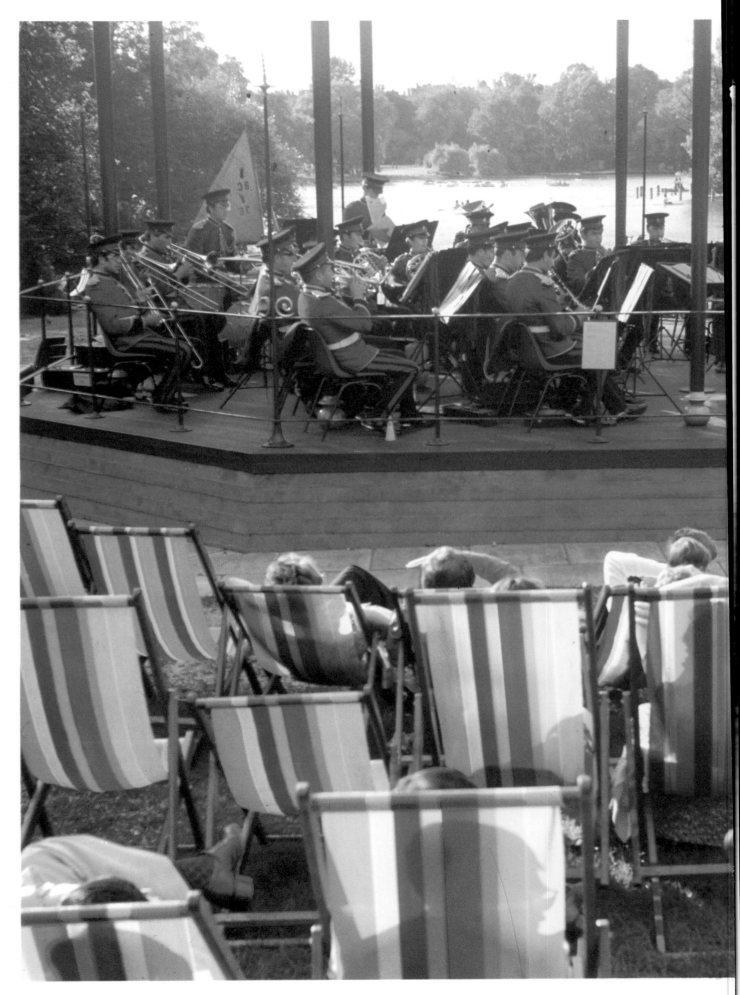

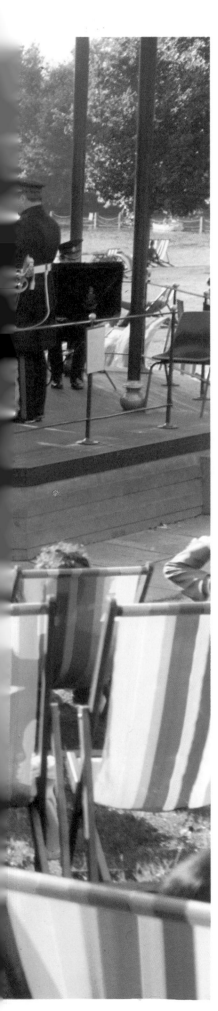

Chapter 3

Sight and Hearing

Our perception and experience of the world about us depend on the correct functioning of our five basic senses: sight, hearing, smell, touch, and taste. Of these sight and hearing are probably the most vital of these senses. Human beings are highly visual animals: they learn by seeing. When sight fails the world suddenly becomes a very different place: it shrinks to objects that can only be touched and noises that confuse. Deafness can be even more isolating as blindness and just as devastating in its impact. But the blind and deaf have bravely learned to compensate for their handicap by developing reserve abilities and using techniques for living that do not depend on their missing senses.

Opposite: among the animals only humans have developed sight and hearing beyond the perception of the environment and communication. We use our ears and eyes to obtain and provide pleasure in the form of music and the arts.

The Eye as a Camera

The eye works like a camera. Light passes through an aperture of variable size (the *pupil*) and a *lens* of variable focus to initiate a chemical reaction on a light-sensitive surface (the *retina*). In black-and-white film a chemical reaction turns fine grains of silver compound gray or black to form a negative image. In the retina chemical reaction causes electrical signals to travel along the *optic nerve* to the brain. We can discriminate between colors because several different types of *receptors* respond selectively to different parts of the light spectrum.

The *cornea* forms the delicate front surface of the eye. It is protected from dust particles by being continuously washed by antiseptic tears. The upper eyelids pass up and down over the front of the eyes, acting like windscreen wipers. But the greatest protection of all is that the front of the cornea is covered by a transparent membrane called the *conjunctiva*, consisting of self-repairing stratified layers of cells. The cornea is a fixed-focus lens and it focuses images roughly near the retina. It is left to the crystalline lens to act as a fine adjuster and to focus the image accurately onto the retina. It does this by means of muscles that cause the lens to alter its shape according to the distance of the image.

The refractive parts of the eye are like any other organ: they must be fed. But they are transparent, so it is impossible to provide nourishment through a network of capillaries. Instead they are nourished by transparent fluids that themselves exchange nutrients and gases with the capillaries of the eyeball. These fluids also maintain a constant pressure against the inside of the eyeball, to keep it in its correct spherical shape and also to exert a necessary pressure on the nerve cells of the retina.

By reducing excess light entering a camera, the sharpness of the image is increased, and exactly the same is true for the eye. Light intensity is regulated by an automatic diaphragm between the lens and the cornea, called the *iris*, and its center is an opening called the *pupil*. In bright light the pupil narrows and in dim light it dilates (enlarges).

Finally light reaches the retina. This consists of

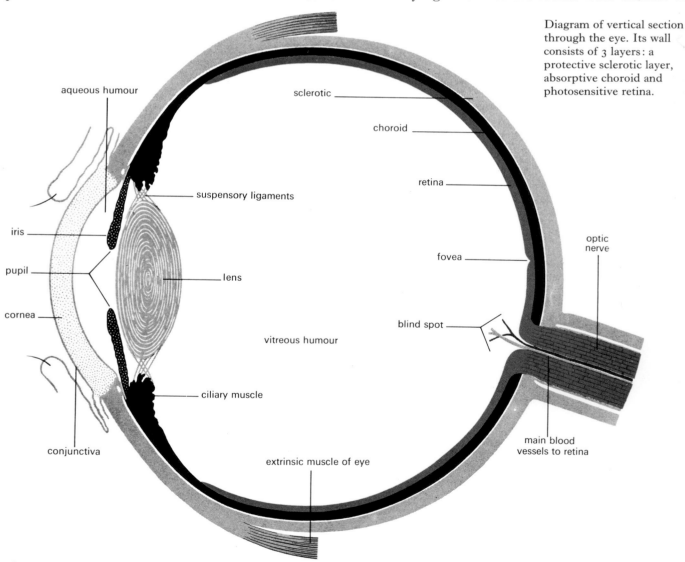

Diagram of vertical section through the eye. Its wall consists of 3 layers: a protective sclerotic layer, absorptive choroid and photosensitive retina.

aqueous humour

sclerotic

choroid

suspensory ligaments

retina

iris

fovea

optic nerve

pupil

lens

cornea

blind spot

vitreous humour

ciliary muscle

conjunctiva

main blood vessels to retina

extrinsic muscle of eye

over 100 million receptors of two kinds – *rods* and *cones*. The rods come into play when the light intensity is low and they give a picture in varying shades of gray. The retina has a pigment called *rhodopsin* that slowly breaks down when it absorbs light of low intensity. When this happens, there is a release of energy that triggers off nerve impulses. But rhodopsin can rebuild itself so that it is ready to receive new stimuli. The rods are so sensitive that on a clear, dark night they can detect a candle flame more than nine miles away. At this distance the eye receives less than 100 million millionth part of the original light.

The other type of receptors in the retina – the cones – are used in daylight vision and are also responsible for our color vision. The pigments in the cones give rise to nerve impulses that depend on color, and the part of the brain called the *visual cortex* then interprets these impulses as color sensations.

The nerve cells that cover the retina terminate in nerve fibers that meet at one point to form the optic nerve. This point is called the *blind spot*, because being devoid of receptors it cannot respond to light. Almost opposite the middle of the lens is a yellow spot, the *fovea*. The fovea is adapted to record the finest detail: each cone from this area is connected to its own individual fiber in the optic nerve and here light is in a better position to reach the receptors because the area is not overlain by the curtain of blood vessels. If we look straight at something, the subject is focused on the fovea. Consequently the image of the object receives intense scrutiny and detailed interpretation, while its surroundings are roughly sketched in.

The line of vision of each eye converges so that they both see the same object, but the eyes are about $2\frac{1}{2}$ inches apart, so the images that fall on each retina are not quite identical. This enables the brain to see the object in three dimensions, that is, we make out its depth as well as its height and width. The brain also uses the two different images to judge the distance of the object, although just how this is done is not fully understood. We know, however, that different groups of cells in the visual area of the cortex deal with a definite part of the retina and with images of a particular shape. An upright square, for example, is "seen" by one set of cortical cells, but if the square is tilted, an entirely new set of cells comes into action. It is not surprising to find, therefore, that the cerebral cortex has a very large area allocated to interpret all this information.

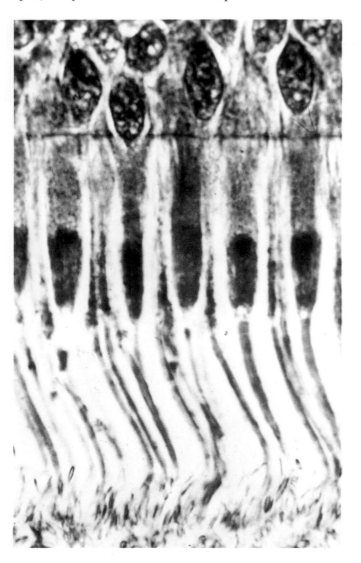

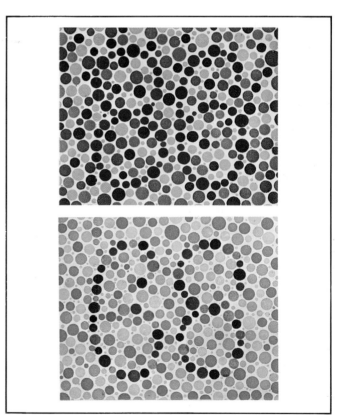

Left: section through the retina. The upper layer contains the cell bodies of the rods and cones, while the lower layer consists of pigment cells which mark the boundary between the retina and the choroid.

Above: diagnostic tests for possible abnormalities of color vision. Top: a red-green-blind subject cannot see green or distinguish between reds, yellows and oranges. Bottom: a red-blind subject cannot distinguish between green and red.

When Sight is Damaged

Few people are born completely blind, but many suffer from serious defects in their vision and nearly everyone has some minor sight defect. Blindness is usually the result of an injury or disease in which the cornea or retina are destroyed. Another common cause is cataract, or opacity of the lens. Distortions and refractive (light bending) errors cause less serious defects in vision.

Nowadays automobile accidents are the main cause of severe eye injuries, the second being injuries from industrial mishaps, such as sparks flying from a grinding machine. In most serious injuries the eyeball is pierced or the lens damaged. Sometimes when one eye has been injured, infection may spread to the other eye and cause total loss of sight.

The nerves of the eyes may be damaged by injury, by an infection of the meningeal membranes, or by a tumor. In these cases a person will lose sight in one eye or some part of the vision of both. The original disease can be treated but the nerves cannot be repaired by any means and the loss of sight is permanent.

Congenital blindness is very difficult to treat and many people with such diseases remain blind throughout their lives. If a mother contracts German measles in the first eight weeks of pregnancy she may give birth to a child with congenital cataract.

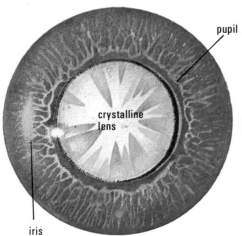

pupil

crystalline lens

iris

Cortical cataract

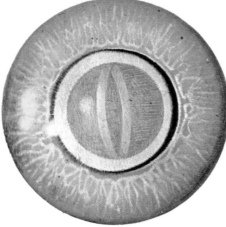

Nuclear cataract

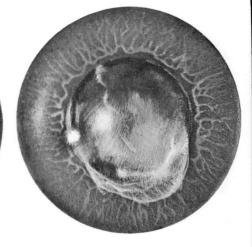

Traumatic cataract

Above: forms of cataract. In cortical cataract the outer part of the crystalline lens clouds over. Nuclear cataract is so called because the opacity develops at the center of the lens. The opacity and swelling of the lens in a traumatic cataract are the results of penetration of aqueous humor between the lens fibers, usually following extensive injury to the eyeball.

Right: a congenital cataract.

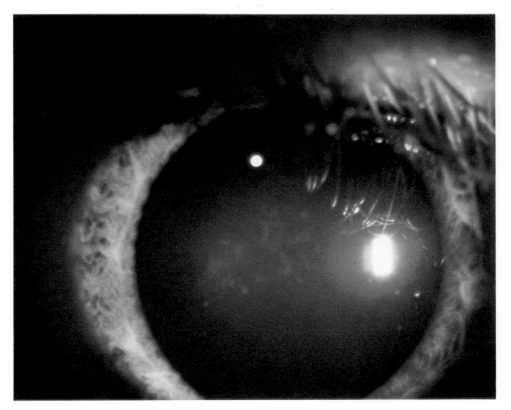

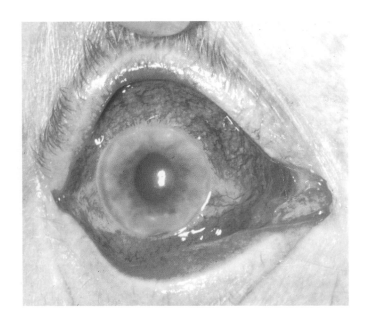

Acute glaucoma. It is a disease more common in people with smaller-than-normal eyeballs. The lens pushes the iris forward and obstructs the flow of the aqueous humor through the pupil. Pressure builds up, causing severe pain, nausea and distortion of vision. The attacks may be intermittent because when the pupil contracts, as for example during sleep, the iris is pulled back, allowing the flow to restart.

There is also a rare hereditary disease called *reticuloblastoma*, in which a malignant tumor appears in the second or third year of life. Unless the eye is removed this tumor can spread along the optic nerve to the base of the brain and cause death.

Blindness later in life often results from cataract or glaucoma. In cataract, the lens becomes opaque and this occurs most often as senile cataract in later life. The condition need no longer cause severe deterioration of vision because it can be successfully treated by surgery.

Glaucoma is another extremely serious eye condition as it can lead to permanent blindness. In this disease the pressure of fluid within the eye rises above the normal level and may damage the nerves transmitting the visual impulses. There are two types of glaucoma. In chronic glaucoma the pressure builds up over a long period; it does not produce symptoms in its early stages and is usually detected during an eye examination. In the early stages of acute glaucoma a sufferer can often see colored rings around bright lights.

Later severe pain and loss of vision occur. Any of these signs demand an immediate consultation with a doctor. Prompt diagnosis and treatment can be life saving. Thanks to instruments such as the ophthalmoscope and tonometer, the miotic drugs (which constrict pupil size), and also to some forms of surgery, the ancient scourge of glaucoma can be treated so that its damage is stopped and blindness prevented. This represents one of the great advances of modern medicine.

A person with *hypermetropia*, or farsightedness, can distinguish distant objects clearly but is unable to focus near objects for reading and close work. With increasing age the lens often loses its capacity to focus on distant objects and during middle age many people come to need glasses to increase the focusing powers of their eyes. Farsightedness is a hereditary refractive error, as is *myopia*, or nearsightedness, which often occurs in early life. This defect of vision makes distant objects blurred. Myopic children need to wear glasses to read the blackboard at school and to see properly in the street.

Farsightedness (right): the eyeball is relatively short and the image is focused behind the retina. Convergent lenses correct this defect. Nearsightedness (left): the converse applies and divergent lenses are prescribed.

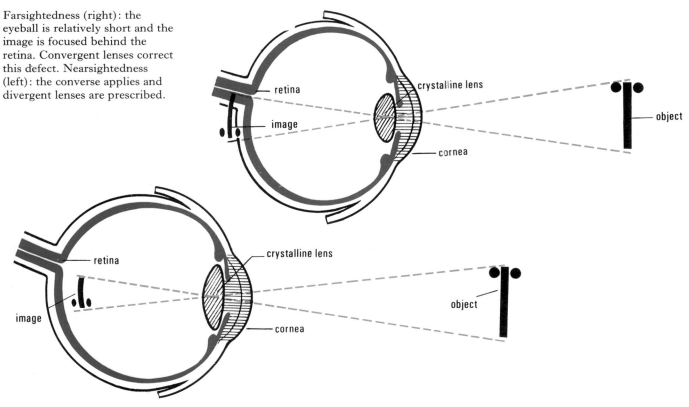

Weaknesses of Vision

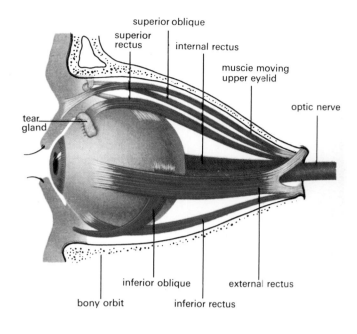

Crossed eyes and other forms of *strabismus* (squint) do not correct themselves. It is very important to realize that if we mistakenly wait for self-correction, some of the damage may become permanent. Perhaps some two people out of a hundred have strabismus in some form, and in practically every case it can be corrected painlessly, without hazard and with no loss of vision, if attended to early enough. If neglected, the eyes can still be aligned, but the damage done to the eyesight can rarely be fully reversed.

A newborn infant has the innate tendency, but not the ability, to coordinate the eyes so that they both turn directly toward the object he or she is looking at. The ability to coordinate usually becomes firmly established within a few months after birth. With such coordination the infant then has the same image focused sharply on the fovea of the retina, and both images are combined to give a clear, unified, three-dimensional picture. This is called binocular single vision, or binocular fusion, and it helps us judge both depth and distance.

If the eyes do not line up, however, each retina

The eyeball is moved by six extrinsic muscles, attached both to the sclerotic coat and the bony orbit. The muscles continuously position the eyeballs so that the eyes converge (both see the same image). If the eyes are wrongly coordinated one of the eyes turns inward or outward.

has a different image focused upon it. This situation, in which the person sees a double image, is common to squint. It is known as *diplopia*, and it can be very disturbing. Not only does each eye look in a different direction, seeing a different object, but depth and distance perception are disturbed as well. Strabismus can take a number of forms, depending upon which

Orthoptist treating a young patient. The earlier an eye defect is diagnosed and treated, the better the chances of normal vision.

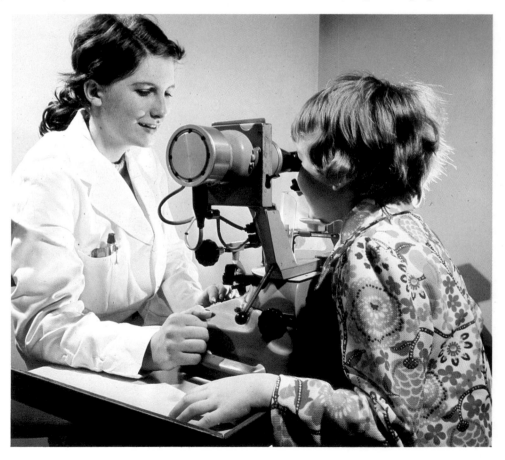

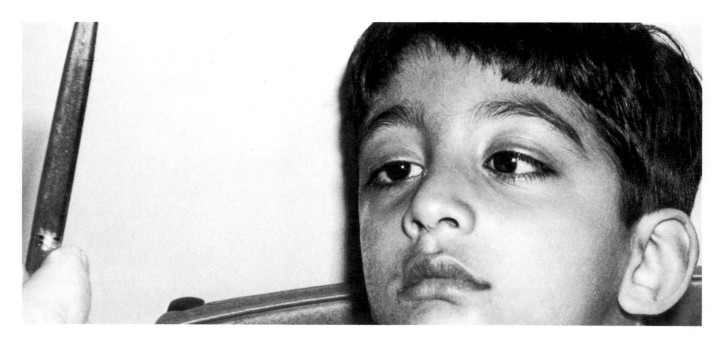

This patient has a convergent squint in his left eye. Most small children are slightly farsighted and when they focus on distant objects the eyes tend to converge slightly. Normally this reflex action of the eye muscles is controlled; a breakdown in coordination results in a squint.

of the six muscles controlling the movement of each eye are involved. Some strabismus is intermittent, the abnormality appearing only under conditions of illness, fatigue or emotional disturbance. Also, when a person has had even moderate amounts of alcohol, the ability to fuse the two images and thus judge depth and distance, is greatly reduced.

For the most part, however, strabismus begins in childhood. Because double vision is very disturbing to the brain it automatically begins to suppress the image of one eye, generally the eye that is off center. This suppression can develop very quickly. It might appear that this image inhibition by the brain is beneficial but it all goes at the cost of the suppressed eye, for that eye is for all practical purposes blind. As time goes by the suppressed eye's acuity (sharpness) of vision diminishes. This deterioration of vision may become so extreme that the affected eye can barely perceive light.

Infants and small children are usually treated for strabismus with *occlusion therapy*: the good eye is simply covered with an eyepatch and the crossed eye has to be used exclusively. The result is usually successful. If not, a simple surgical operation can correct the defect. Older children who develop strabismus generally receive special glasses that will help straighten the deviating eye. Should the eyes continue to remain crossed despite occlusion therapy, surgery is necessary to correct the orbital muscles. These operations are safe, but they may have to be repeated until the precise adjustment is made to straighten the eye.

A number of people are affected by *amblyopia* – partial or complete blindness without any apparent structural defect in the eyeball itself. Sometimes this condition develops when the retina is not stimulated enough during infancy. The human eye is rarely injured by overuse, but it can be harmed by not being used enough. Or the condition may be caused by an infantile cataract: a cloudy or opaque lens prevents adequate light from reaching the retina. Poisoning by lead, nicotine, alcohol or other toxins is another cause.

In the most common form of amblyopia the images formed on each retina are so unequal or confused that they cannot be combined by the brain into a single image. Another form of common amblyopia is generally due to one of two forms of interference with normal fusion of the images we see with each eye: strabismus, resulting from an imbalance of the eye muscles, and *anisometropia*, which means "not having the same size." Anisometropia occurs when the focusing power of the two eyes is different or when the same image is seen in two different sizes. This condition can result from marked variation in curvature of the corneas of each eye, differences in eyeball length, or the removal of a lens due to a cataract.

The techniques and training methods for adjusting deviated and weakened vision is known as *orthoptics*; and its most recent system of exercises and conditioning methods designed to retrain the eye so that the fovea can become useful once again is called *pleoptic therapy*. This helps children whose amblyopia has been allowed to become too advanced for correction by occlusion therapy. In many cases it can also help to improve the vision of adults.

Practically all deviating eye conditions can be corrected, and this should be done at the earliest possible moment. Good results are obtained in 80 percent of children from two to four years of age, but in only 40 percent of those from four to seven. Double vision at one year of age can often be eliminated within a few weeks. Early detection and treatment remain the best insurance against permanent damage.

Coping with Blindness

Paul Mussgay was a World War II fighter pilot. During a mission his plane caught fire but he managed to return to base. He was pulled unconscious from his blazing aircraft. The medical team were able to save his life but not his eyesight: his corneas were badly burned. Despite his handicap he was determined to study economics. He learned Braille and his wife read textbooks to him. Against all the odds he succeeded and eventually became a university lecturer and later professor of social economics. Today he is the author of over a dozen books and an authority on the problems of social economics. For relaxation he plays chess and swims. And yet he is still only able to read Braille, walks with a fine white

The invention of Braille revolutionized the possibilities for the blind to participate in a sighted world. This telephone operator is able to record notes by means of the Braille shorthand machine (on his left).

cane, and needs a guide dog to help him get around.

The ability to communicate with others is most important to blind people. First of all Paul Mussgay had to learn the Braille alphabet. His wife also became familiar with this system of raised dots so she could write to her husband without another person having to read her letters to him. Later he made great use of the tape-recorder. The radio was also a tremendous help to him as he found it most important to keep up with current events. As a student and later as a teacher he never let his handicap prevent him from taking part in social and athletic activities. He went on long walks and obtained relief from the tensions of daily living by swimming and physical exercises. He learned to develop other senses as a substitute for his lost sight. He became an expert on how to use his ears as guides for movement. He trained his memory to work hyperefficiently – always at a disadvantage when playing chess against a sighted person, he is nevertheless a formidable opponent.

Paul Mussgay's story is one of an extraordinarily talented and determined man who, despite a great physical handicap, was able to achieve a great deal. But most blind people just have average abilities – and basically want to lead as "normal" and happy a life as possible.

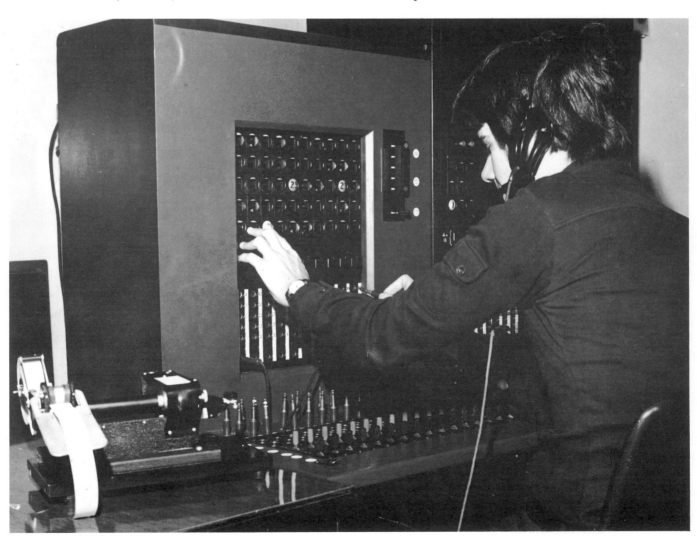

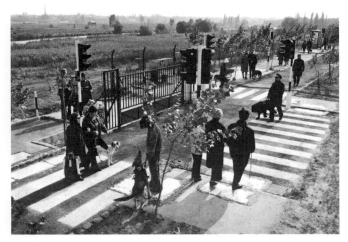

These mock pedestrian crossings in Budapest, Hungary, are used to train guide dogs to help the blind cope with traffic situations.

college education and pursue a professional career.

Problems are no less acute for the partially-sighted. They are able to move freely around by themselves and some are able to read normally. Partially-sighted children can usually manage at kindergarten schools, where they are given a great deal of personal teaching. They often go to ordinary schools, where the brighter ones can – with the help of their teachers – keep up with the fully-sighted children, but many find the struggle beyond their powers and fall behind the rest of the class. At the age of six or seven they may need to go to a school for the partially-sighted where they do not have to compete with sighted children and where special teaching techniques are used. Children who attend these schools learn best if they live at home, or at least spend weekends with their parents. Unfortunately this is not always possible as not every town has a special school. Sometimes it is difficult for parents to accept that their child is handicapped and they may insist that he or she should go to an ordinary school. But the partially-sighted child invariably benefits from a special education.

Over the years the blind have devised patterns of living that set them off from their sighted friends. But they can still be integrated into normal society, earning their keep and running their own lives.

The more difficult problems arise with the small number of people who are born blind and have to be brought up and educated without the help of vision. Special education is given at residential schools where from an early age blind children are taught the special skills that will enable them to live in the community at large and to find employment. Many pass ordinary school examinations; some go on to a

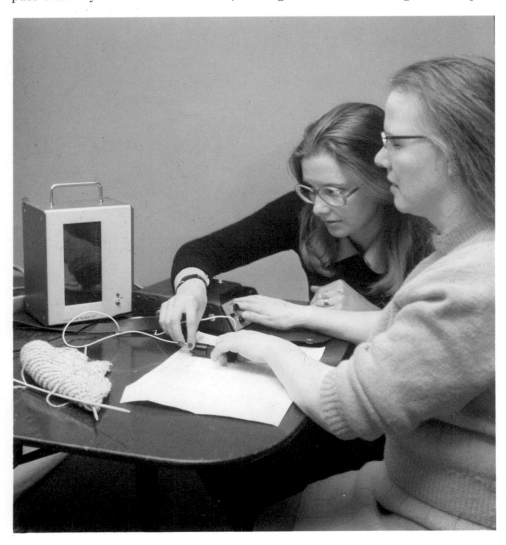

This "reading" machine, about the size of a small taperecorder, scans and converts printed words into vibrations of the shape of the letters, which the blind person can "read" with the fingertips.

Correcting Eye Defects

Glasses and contact lenses have a simple purpose – to correct defects in vision so that we can see as normally as possible. The way this is done is relatively simple in concept, but considerably more complicated in execution. The lenses used alter the focus of the light rays that enter the eye in such a way that they compensate exactly for the distortion caused by the sight defect.

Eyes are tested by an *optometrist*, who examines eyes and prescribes lenses and exercises; or an *ophthalmologist*, a doctor who diagnoses and treats eye diseases and defects. First the visual acuity (sharpness) of each eye is tested, and then both together, using a Snellen chart. This test helps show the furthest distance at which we can see clearly. Jaeger's test determines near vision: the person reads paragraphs printed on a card in various sizes of type and a record is made of the smallest type that can be read, as well as the distance at which the type can be distinguished. Next the examiner determines, by using a *retinoscope* (looking through a tiny hole in the center of a mirror), the changes in the light beam as it is reflected back from the retina to the pupil. In this way the presence and extent of any refractive error in the eye, and the amount of correction needed to restore the condition to normal, can be determined.

Another frequently used test actually allows the patient to select his own glasses. This is the *manifest refractive* test in which the person being examined wears frames with removable lenses. As the optometrist studies the eyes he keeps changing the lenses for each eye until the test chart can be seen with greatest clarity. When this point of sharpest vision for each eye is obtained, the eyes are tested together. If no further problem presents itself, the final lenses are the ones that will be prescribed for the patient.

Lenses to correct nearsightedness must prevent the light rays from coming into focus until they reach the retina. This is accomplished by a concave lens. Since these glasses are designed only to correct for distant vision, they will create distorted images close up. Consequently, nearsighted people have to remove their glasses when reading. Lenses for farsightedness are convex.

An ophthalmologist examines a patient's eye with a tonometer. This instrument measures the pressure within the eyeball and is a routine test for the diagnosis of possible glaucoma.

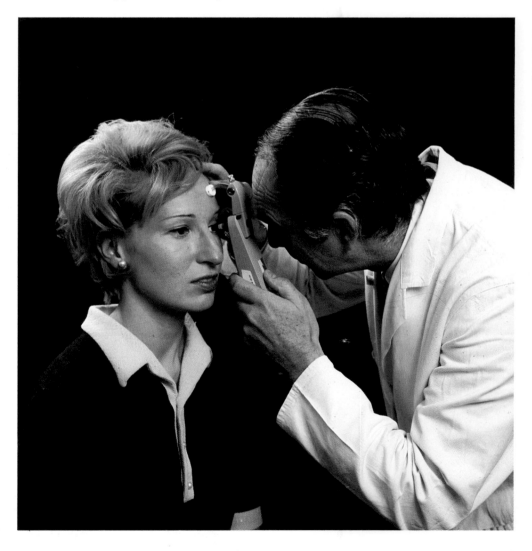

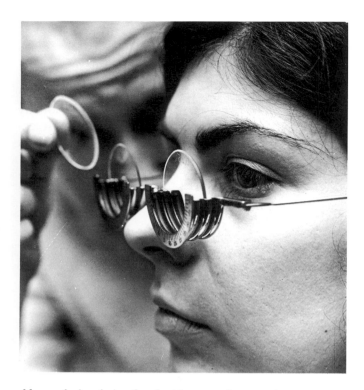

the lens maintains the same relative relationship to the retina that the normal crystalline lens would.

The corneal lens is the most popular type of contact lens worn today. It is the simplest to wear, but each lens has to be specially designed for the individual eye. It fits over the cornea, held in place by the surface tension of the thin film of tears on which it floats. The *scleral* lens is the oldest type of contact lens. It is molded to fit flush against the contour of the eye and today is not used at all for visual correction but as an aid to healing.

Contact lenses have many advantages over glasses. Apart from cosmetic reasons, they are not very easily dislodged by running, jumping, or any other physical activity. But they should not be worn by swimmers, because the lenses may float away when the eyes are open under water. However, as more and more people wear contact lenses, their potential dangers become more apparent. Poorly designed or badly fitted lenses can irritate, inflame, and damage the cornea. Another danger arises from simple human error. Wearers may wear them for too long a period, forget to remove them at bedtime, or are careless about cleaning them properly.

Glasses still remain the most popular method of wearing remedial lenses. There are several reasons for this. Some people simply cannot tolerate any

Above: before being fitted with spectacles, a patient undergoes the manifest refractive test. The frames have removable lenses which the optometrist keeps changing until a suitable one is found. Each eye is examined in turn, and then both lenses are tested together.

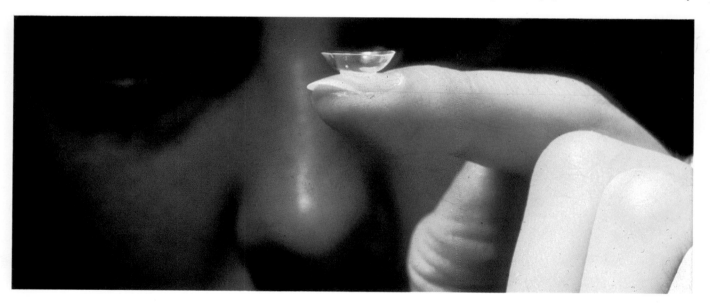

Above: bifocal contact lens. The eye focuses for near vision through the inner circle of the lens. When the eye accommodates for far vision it looks downward and the lower eyelid supports the lens in such a way that the eye can focus through the outer circle, which is adjusted for this purpose.

Astigmatism is caused by an unevenness of the lens or cornea and as a result the image focused on the retina is somewhat distorted. This defect can nevertheless be corrected by employing a cylindrical lens – one that is a section of a cylinder rather than a sphere.

An estimated ten million Americans are currently wearing shatterproof plastic contact lenses. The idea of the contact lens is extremely simple. The plastic surface of the contact lens itself takes over the function of the cornea. The contact lens floats upon the eye on a layer of tear fluid which, by filling the open space behind the curved lens surface, forms the liquid portion of the lens. By moving with the eye,

foreign substance in their eyes. Others are only able to tolerate contact lenses for a short period of time, and they must remove them to rest their eyes. The insertion of contact lenses into the eyes requires a certain amount of manual dexterity which some people do not have. Expense is another possible reason, since contact lenses are substantially more expensive than glasses. Furthermore, contact lenses are easy to lose but very difficult to find.

Eye Surgery Today

Eye surgery today is performed mostly on the front part of the eye to deal with cataracts, corneal disease, and glaucoma. Occasionally it is used to improve squints and structures actually outside the eye, such as the muscles which move the eyeball.

Cataract surgery is believed to have been practiced 2000 years ago by the Hindu surgeon Susruta; but the first account of the procedure to remove lenses

ments, in particular stitching with extremely fine sutures. Today the extraction of a cataract has become a safe operation, and the use of *cryotherapy* in the eye makes this much easier and safer. In this procedure the tip of a probe is cooled to up to minus 14 °F. When the probe is applied to the lens a ball of ice forms, which 'fuses" the cataract to the probe. Then the cataract can be pulled out of the eye in one piece and the risk of its breaking on extraction is negligible. Previously pieces of cataract left behind had often to be removed by a second or even third operation. The "longsightedness" following cataract extraction is sometimes corrected by contact lenses, or more commonly by thick lenses worn in spectacle frames. Relatively few surgeons have even attempted to put a new lens right into the eye.

At the time of the amazing results of heart trans-

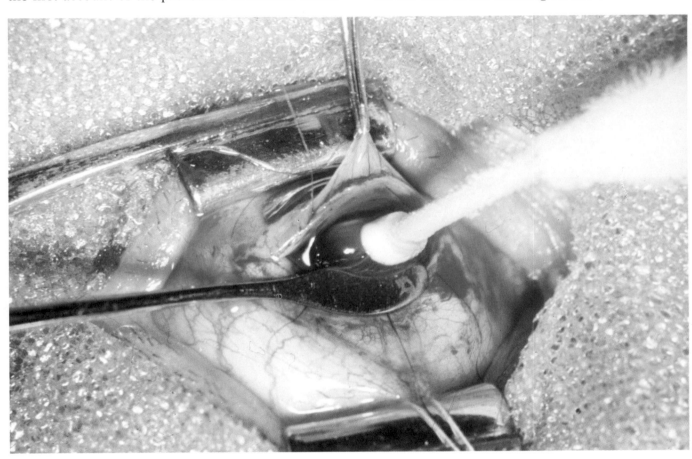

Removal of a cataract by cryotherapy. The surgeon uses a probe which is cooled down to an extremely low temperature. When the probe is applied to the cataract it fuses to the instrument and can be removed simply, without damage to surrounding tissue.

that had lost their transparency was provided by the Roman medical writer Celsus in the 1st century AD. However, the first surgeon who actually opened the eyeball in a manner comparable to that employed by surgeons today was the Frenchman Daniel in 1745.

Advances in cataract surgery technique were brought about by the advent of anesthetics and antibiotics, as well as the development of new instru-

plant surgery in the 1960s, few people realized that corneal transplants had been a common practice for several decades. In animals of the same species, the first successful corneal transplants were performed in 1835. For a time, when donor material from animals was used on humans, rejection of the newly introduced tissue invariably led to failure. In 1905 a surgeon succeeded in performing a corneal graft using an eye from another human being. Corneal grafts are often successful because the cornea is normally completely devoid of blood vessels and the reaction to a foreign body is extremely mild. Also the longer survival of the corneal tissue after death undoubtedly adds to the more favorable result compared with other

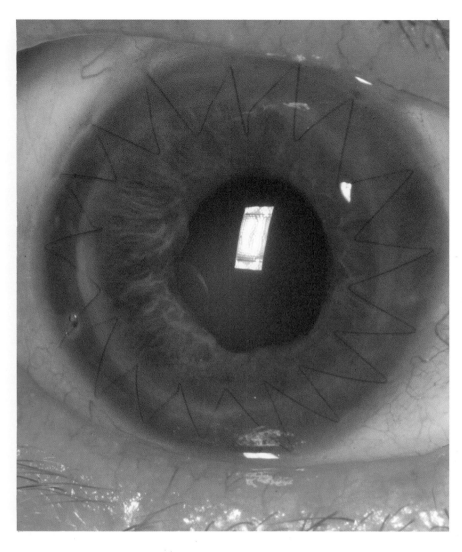

A corneal graft. The starlike pattern marks the position of the sutures. The cornea has no blood vessels and therefore there are no problems of tissue rejection with this particular graft.

tissue transplants. In many countries there are now eye banks set up to take care of the removal and storage of donor eyes. Recently attempts have been made at inserting an artificial, plastic cornea.

Surgery has also been used successfully to treat acute glaucoma, a major cause of blindness. The surgeon makes a small incision in the outside of the iris to effect a bypass of the watery aqueous humor, removing a build-up of pressure. Treatment of chronic glaucoma is still mainly confined to drugs.

The retina is a delicate structure and has no regenerative powers. Retinal detachments are nearly always associated with breaks in the retina and surgery is extremely difficult as it is not easy to locate the holes with accuracy. The operation consists of forcing out the fluid which separates the retina from the underlying tissue. Heat, extreme cold, or a laser beam are applied to produce an inflammatory reaction which causes the retina to adhere to the choroid. Laser beams produce very small burns, and can be accurately focused. These "welding" techniques are useful in preventing major retinal detachment and treating them in the very early stages.

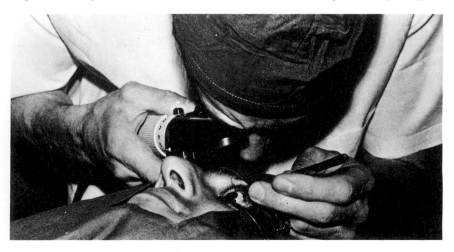

Using a laser ophthalmoscope to repair a detached retina. Very little heat and no pain are produced; therefore no anesthetic is required. It takes a fraction of a second.

How the Ear Works

Each ear consists of two distinct organs: one for hearing and one for balance. The visible part of the ear is called the outer ear or pinna, which in human beings is not very well developed. It helps to collect and guide vibrations (sound waves) to the eardrum, or *tympanic membrane*. Vibrations set up in this membrane travel along three linked bones (*ossicles*) in the *tympanum* (middle ear) to another membrane called the *oval window*. These bones form a system of levers which magnify the intensity of the vibrations in the tympanum. In addition, the oval window is very small so that it vibrates more intensely than the larger tympanum.

If the tympanum is to vibrate efficiently there must be an adequate atmospheric pressure on either side of it. We realize the importance of this when we change altitude quickly in an elevator or in an aircraft. At such times it is often difficult to hear, but a ventilation shaft (*the Eustachian tube*) links the middle ear with the back of the throat so that when we swallow air passes into or out of the middle ear to equalize the pressure.

The organ of hearing, in the inner ear, is a spirally wound tube called the *cochlea*; it is lined with groups of sensory cells mounted on a membrane. Vibrations of the oval window pass first through the fluid surrounding the cochlea and then through fluid inside it, finally spreading along the membrane. Much of the membrane vibrates at all audible frequencies, but a particular note makes one part vibrate more strongly than the rest. When the membrane vibrates it has an effect on hairlike sense cells; impulses set up in all the sense cells transmit information along about 30,000 nerve fibers. This, however, is apparently only one factor in the complex process of hearing. Both the ear and the brain must further analyze the sound, but how this is done is still obscure.

Sound is the result of wavelike vibrations in the air. The *amplitude* or height of the wave determines the loudness: the greater the amplitude the louder the sound. Pitch is determined by the *frequency* or number of waves in a given period of time, usually

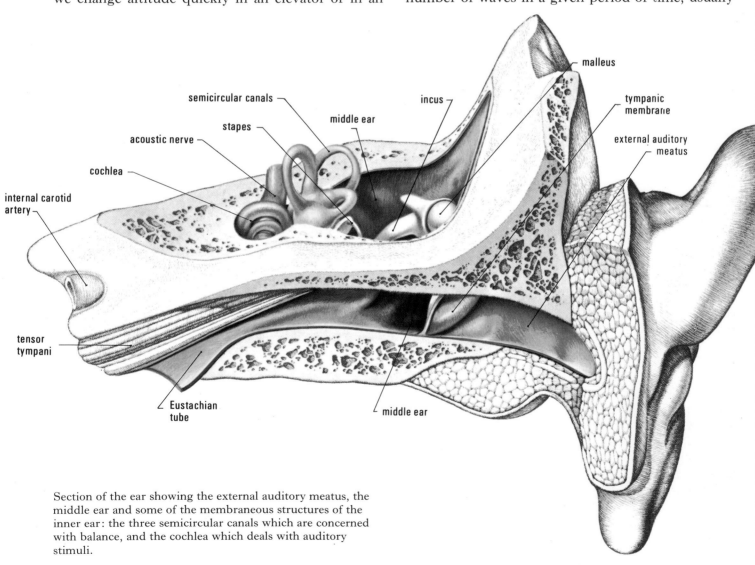

Section of the ear showing the external auditory meatus, the middle ear and some of the membraneous structures of the inner ear: the three semicircular canals which are concerned with balance, and the cochlea which deals with auditory stimuli.

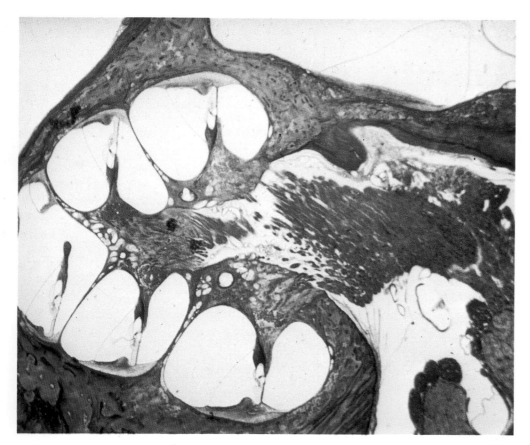

Left: photomicrograph through the cochlea and surrounding bone. The five white areas are sections through the spiral turns of the cochlea, with the organ of Corti in the center.

Below: the organ of Corti. These sensory cells with hairlike projections receive vibrations, corresponding to sound vibrations transmitted by the ossicles, from the surrounding fluid and convert them into electrical impulses which are then conveyed to the brain.

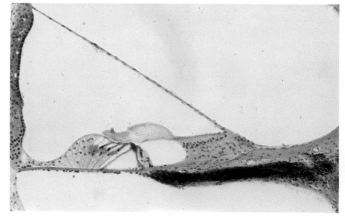

expressed as cycles per second (c/s). The average person can hear frequencies of between about 20 and 20,000 c/s. The ear is more sensitive to variations of pitch than to those of volume; we can distinguish some 2000 changes in pitch but only about 370 changes in volume.

The ears are also capable of distinguishing the direction from which the sound has originated. When listening to a sound coming from the side, one ear receives a wave at a certain amplitude, while the other receives it at a different amplitude – that is, the waves are "out of phase." The impulses in the auditory nerves are therefore out of step. Also, the loudness of the sounds arriving at the two ears are unequal. The brain interprets the minute differences between the signals coming from the two ears, so that we know from which direction the sound is coming. But if the sound comes from directly in front or behind, both ears receive waves in phase and this, too, helps the brain to locate the origin of the sound.

Serious hearing defects can often be corrected by a hearing aid that fits neatly behind the ear. With the help of transistors, it picks up sound waves, amplifies them, and transmits sound to the cochlea through the bones of the skull itself. This is why a hearing aid works even when the drum or the ossicles are seriously damaged.

The part of the inner ear concerned with balance is connected to the cochlea, but we must remember that hearing and balance are two quite distinct senses. The parts that respond to changes in motion – that is to acceleration and deceleration – are called

the *semicircular canals*. These lie in three different planes at 90 degrees to each other; each canal is swollen at its base and contains hairlike sense cells (*receptors*). When your head or body moves, the canals move as well, but due to inertia, the fluid inside them is momentarily left behind so that it presses on the receptors. As the canals are in three different planes, a movement in any direction will stimulate the hairs in one or more of the canals; the greater the acceleration or deceleration of the body, the faster the receptors send impulses to the brain.

The semicircular canals lead into two connected sacs, each containing groups of hairlike sense cells on which rest particles of chalk. This is the part of the inner ear that senses the body's position in space. As the position of the body and head alters, the pressure of the particles on the receptors varies. As the body tilts away from its normal vertical position, the speed of the impulses traveling to the brain increases.

Disturbances of Hearing

Defective hearing is more common than most people realize, largely because many people are not aware of their own slight loss of hearing when it occurs. The totally deaf suffer from a greater isolation than the totally blind, and the more distressing loss to the partially deaf is that of being able to understand speech clearly. *Tinnitus* (ringing in the ears) and deafness are frequent symptoms of hearing disturbance and invariably indicate disease of the ear or of the auditory nerve and its central connections.

Tinnitus is a purely subjective phenomenon and may also be experienced as a buzzing, whistling, hissing, or roaring sound. Transient tinnitus is a common symptom in adults; it may be of no signifi-

Examining the ear with an otoscope. It consists of a battery-powered light which illuminates the inside of the external ear, and a lens which magnifies it about six times. The otoscope is used for observing changes and infections in the external auditory canal and eardrum.

cance and due only to wax in the outer ear or to a blocked Eustachian tube. On the other hand, it is regularly associated with disease of the auditory nerve, inner ear, or ossicles; certain drugs, such as salicylates and quinine, produce tinnitus and transient deafness, as can a rise in blood pressure.

There are two main types of deafness. *Nerve deafness* is due to a damaged or incompletely developed inner ear. *Conduction deafness* is caused by diseases or blockages in the outer and middle ear. Doctors distinguish between these two types by using a tuning fork. When a vibrating fork is held several inches from the ear, sound will only be heard if the waves are transmitted through the middle ear and will be reduced if this area is diseased or blocked. When the fork is struck and applied to the skull, the sound waves are conveyed directly to the cochlea, without the intervention of the middle ear. With diseases of the cochlea or of the auditory nerve, both air and bone conduction will be reduced or lost.

The common causes of conduction deafness are a blockage of the auditory canal (usually by wax), inflammation or abscess in the middle ear, defective bone growth, fluid in the ear, and rupture of the eardrum. *Hereditary otosclerosis* (hardening of the tissues of the middle ear) is the most frequent cause of deafness in adults. Nerve deafness has many causes. The internal ear may be underdeveloped

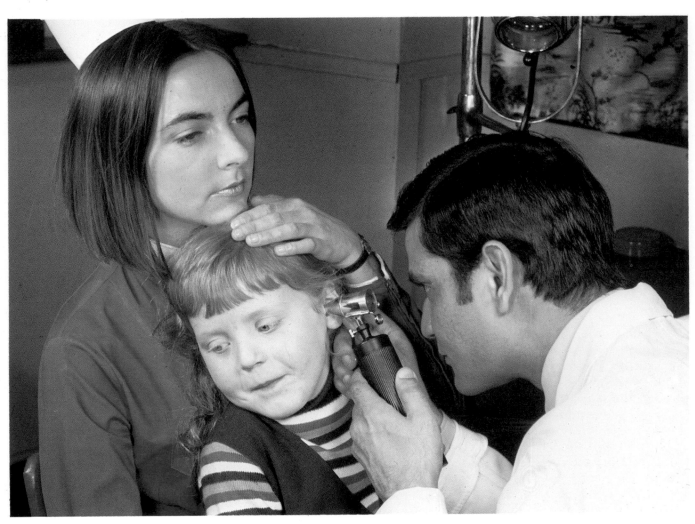

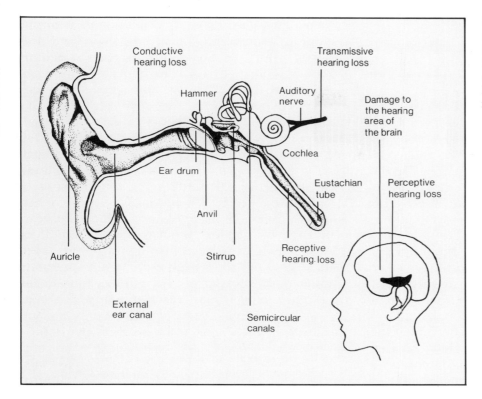

Damage to different parts of the ear results in different types of deafness. Conductive deafness is caused by a defect in the outer or middle ear. If the inner ear or nervous tissue connected with hearing are damaged, then the result is nerve deafness or perceptive hearing loss.

from birth (hereditary deafness, or mutism), or it may be damaged because the pregnant mother had German measles. Acute inflammation of the meningeal membranes (*meningitis*), or chronic infection spreading from the middle ear, are common causes of nerve deafness in childhood. The auditory nerve may be affected by brain tumors or by syphilis. Hereditary deafness might accompany various combinations of mental backwardness or skin abnormalities.

Excessive noise is not a new problem, but industrial, electronic and military developments have enormously increased the aggravation and distress. The din made by boilermakers riveting inside resounding boilers has long been known to damage their hearing. Noise is a hazard near aircraft and people working at airports often wear earmuffs for protection. Steady noise should not exceed a sound intensity of 85 dB (decibels) over eight hours. Exposure to 120 dB should never occur for more than half a minute per working day. A jet aircraft at takeoff can have an intensity of up to 140 dB; a train around 75 dB; and normal conversation about 50 dB. In practice noise is very rarely constant for long periods, but occurs in bursts or with frequent changes of intensity. Hearing loss due to excessive noise is doubly treacherous. Firstly because the noise very quickly produces an initial temporary deafness it seems to diminish. Secondly, any damage done in youth may only become apparent much later in life when the condition is too advanced for successful treatment.

A frequent and permanent disability resulting from continual exposure to excessive noise is high-tone deafness. The tragedy is that the disease takes a long time to develop, cannot be reversed, and yet can be prevented by protective ear covering.

Even if it does not produce actual deafness, noise can block conversation, cause accidents when warnings are not heard, ruin sleep, engender ill temper and fatigue, and impair industrial productivity.

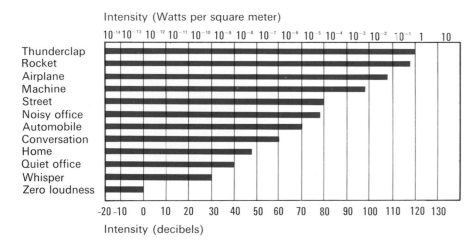

Comparative intensities of a variety of common sounds, from top to bottom in order of increasing sound pressure. 85 decibels is considered to be the upper safety limit for continuous exposure.

Deafness in the Family

Deafness is sometimes hereditary. It may be the result of a defect in the parents' genes that prevents normal development of the cochlea. When this happens there is often more than one deaf child in the family. However, sometimes the children of a deaf person have normal hearing. Intermarriage between people with hereditary deafness should be considered very carefully, since the likelihood of their having deaf children is greater than that of other people.

There are many types of hereditary deafness. One large group is connected with abnormalities in other parts of the body. Eye conditions, albinism (a congenital absence of pigment in the skin, hair, and other places), skeletal disorders, and disorders of the nervous system, may be associated with hearing loss.

If hereditary deafness is associated with nephritis (kidney inflammation), the condition is known as Alport's syndrome. Sometimes deafness is accompanied by goiter. Types of hereditary deafness not associated with other abnormalities include dominant types of severe congenital deafness, progressive nerve deafness, low-frequency hearing loss, and mid-frequency hearing loss.

Deformities of the ossicles in the middle ear, such as an absent *incus* (anvil) or *stapes* (stirrup), or a fused incus and *malleus* (hammer), are commonly associated with a congenital blockage of the external auditory canal. *Otosclerosis*, a common cause of conductive hearing loss, is a hereditary defect of unknown cause and twice as common in women as in men. It does not show itself at birth but appears in adulthood. In otosclerosis the normal bone in the ear is replaced by a highly vascular bone which tends

The ossicles, or bones, of the middle ear. From left to right: stapes (stirrup), incus (anvil) and malleus (hammer). They are linked together and transmit sound vibrations from the tympanic membrane to the oval window. These can be damaged through injuries to the skull, with resulting deafness. With the increase in motor accidents, these injuries are now more common.

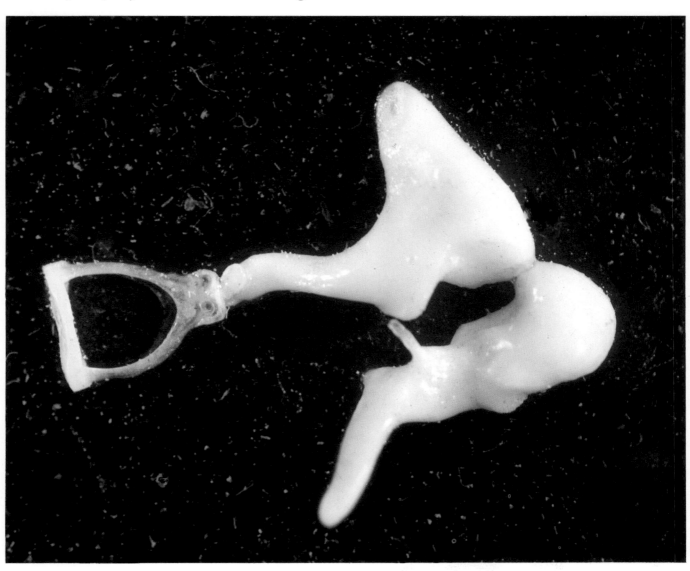

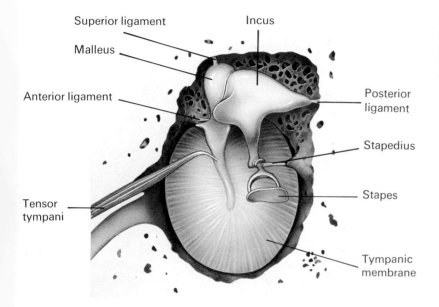

Superior ligament
Malleus
Anterior ligament
Tensor tympani
Incus
Posterior ligament
Stapedius
Stapes
Tympanic membrane

Left: a view of the tympanic membrane (eardrum) seen from the inside. The membrane vibrates in sympathy with sound vibrations in the external auditory meatus (canal).

Below: a plastic tube or grommet, inserted through a puncture in the eardrum, helps to drain the fluid which accumulates in the normally air-filled middle ear. This condition, known as glue ear, is the most common cause of deafness in children. Because the eardrum has a tendency to heal very quickly, it pushes out the tube and the hole heals up of its own accord.

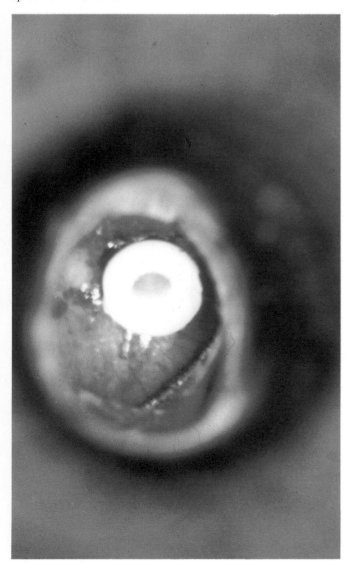

to overgrow the normal bone. Otosclerotic bone causes progressive fixation of the footplate of the stapes, which becomes evident by a slowly progressive hearing loss. In women it may progress more rapidly during or immediately after pregnancy. If the cochlea is functioning normally, the condition may be improved by surgery.

Not all congenital deafness is genetically transmitted. In addition to hereditary deafness, there are two other groups of congenital disease: the prenatal group, in which deafness results from damage to the embryo; and the perinatal group, in which a trauma or disease in the periods directly before, during and just after birth causes deafness.

The prenatal category includes deafness as a result of a German measles infection in the mother during the first three or four months of pregnancy. The embryo is susceptible because this is the period during which the cochlea is developing. Another disease of the pregnant mother which can cause subsequent deafness in the child is syphilis. Generally, the deafness is not present at birth. The time it takes to develop depends on the form of the disease. In the early form deafness will occur in the first two years of the child's life, while in the late form it manifests itself at about the time of puberty.

Certain drugs taken by the pregnant mother have been shown to be responsible for congenital deafness, and it cannot be stressed often enough that all medication taken during pregnancy should be done so with extreme caution. Thalidomide, in addition to many limb deformities, produced conduction deafness in some of its victims.

Unlike the prenatal group of congenital deafness, which affects hearing across the whole frequency band, deafness due to perinatal causes is often high-tone. This is because the area of the brain responsible for high-tone hearing has not fully developed at birth and is thus more susceptible to perinatal factors such as anoxia (lack of oxygen), prematurity or neonatal jaundice.

Living with Deafness

Although today many people with a hearing loss benefit from medical and surgical treatment, there are many others whose hearing cannot be improved. It is estimated that in Europe over 20 million people will need help for a hearing problem sometime during their lives. Of these a minimum of five million have a permanent hearing loss great enough to handicap them. For these people help must come from the use of hearing aids and speech therapy, but in no other field of medicine is rehabilitation considered so important. Under the guidance of *otologists* (specialists in ear diseases), and with the help of educators of the deaf and community organizations, a large number of audiologists, speech therapists, and speech teachers are available to help those with a hearing handicap.

From the time the human held a cupped hand to the ear to aid hearing, there has been a constant search for better methods to amplify sound. An early (and still excellent) device is the ear trumpet.

Early electric hearing aids were like telephones; their development progressed from the use of vacuum tubes to the use today of transistors which make it possible to reduce the size of hearing aids so they can be concealed in the hair, worn behind the ear, or incorporated into the frames of glasses.

The people who benefit most from the use of a hearing aid are those who have a purely conductive hearing loss. They can receive sound over a wide range of intensities without discomfort. The person with a mixed or sensory-neural hearing loss has more difficulty in using a hearing aid. This loss involves the high tones, or the high and the middle tones, and it has not yet been possible to build a hearing aid that will selectively amplify only certain tones. The person who had damaged cochlear sense cells is the most difficult to help with a hearing aid. He or she hears weak sounds poorly or not at all, and loud sounds cause distortion and are accompanied by pain. The intolerance of a person with this type of disability to minute increase in volume, and the narrow range between comfortable loudness and uncomfortable loudness, creates problems that sometimes cannot be solved, although a simple ear trumpet can help

Rinné's test. The tuning fork is struck and held alternately on the mastoid process and at the external canal until no longer heard by either. In normal hearing and nerve deafness the sound is heard for longer by air conduction; in conduction deafness the converse occurs.

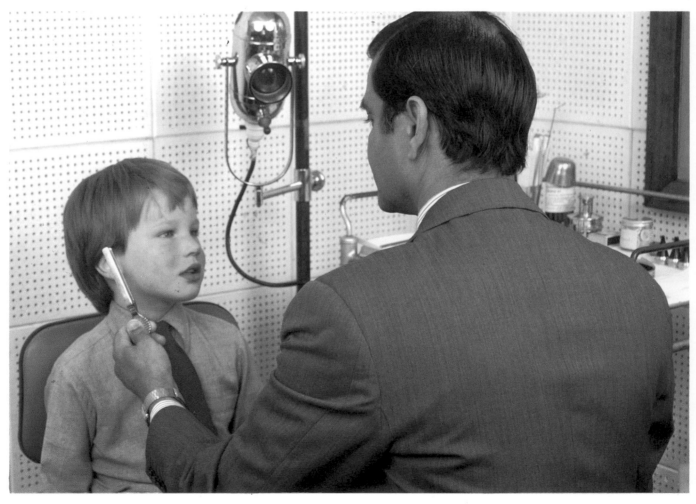

such people considerably.

A recent device picks up the auditory signals in a microphone placed near the poor ear and electrically routes them across to an earphone mounted beside the good ear. This has been designed to reduce the listening problems of those with the use of one ear only.

The ability to understand speech through the observance of lip and tongue movement and facial expression is known as *speech reading* or *lip reading*. This can be an additional aid to anyone with hearing impairment. Although some people can learn it by themselves, help from a teacher is usually necessary. The combination of a well-fitted hearing aid and good lip-reading ability is the ultimate in hearing rehabilitation.

No child born deaf is intrinsically mute because the larynx and vocal cords function normally. A deaf child is mute only because he or she cannot hear sounds and words. But the educational problem presented by the deaf or profoundly hard-of-hearing child is a serious one. The mute child produces sound, a lot of it, but it is unintelligible unless years of special training are provided. "Early warning" tests for deafness are part of a routine medical examination, because early recognition of hearing loss is essential if the child is going to receive the right kind of teaching – from about the age of two or sooner – that will enable proper speech to develop.

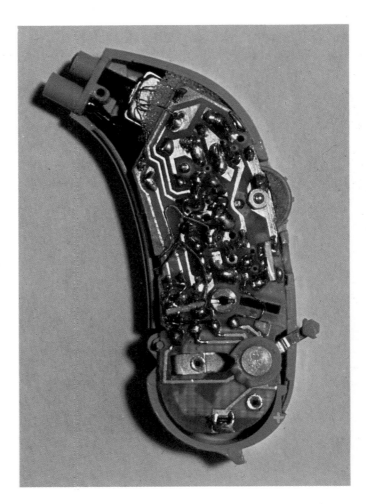

Above: interior of a hearing aid. It weighs 5 grams and fits neatly behind the ear.

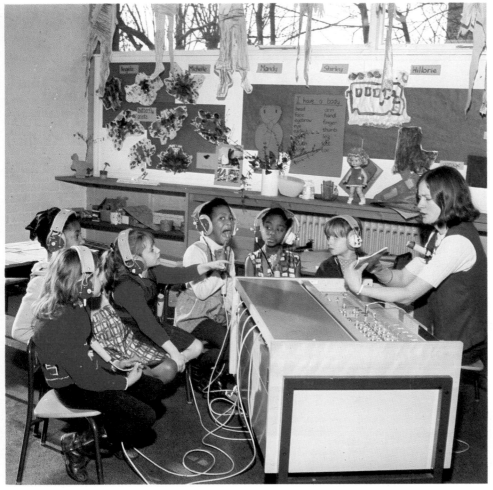

Left: children born with congenital deafness require special educational facilities. The majority have some residual hearing which responds to auditory training.

75

The Ear's Role in Balance

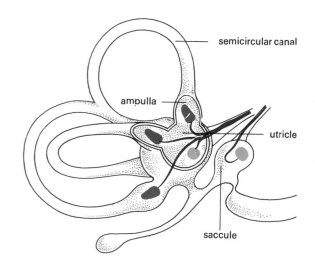

Equilibrium is a state of balance or equipoise in which opposing forces, such as gravity and the reflexes that keep our bodies erect, so-called *postural reflexes*, counteract each other exactly. But people often have difficulty in describing sensations of imbalance. Usually the term "dizziness" indicates

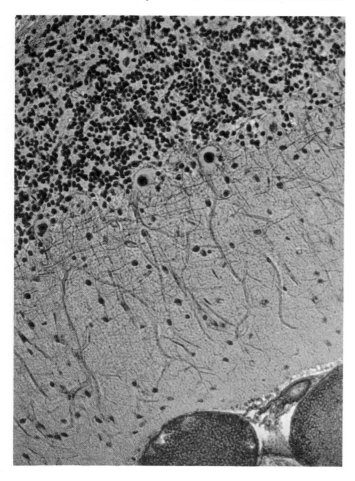

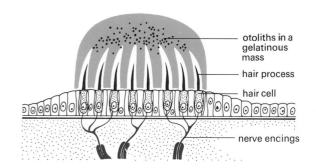

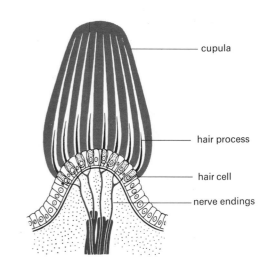

The saccules and utricles of the semicircular canals (top) contain a macula (center) whose receptors register the head's position. The swellings at the canals' bases contain a crista (bottom) which registers the head's movements.

Section through the cerebellum. It controls posture and balance, and consists of a left and right half, connected by a bridge of fibers called the pons. This permits muscular coordination between the two sides of the body.

not only a sense of rotation, but also vague experiences such as unsteadiness, insecurity, weakness, faintness, and lightheadedness. *Vertigo* literally means "sense of turning," either of one's body or of the surroundings.

In disturbances in which vertigo is a leading symptom, the person's medical history is of special importance in diagnosis, for this symptom may be accompanied by no visible signs. A feeling of near panic is particularly characteristic of vertigo: the sufferer feels as if the floor or walls are undulating,

or sinking or rising up, or that he or she is pulled to one side or to the ground, as though drawn by a strong magnet. Stance and gait are almost invariably affected during an attack of vertigo.

Vertigo may sometimes be caused by disorders of the cerebral cortex, eye muscles, cerebellum, ear mechanisms, and also by a disorder of the brain stem. Vertigo of the inner ear is common and it may accompany an ear infection (*labyrinthitis*), or occur as a symptom of an ear disease called Menière's syndrome.

The way people walk is always of interest, although a normal gait seldom attracts attention. The body is erect, the head straight, and the arms hang loosely and gracefully at the sides, each moving rhythmically forward with the opposite leg. With each step there is a coordinated flexion of foot and a barely visible elevation of the hip so that the foot clears the ground.

There are many variations of gait, and it is a commonplace observation that the sound of an individual's footsteps, notably the pace and heaviness of tread, may identify them. The manner of walking and the carriage of the body may even provide clues to character, personality and occupation. The sailor's rolling gait is an obvious example.

(proprioception) can also often abolish for a long time the capacity for independent locomotion.

A large number of abnormal gaits are recognized and classified by doctors. Cerebellar gait is most commonly seen in people with multiple sclerosis, cerebellar hemorrhage, or a tumor in the cerebellum. In people with *hemiplegia* (paralysis of one side of the body), one leg is held stiffly and does not flow freely and gracefully at the knee and hip. It tends to rotate outward, describing a semicircle. The hemiplegic gait can be "heard" by the slow rhythmic scuff of the foot along the floor. Paralysis of the fibular muscles causes a horselike gait. The leg must be lifted abnormally high so that the foot can clear the ground. There is a slapping noise when the

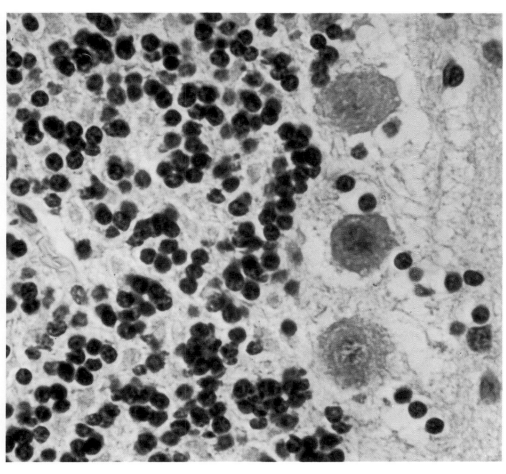

Cells in the cerebellum. The size of this area of the brain is related to muscular activity. It is larger in animals whose movements involve complex muscular coordination, for example, birds.

Certain female characteristics of gait, if observed in a man, immediately impart an (often false) impression of femininity.

Since normal body posture and locomotion require good visual information and correct functioning of the inner ear and of the skeleton and muscles, it is obvious that any breakdown in these functions will have an effect on the way we walk. A blind person or a normal one who is blindfolded, may walk very well, but they move cautiously to avoid collision with objects. A person with a middle ear that is not functioning efficiently shows a slight unsteadiness in walking and cannot descend stairs without holding on to a banister. They also find it difficult to run. A loss of response to internally produced stimuli

foot strikes the floor. Staggering or drunken gait is characteristic of alcohol or barbiturate intoxication. The drunken person totters, reels, tips forward and then may lose his balance and fall. Control over trunk and legs is greatly impaired. The steps are irregular and uncertain.

One curious irregular gait is neurotic. It imitates the gait of people with certain paralytic disorders. Usually a hysterical paraplegic depends on a crutch or remains helpless in bed. Some lurch wildly in all directions, actually demonstrating by their gyrations the most remarkable ability to make rapid postural adjustments. There are other gait disorders that are still poorly understood, such as senile gait and festinating gait (Latin *festinatio*, haste).

Your Children's Speech

The first year of a child's life is extremely important for the growth and development of language. Babbling, which begins at about four months, appears to be a rehearsal for the first simple words,

Talking regularly to your child increases his or her vocabulary and is one of the most important ways of enabling intellectual development to take place.

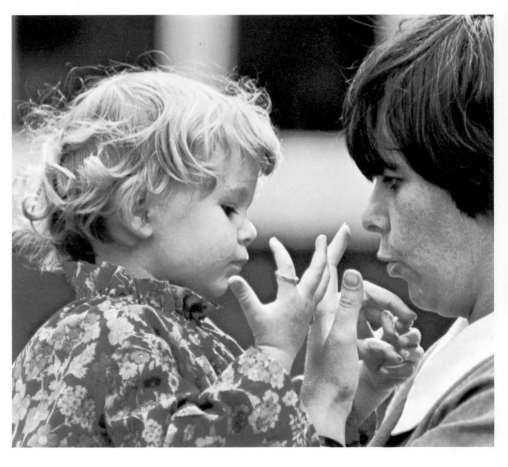

babbling as well as other prelanguage activities.

Up to the age of approximately 12 to 18 months little language development occurs and speech may come to a virtual standstill. The child's time and attention during this period are directed toward an exploration of his or her physical surroundings and learning how to walk. But after the age of 18 months language usually develops rapidly. A vocabulary of 20 words at 18 months of age may increase to 250 words by the age of two years.

During the period from two to four years of age, children attempt to use a rapidly increasing, and often inadequate, vocabulary to meet their expand-

which are usually spoken between the ninth and twelfth months of age. During this time children learn to enjoy sounds and to make a variety of their own. This not only exercises the speech organs but is also the beginning of ear training.

During this period, variations in pitch, inflection and volume will begin. Some sound combinations that sound like words are produced. The word "mum" or "mamma" is often the first combination. After the mother hears it and repeats it back to the child a few times, the child soon learns that by saying the word "mamma" it may get what it wants.

The normal development of language can be delayed by conditions that interfere with usual prelanguage activity. Congenital anomalies, such as cleft lip or palate, birth and emotional traumas, delayed physical development, mental retardation, serious illness, or a hearing impediment, may prevent

ing needs. A lack of fluency is quite normal for many children at this time and if parents are constantly correcting their child then this may create more problems than it solves. It is often during this period that parents become worried and seek the advice of a doctor. Their chief complaint is: "My child is stuttering, What shall we do?" The usual – and good – advice is: do nothing. This stage of speech development is normal.

Most children have an adequate vocabulary for most situations when they are ready to start school. A few have not. A child is suddenly confronted with a strange adult and a large group of unfamiliar children. The language that has previously met his or her needs in the family may now be insufficient, with the result that he or she may begin to stutter. Many cases of stuttering begin in the kindergarten, or first or second grade. Again the proper handling of this problem should be to accept it, provide security, and avoid stress until the child's language matures.

If there is a real problem, then a speech specialist should be consulted. In order to make a proper diagnosis of a speech disorder the specialist must know as much as possible about the probable causes – both physical and emotional – underlying the defect. Only then can it be decided how much of a problem the speech disorder will be to the child and what the child's and parent's potentials are for over-coming it. After the specialist evaluates all the find-ings, speech therapy may begin, or it may be delayed until the child is older. Ordinarily speech therapy is of long duration, often extending for several years. If the therapy is to be a success, the parents must cooperate actively with the therapist until it is decided that the speech defect no longer exists or no further improvement can be made.

As a rough guideline, parents should seek medical advice about speech development if their child is not talking at all by the age of two, if speech is largely unintelligible after the age of three, if the child uses mostly vowel sounds, if he or she is not forming sentences by three, if there is a noticeable non-fluency after age five, or if the child's voice is monotonous, extremely loud, or largely inaudible.

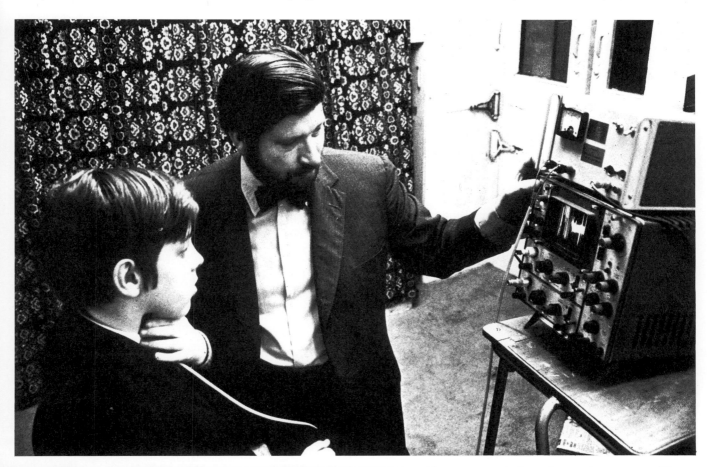

Above: a speech therapist treating a stutter. The pickups attached to the patient's throat are linked to a voice pattern machine. The patient can see the difference between his normal and abnormal patterns and adjust the latter.

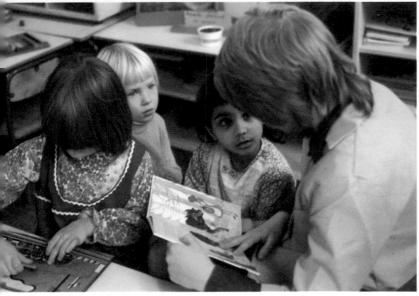

Left: when a child starts school he or she is suddenly confronted with a large group of strangers. A shy child, or one with an inadequate vocabulary, may become confused and develop a speech disorder.

79

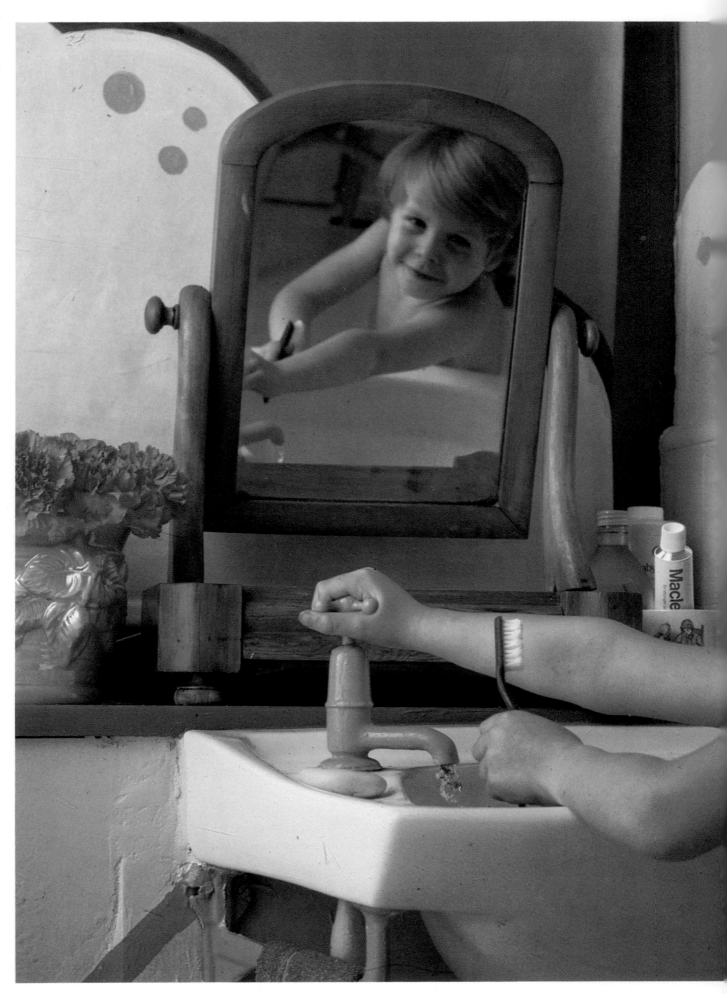

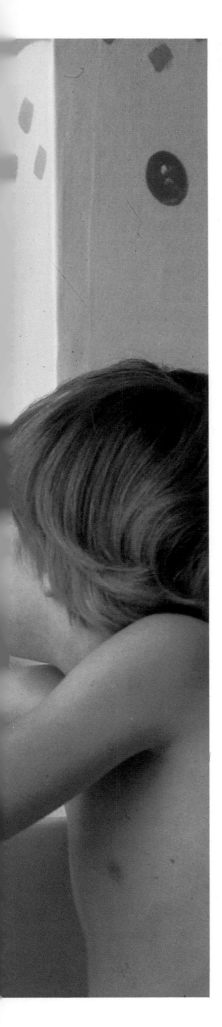

Chapter 4

Dental Health

In certain communities not so many years ago a young woman who wore a full set of dentures was considered a better marriage prospect than one who still had all her own teeth. She was thought to be a less troublesome and less expensive proposition! Although such attitudes have now disappeared, we still tend to think that our teeth are a problem only when we are suffering the agonies of toothache. We should be much more aware that effective prevention of decay – especially for our children – can be achieved by the use of fluoridation, by correct brushing, by avoiding certain kinds of food, and by having regular checkups.

Opposite: the majority of adults have extensive tooth decay and gum disease, the results of bad eating habits and poor dental hygiene. We should learn by our experiences and insure that our children have healthy teeth.

A Full Set of Teeth

A baby's 20 *deciduous* or milk teeth, and the elements of the permanent teeth, are formed before birth; they lie hidden beneath the gums. Approximately one child in 2000 is born with a visible tooth; among the few said to have been born with one were Julius Caesar, Hannibal, and Napoleon. In some countries a baby born with a tooth was once viewed with superstition – and in parts of Africa it was killed! The milk teeth begin to erupt at about six months, and it will take another two years for the full set to appear.

The milk teeth begin to fall out from the age of about six onward. By age 12 all the 32 permanent teeth will have erupted, with the exception of the molar teeth known as the "wisdom" teeth, which are cut between the ages of 18 to 25. A full set of permanent teeth consists of eight incisors for cutting, four canines for biting, eight premolars and twelve molars for grinding.

The bulk of the tooth consists of a substance called *dentine*, which is covered in the part projecting out of the gum (the *crown*) by hard *enamel*, and in the root by *cementum*. The enamel and cementum come together at the *neck* where the mucous membrane of the gum meets the tooth. The dentine surrounds the pulp cavity, which is filled with loose connective

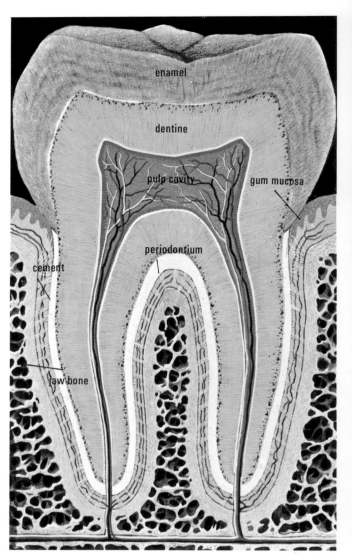

Above: longitudinal section of a lower molar. The tooth is hollow internally and lies in a cavity of the mandible (alveolus) covered by the gum mucosa. The exposed part of the tooth is covered by enamel (the crown), while that in the alveolus is covered by cement (root and neck). The root is attached to the alveolus by the gum.

tissue, the *dental pulp*. This contains blood vessels, lymph tissue, and nerves which enter and leave the root of the tooth by means of the *apical canals*. Survival of any tooth depends upon the healthy functioning of the pulp. When teeth erupt, the crowns are fully formed and do not increase in size. The roots, however, are not fully grown and in the permanent teeth take about three years to reach their maximum size.

Because most tooth formation occurs before birth, it is essential that the mother's diet contains plenty of the substances needed for the building of healthy teeth. The most important of these are vitamin D and calcium, both of which are present in large quantities in dairy foods, such as milk, butter, oily fish, and cheese.

Teething must be looked at as a natural – though sometimes painful – process. If a teething baby becomes reluctant to eat hard foods for a short

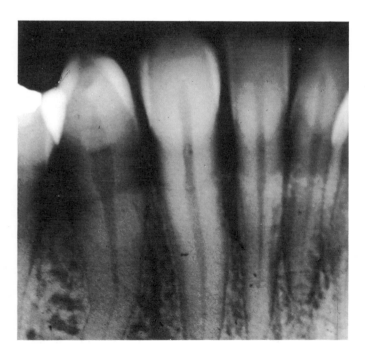

X-ray of the teeth showing the dental pulp. The pulp contains specialized cells called odontoblasts which form the dentine and grow out from the pulp as long processes. The pulp also contains nerves which provide the sensations of toothache when the pulp is damaged.

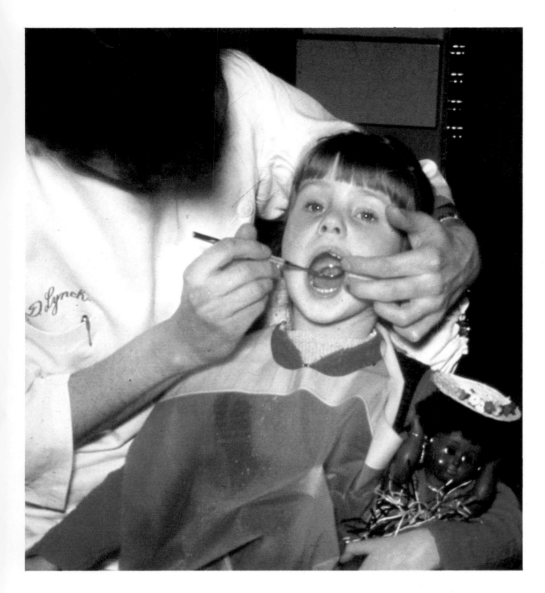

Although deciduous teeth eventually fall out, their health is still important and 6-monthly checkups are advisable. If the deciduous teeth are allowed to decay their permanent successors may develop crookedly.

period, the diet should be suitably modified. If the baby is in considerable pain at night, a small quantity of junior aspirin can be given. Plastic "teething rings" give the baby something to "bite" on and can be a great comfort. They should be choke-proof and be

Below: dentition of a young child, showing the permanent teeth developing beneath the deciduous dentition. Humans have 20 deciduous teeth, and 32 permanent ones. The first permanent teeth to erupt – the molars – do so at age 6–7.

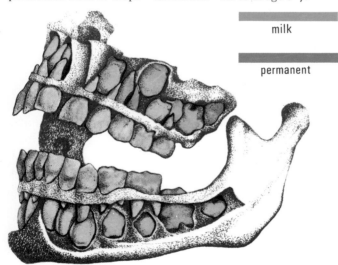

milk

permanent

kept scrupulously clean. Iced water may be used to "cool the gums," and proprietary teething jellies are also available.

By the age of 18 months old, children should be encouraged to brush their teeth after each meal. In addition the child should be encouraged to eat crisp fruit or vegetables such as apples, celery or carrots after a meal. These have rough fibers that perform a brushing action on the teeth. Regular six-monthly visits to the dentist should begin as soon as the child is three years old. The time to get cavities filled is when they are small – it saves the teeth and hurts the child less.

Parents sometimes wrongly believe that they do not have to worry about the decay of milk teeth, because they are going to be lost anyway. But a decayed milk tooth may cause a child a great deal of pain, and can lead to jaw infection. If it has to be extracted the resultant space allows nearby teeth to grow out of position. This means there is not enough room for the permanent tooth when it is ready to come through. As the last baby teeth are not lost until the child is about 12 years old, they should be looked after with as much care as the permanent ones.

The Scope of Dentistry

It seems that as long as human beings have had teeth, they have suffered from toothache. Around 5000 BC, Sumerian texts gave instructions for the treatment of dental disease, and in ancient India tartar deposits were removed and loose teeth splinted. There are Egyptian mummies with fillings and artificial teeth, though probably the work was done after death. In northern Italy, the ancient Etruscans of 500 BC constructed partial dentures by fixing teeth in vacant spaces with gold splints attached to neighboring teeth. But after the fall of Rome, dentistry, like medicine, languished for hundreds of years.

The first authoritative book on dentistry was written by Pierre Fauchard in the first half of the 18th century. He mentions tin, lead and gold as being suitable materials for filling teeth. The fact that metal could be mixed with mercury to form a soft mass which would then set solid, was recognized in 1826, and such amalgams were a great improvement on molten metal.

The beginning of the 20th century saw the introduction of porcelain for filling the front teeth, improved amalgams, and the development of gold alloys for the casting of inlays that did not shrink or warp, thereby making the precision inlays and bridgework of today possible. In the 1940s natural looking plastics took the place of · porcelain for dentures.

From barbaric remedies, painful operations and crude replacements of missing teeth and tissues,

Skilled dental treatment can make a vast improvement to personal appearance. Top: irregular, misplaced teeth. Bottom: the same set after the teeth have been crowned.

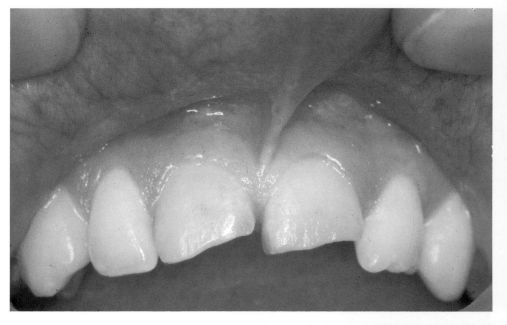

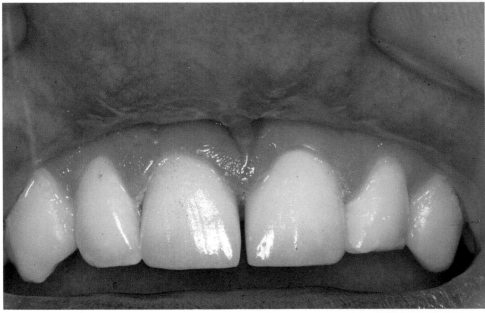

dentistry has evolved to the position where any dental ailment can be treated effectively and painlessly. It is a far cry from the itinerant tooth-puller to the dentist of today performing delicate operations with the aid of complicated equipment and shadowless lighting. The dentist in general practice conducts a hospital in miniature, with facilities for radiography, anesthesia, sterilization of instruments and dressings, operating chairs that can accommodate the patient either sitting or lying, equipment powered by electricity and compressed air, water and air sprays, electric cautery, tungsten and diamond drills, and materials of natural appearance for replacing lost teeth and the tissues in which they are set.

What can dentistry accomplish today? The crowns of teeth attacked by decay can be rebuilt, and the inflamed pulp can be treated medically, destroyed or cut out. The ends of diseased roots can be amputated through windows cut in the bone.

Artificial crowns can be made either to replace the entire natural crown or to envelop a core protecting the vital pulp. Gum diseases can be treated either surgically or with drugs. Irregular teeth can be straightened and even deep-rooted diseased teeth extracted painlessly; unsightly spaces where the teeth have been lost can be eliminated, and a complete set of dentures can give back to a person a normal appearance and the ability to enjoy food.

Modern dentistry has become highly specialized, each branch often requiring special skills and techniques. *Operative* dentistry deals with the preservation of natural teeth, and is closely associated with *endodontics*, which deals with the treatment of the soft tissue space between the teeth. The replacement of missing teeth by means of artificial substitution is called *prosthodontics*. *Orthodontics* involves the realignment of faulty tooth positions, often with the use of braces. And there are many more specializations.

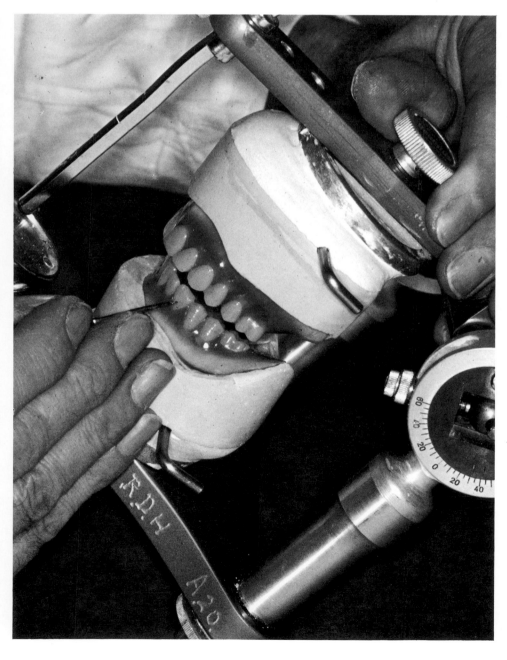

Prosthodontics is the branch of dentistry which deals with the restoration of dental health and structure by the use of prostheses. It includes the fitting, design, and manufacture of dentures.

Correct Brushing

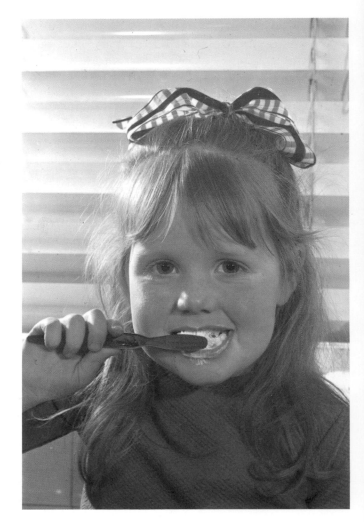

A beautiful smile can come only from a healthy person who has healthy teeth. This end result alone would be enough to justify *oral hygiene*, but there are many other reasons why it is practiced. Oral hygiene is the science that deals with the preservation and health of the hard and soft tissues of the mouth. The marked increase in the consumption of refined carbohydrates, especially sugar, by people of all ages during the past 25 years, with the resulting tooth destruction, makes the practice of oral hygiene vital for the preservation of general bodily health.

An important aspect of oral hygiene is concerned with the best way of brushing your teeth. There are several acceptable methods of toothbrushing and different dentists will sometimes give different instructions, often depending on the general state of your mouth. But it is generally agreed that considerable wear of the teeth can be caused by toothbrush abrasion if brushing is habitually and vigorously done from side to side instead of up and down or forward and backward in a scrubbing manner.

Your dentist is the best person to advise you about

Above right: correct brushing after meals is the best form of preventive dentistry. It staves off tooth decay and keeps the gums healthy.

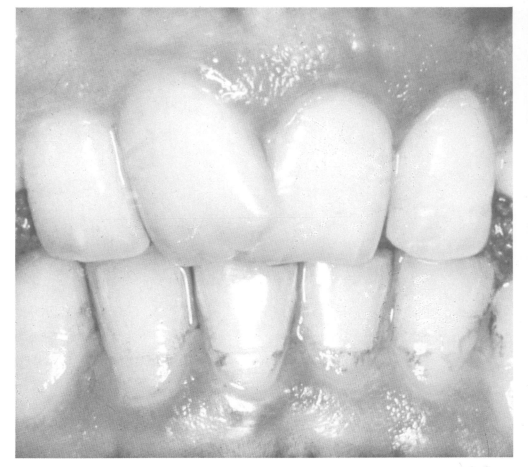

Right: these teeth appear clean because plaque deposits, being the same color as the teeth themselves, are difficult to see.

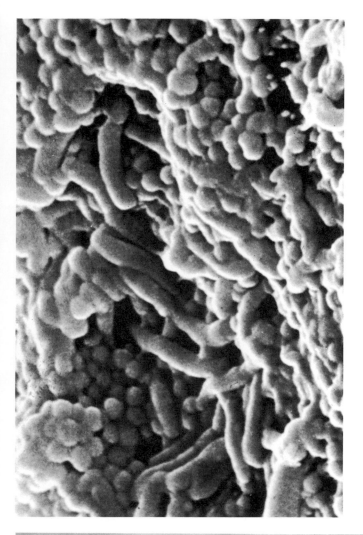

the type of brush that will suit you best. Remember that an old, worn out brush cannot do an effective job. The type of toothpaste you use does not matter greatly as long as you find its taste pleasant, but abrasive tooth powders should be avoided.

Try to brush your teeth three times a day, and especially last thing at night. Since the greatest amount of acid is produced in the mouth a few minutes after eating, it is essential that in order to prevent decay that brushing should be done as soon as possible after a meal. However, where this is not possible it is highly advisable to rinse your mouth thoroughly with water.

Sometimes brushing is not enough. Where disease has destroyed the tissue between the teeth, it may be necessary, following proper treatment of the gums, to use additional cleansing devices recommended by a dentist. They might include the use of a tooth pick, or cleaning in between the teeth with dental floss.

Mouthwashes help remove food particles from the teeth and mouth, and tapwater is perfectly satisfactory for this purpose. Some people prefer a dilute solution of common salt (half a teaspoonful to half a glass of water), or baking soda (quarter of a teaspoonful to half a glass of water). Medical mouthwashes should not be used unless they are prescribed by the dentist. In addition, it is advisable to pay a visit twice a year to a dental hygienist to have your teeth thoroughly cleaned and the scaly deposits of tartar removed.

Above left: plaque consists of millions of bacteria enmeshed in tartar and food particles.

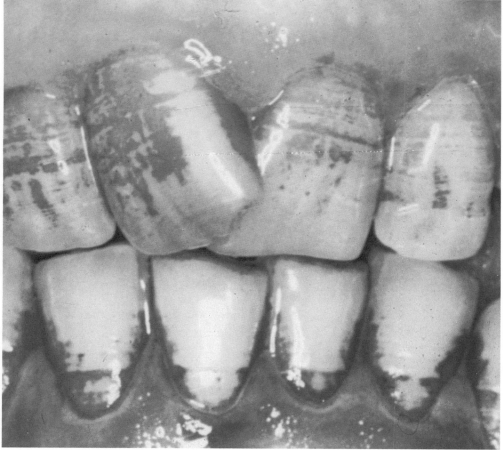

Left: the same set of teeth as those on the opposite page. The harmless red vegetable dye shows up the extent of the plaque.

Preventing Dental Caries

We are all given healthy teeth in childhood, and it is therefore obvious that despite the wonders of modern dentistry, prevention of decay must be aimed at in the young. Damage caused by dental disease cannot be rectified naturally. Lost teeth will not replace themselves and teeth, unlike many other body tissues, cannot repair themselves once damage has been done.

It is now well established that dental *caries* (decay that leads to the destruction of tooth tissue) is especially rife in countries where people eat a great amount of refined foods containing large quantities of sugar particularly in a sticky, retentive form, and other carbohydrates. It is also well known that caries can be drastically reduced by the use of simple but effective measures, including the fluoridation of drinking water. But although it is estimated that fluoride in drinking water can cut the number of cavities in children's teeth by two thirds, experiments have shown that the fewest cavities of all occur among children who eat little sweetened foods. No amount of fluoride can make up for a poor diet.

Caries begins with the breakdown of carbohydrate foodstuffs caught in the dental *plaque*. Plaque is a white gelatinous film of bacteria and food that sticks to the teeth. The carbohydrates are turned into acid by the action of the bacteria, and it is this acid that eats away the tooth's protective enamel layer. The decay spreads to the whole tooth which then dies.

Caries occur in certain well-defined "danger areas," common sites being the pits and fissures of the molars and premolars and the contact points between the teeth. Once the enamel is destroyed it cannot be repaired. As the disease progresses it destroys the dentine beneath the enamel, invades the pulp and finally spread down the root canal. This is when toothache usually starts and abscesses can form round the root, causing swelling and pain. This situation is potentially dangerous since the root canals are infected and biting on the tooth may cause

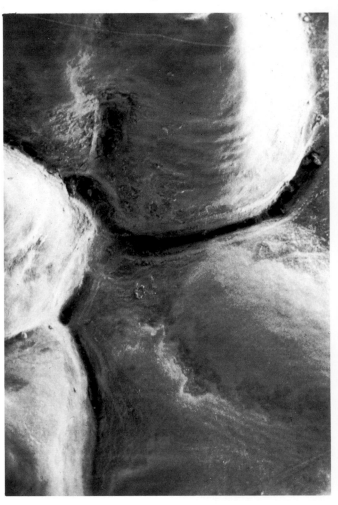

Above: electron scanning micrograph of a molar. The pits and fissures are the danger areas. Food particles, especially sugar, get trapped and provides a breeding ground for bacteria which secrete acids and dissolve the enamel.

Below: the process of tooth decay. A: a healthy intact tooth. B: a cavity develops; the enamel is worn through and the pulp becomes inflamed. C: there is active inflammation of the pulp. D: a chronic ulcer develops.

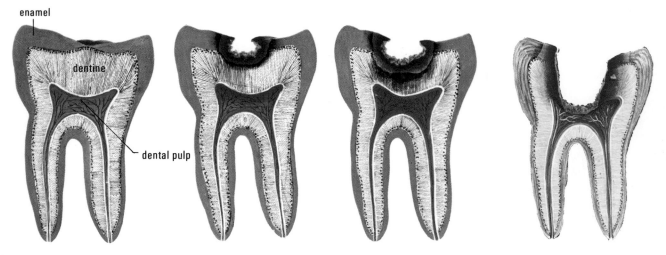

enamel

dentine

dental pulp

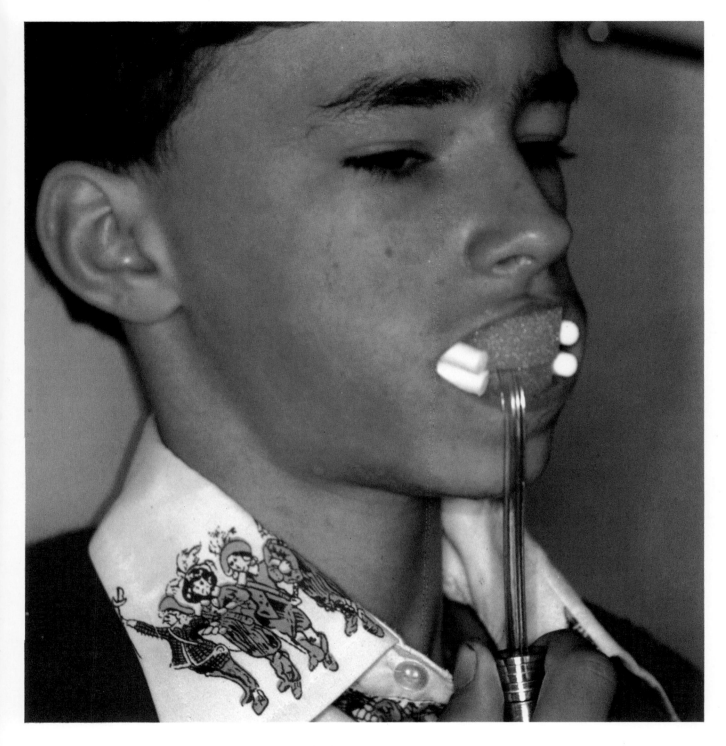

repeated invasion of disease-carrying bacteria into the bloodstream.

Bacteria in dental plaque, or the presence of an encrustation of tartar on the teeth, can often cause inflammation and infection of the gums. If this is not treated promptly the gums will shrink – causing the teeth to loosen and eventually fall out.

The action of sodium fluoride on the teeth results in stronger enamel and increased resistance to decay. Since this beneficial action was first discovered in the 1930s, fluoride at levels of one to two parts per million has been added to the water supplies in many areas of the world – with the result that the occurrence of caries has been significantly reduced.

Other methods of floridation are also used. One

Topical application of fluoride. Fluoride gel is poured into each application tray, one for the upper set, and one for the lower, and these are fitted over the teeth for 4 minutes. The tube between the teeth is a saliva ejector.

employed by the dentist is periodically coating the teeth with a strong fluoride solution. In the United States this method of prevention has shown some 40 percent reduction in the incidence of caries in children. Fluoride is often added to toothpastes and mouthwashes, and while extravagant claims are made for the efficiency of fluoridated dentifrices in stopping dental caries, the benefits derived seem to depend to a great extent on regular correct brushing and less on the therapeutic properties of the added fluoride.

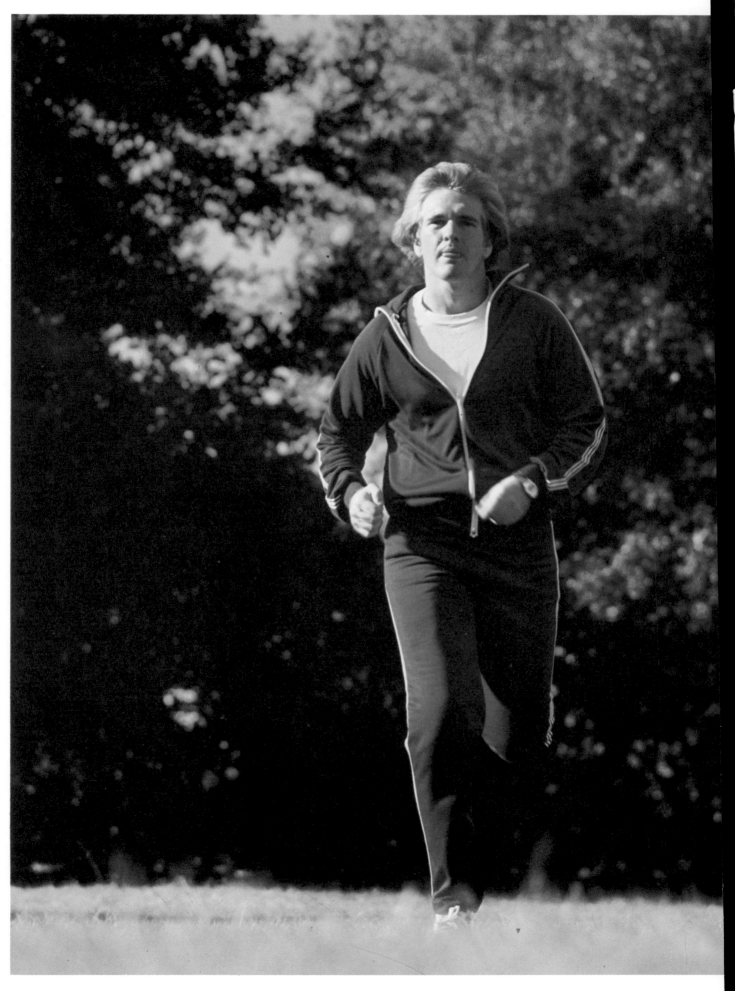

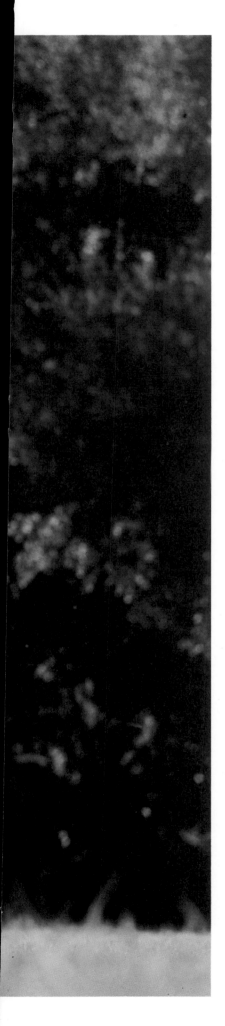

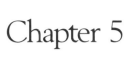

Chapter 5

Why Your Heart Matters

Your heart is among the most remarkable machines in the world. It is a highly efficient pump that every day does enough work to lift a person weighing 155 pounds almost 1150 feet into the air. Every day some 14,000 pints of life-giving blood pass through this pump, circulating the body again and again. The heart's Herculean task is to keep the body's 60,000-mile network of arteries, veins, and capillaries supplied – perhaps for up to 100 years without a pause for servicing or repairs – with the fluid that brings nourishment to every living cell.

Opposite: regular exercise has been shown to guard against heart disease. In our unnatural environment it keeps this essential organ functioning at its optimum capacity. Exercise also aids recovery after a heart attack.

When a Heart Attack Strikes

Philip, a 42-year-old successful architect, had for some time been deeply involved with planning a large urban development project. One hot summer's day he had to drive more than 500 miles to attend an architect's meeting. There he had to present a report to the people who were funding the project – so a lot depended on its success. The highways were heavily congested and after hours of frustrating delays he was a bit late for the meeting. But his report was well received and he had no difficulty in persuading the meeting that his ideas solved a number of important town planning problems. On his return home he discovered that his mother had been trying to contact him urgently for the previous three days as she had suddenly been taken ill with an intestinal disorder. As she lived only about 50 miles away, he drove immediately to his mother's place. The added journey proved to be unnecessary: in the meantime his mother had recovered, but was glad to see him. As he wanted to talk to a friend about the results of his architect's meeting, he telephoned him and arranged to have dinner with him that evening after returning from his mother's. As he was driving home

he became unexpectedly quite breathless. He stopped at a drive-in and had a cup of coffee. He seemed to improve and his breathlessness finally disappeared during a pleasant meal with his wife and friend. Before going to bed he had a glass of whisky – not an unusual thing for him to do. During that night he woke up with a severe tightness in his chest, which soon became unbearable; he felt as if he was being crushed beneath some very heavy weight. He could not walk to the bathroom and he called out to his wife. Suddenly he felt very frightened and he knew that he was seriously ill. An ambulance was called and on arrival at the hospital, a doctor told him that he had had a "coronary."

Today nearly everyone's circle of friends, relatives, or acquaintances includes at least one person who has undergone such an attack, and yet to many it remains a somewhat mysterious – even frightening – phenomenon. Some people, as they grow toward late middle age, get increasingly worried and ask themselves: "Am I the next in line for a coronary?" What, then, is this condition that annually affects approximately 100,000 people in the United Kingdom alone?

"Coronary" is actually shorthand for "coronary thrombosis," which means a clot in one of the coronary arteries. These arteries bring blood – and thus vital oxygen – to the heart muscle tissue. This blood and its oxygen supply are necessary if the heart muscle cells are to do their work of pumping blood through the vessels of the entire body.

The coronary arteries, like all the other arteries of the body, have a smooth lining called the *endothelium*. As people grow older, deposits of fats and other material are built up on the endothelium. This both narrows and hardens the arteries, and roughens

Posterior (left) and anterior views of the heart. Blood enters the right ventricle and auricle through the vena cava and the pulmonary vein, respectively. It leaves the left side through the pulmonary artery and aorta.

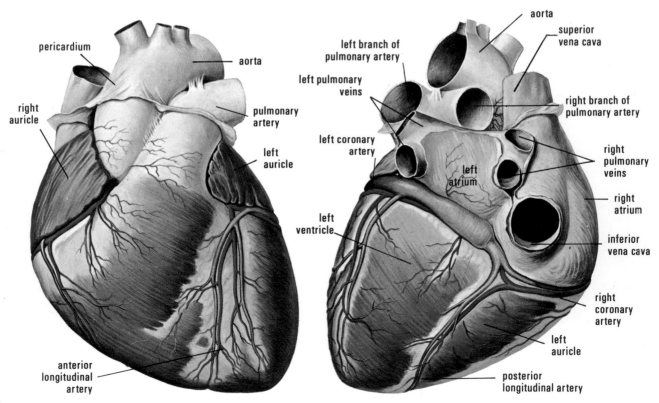

92

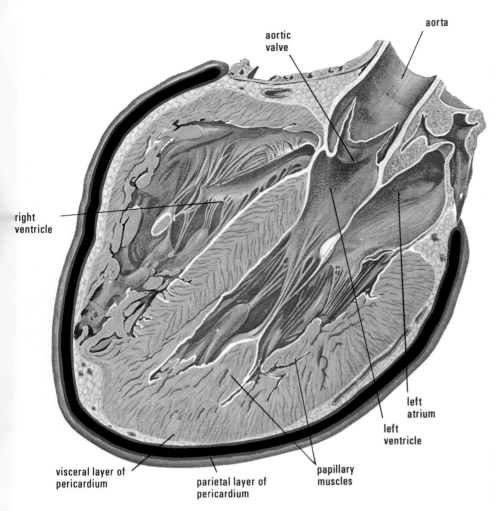

aortic valve

aorta

right ventricle

visceral layer of pericardium

parietal layer of pericardium

papillary muscles

left atrium

left ventricle

Left: section through the heart. It is enclosed in a sheath called the pericardium, the inside of which is moist to allow the heart to beat without generating friction.

Below: this patient is attached to an electrocardiogram, a machine which records the beats of the heart graphically and can thus show up damage.

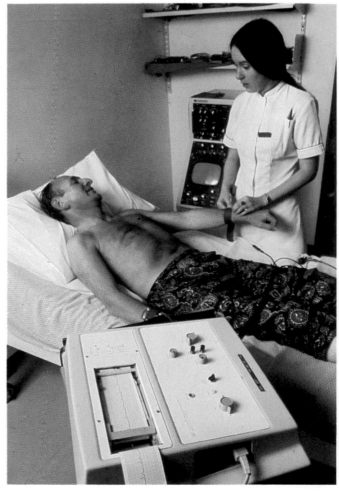

the surface to such an extent that blood flowing through them may clot and a complete blockage may occur. Heart tissue served by the blocked artery dies. The technical term for this is *infarction* and the whole process is known to doctors as *myocardial ischemic disease*. When some part of the heart is put out of action in this way, the heart becomes less efficient – at least for a time – in its vital work of pumping blood around the body.

Most people think of a coronary as occurring "like a bolt from the blue," but there are often warning signs. At a stage when one of the arterial branches is narrowed and before it is actually blocked, the blood supply may be sufficient for the heart while a person is at rest or exerting himself only slightly. If he tries to work harder, or to climb a steep hill, or walk fast up stairs or into the wind on a cold day, the heart will require more blood. But the stiff, narrow vessels cannot accommodate a greater blood supply and a greater flow. At this point the person will experience a sharp pain across the chest, resembling that of a coronary, but vanishing as soon as he stops his exertions. Doctors call this type of pain *angina pectoris*, and although such an attack can be relieved by the use of drugs that make the arteries widen, it should be a warning to the individual that he needs to change his way of life. This is probably his last chance to take his own preventive measures: to give up smoking, cautiously reduce excess weight, and take regular exercise.

Why Your Heart Matters

Every cell in our bodies is surrounded by tissue fluid from which it obtains the necessities of life and into which it discharges both waste and useful products. Cells are like the customers who rely on a local store (the nearest tissue fluid) for their immediate needs. But the store must be restocked by a delivery service; and such a system needs, in turn, a powered vehicle to bring in new supplies and remove waste, and a reliable network of roads.

One of the most economical methods of transporting raw materials is to immerse them in fluid and then pump them through pipelines. In the last few decades this method has been used increasingly by industry. The vehicle of supply and removal in man is blood; the route it follows is the complex network of blood vessels; and the driving power is provided by the pumping action of the heart.

The human body contains approximately five quarts of blood. Of this volume about half is an almost watery fluid called *plasma*, which contains a great variety of simple substances in solution (such as sodium chloride and sodium bicarbonate), and more complicated ones (such as the proteins globulin and albumin, and carbohydrates). In solution blood also contains ingredients that are in transit, continuously entering and leaving the blood vessels and every cell in the body. These include the gases oxygen and carbon dioxide; mineral salts for such purposes as bone building; nitrogenous substances from which proteins are built; sugar in the form of glucose; hormones, enzymes, and many more. The other half of the volume of blood consists of cells that are suspended in the plasma. The red cells contain fluid and a protein called *hemoglobin* that combines with oxygen in the lungs, where its pressure is high. But it can easily part with the oxygen in the tissue where its pressure is low. Blood with a normal number of red cells is capable of carrying 20 parts by volume of oxygen for every 100 parts of blood.

In order to keep eight pints of blood in constant circulation within a closed circuit, there must be a continuous propulsion. A single pump equipped with suitable valves could do the job were it not for the fact that the body needs to pump blood around two circuits simultaneously. The *systemic* circulation

Right: cardiac muscle. It consists of columns of cylindrical cells which resemble striped muscle in appearance but smooth muscle in their autonomic innervation. Functionally the cells behave as a single unit.

Below: coronary arteries supply the heart's muscle with blood.

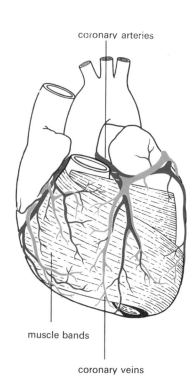

coronary arteries

muscle bands

coronary veins

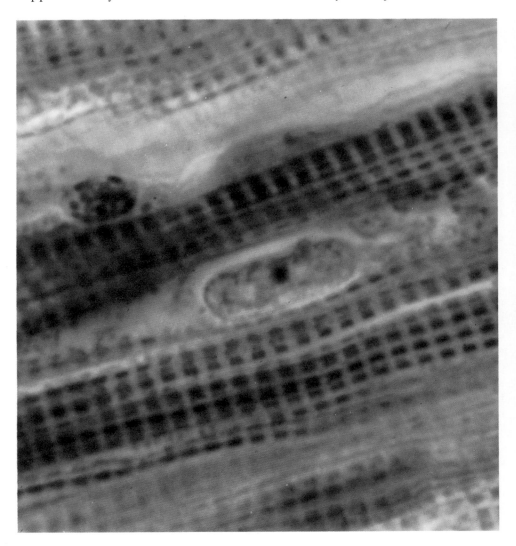

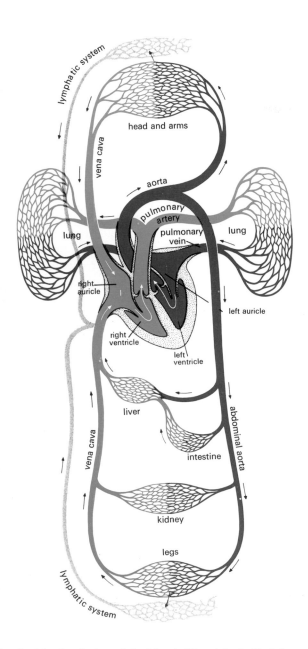

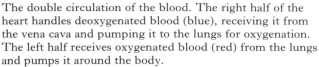

The double circulation of the blood. The right half of the heart handles deoxygenated blood (blue), receiving it from the vena cava and pumping it to the lungs for oxygenation. The left half receives oxygenated blood (red) from the lungs and pumps it around the body.

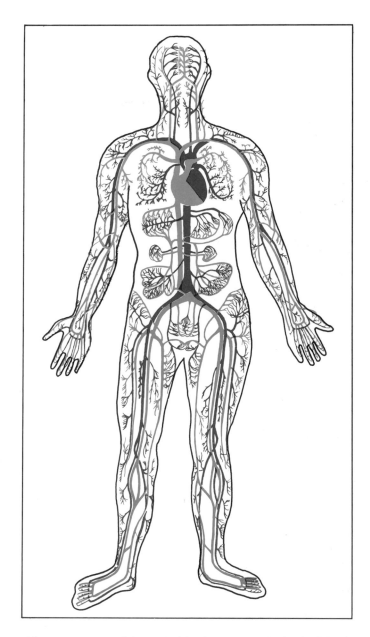

Above: diagram of the main blood vessels of the body. The arteries are colored red, the veins blue. They subdivide to form arterioles and venules, respectively, and eventually capillaries, which have walls one cell thick. This system insures that blood reaches every part of the body.

carries blood to all parts of the body except the lungs and brings it back to the heart again. The *pulmonary* circulation carries blood to the lungs and is operated by a separate pump. Thus the heart is a synchronized double pump – literally "two hearts that beat as one." This double pump begins its cycle when oxygenated blood enters the heart from the lungs and is then pumped to the rest of the body. When this blood has given up its oxygen to the tissues, it returns to the heart, after which it goes to the lungs. The cycle is then repeated.

The tissue that provides the heart's driving force is called *cardiac muscle*. It differs from other types of muscle in that it is arranged as a continuous network of fibers. This explains how a contraction starting at one point can spread throughout the rest of the heart. Waves of alternate contraction and dilation

are repeated rhythmically throughout a person's life, at the rate of about 70 times a minute, or 100,000 times a day. During the course of a day about 14,000 pints of blood are ejected from the heart.

The heartbeat is regulated by two nerves, one of which makes the heart beat faster and the other slower. Various factors affect the rate at which the heart beats. Emotions influence it strongly, especially fear and excitement. The concentration of carbon dioxide in the blood also affects the heart. This concentration is registered by the brain, and the higher the concentration the faster the heart pumps blood to the lungs. Also there are devices, called *receptors*, in various parts of the circulatory system that register the local blood pressure so that the rate of heartbeat and pressure of blood in the vessels is always balanced.

95

The Function of Blood

The blood is a complex transport system. It consists of cells suspended in a fluid known as the plasma. The majority of the blood cells are red and are called *erythrocytes*. They are manufactured in the red marrow of the bone, especially in the backbone, the breastbone, the long bones of limbs, and the ribs. The red cell is a disk that is concave on both sides, which means it has a larger surface to volume ratio. This feature enables gases to diffuse in and out of the cell very quickly.

The oxygen-carrying capacity of the red cells depends on the amount of hemoglobin they contain, and the hemoglobin in turn requires a supply of iron. A man with a severe iron deficiency becomes extremely pale and may develop "air hunger," taking deep, anxious breaths in an effort to get more oxygen into his body's cells. Air hunger also develops at high altitudes, where the air pressure is not great enough to saturate hemoglobin with oxygen. People who live at sea level begin to feel the effects of oxygen shortage at altitudes of about 6000 feet. At altitudes above 9000 feet even a small exertion can make a person feel faint.

The five quarts of the body's blood contain 25 million million red cells, each having an average life of 120 days. This means that the destruction and renewal of red cells goes on at the rate of 210 thousand million per day, or 2.5 million each second. This prodigious destruction and renewal goes on throughout our lives for the sole purpose of insuring a supply of oxygen to every part of the body.

If our body becomes infected, it reacts immediately, isolating and destroying the invading germs. The first sign of counterattack is often an inflammation: a hot, reddened, swollen area, like that surrounding a boil. Inflammation signifies that tiny capillary blood vessels are expanding as blood rushes

Human erythrocytes (red blood cells). They contain the pigment hemoglobin which combines with oxygen at high concentration and releases it at low oxygen pressure. The cells have no nucleus, and are biconcave – a shape which presents the greatest surface area for absorption.

Threads of fibrin, a primary constituent of blood clots. It enmeshes red blood cells and forms a tight plug which prevents further bleeding. Fibrin is formed from a soluble protein in the plasma called fibrinogen, by a complex series of reactions involving the disintegration of platelets.

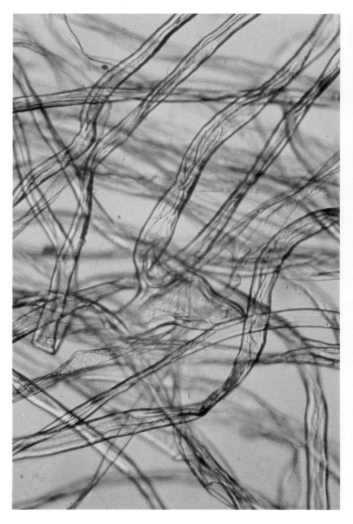

to the area of attack. The increased blood supply brings in great armies of white cells, called *leukocytes*, the natural enemies of disease-causing bacteria. The concentration of *fibrinogen*, a substance in the plasma, is increased too. When it filters through the thin capillary walls it is converted into strands of a protein called *fibrin* that wall off the harmful organisms from healthy tissues and the bloodstream.

White cells known as *granulocytes* also escape from the dilated capillaries into the tissues, where they actively seek the invading organisms. Like tiny amoebas they crawl about and stretch out footlike projections that they use to engulf bacteria and digest them. Each granulocyte can consume about a dozen bacteria this way – a process called *phagocytosis*. Phagocytic cells constitute a large proportion of pus, the creamy fluid that gathers about inflamed areas.

Other white cells, called *lymphocytes*, secrete special proteins, called *antibodies*, which have the power to inactivate the germs. These antibodies are made by cells in the same way as any other proteins – under genetic instruction. The production of anti-bodies is triggered by the presence, in the germs, of *antigens* – proteins foreign to the body. At some time during the development of the embryo in the womb, the body comes to possess cells capable of making all the antibodies that the body could possibly need.

Antibodies can occasionally act as a two-edged weapon. For example there is a disease in which certain proteins leak out from their proper location and enter the bloodstream. The defense mechanisms treat these proteins as hostile antigens; and antibodies are produced to neutralize them. These find their way to the tissue and destroy it. Such responses produce what are known as *autoimmune* diseases. Some blood and rheumatic disorders are believed to be produced in this way.

Red blood cells adhering in groups called rouleaux. The membranes contain systems of antigens which confer blood-group specificity. These antigen groups include the ABO system and the Rhesus factor. Blood-group A subjects have A antigens; group B subjects, B antigens; group AB both A and B; and group O neither. Also, the serum of individuals has antibodies against the antigens they do not possess. Group A have anti-B antibodies, group B have anti-A antibodies, group O anti-A and B, and group AB neither.

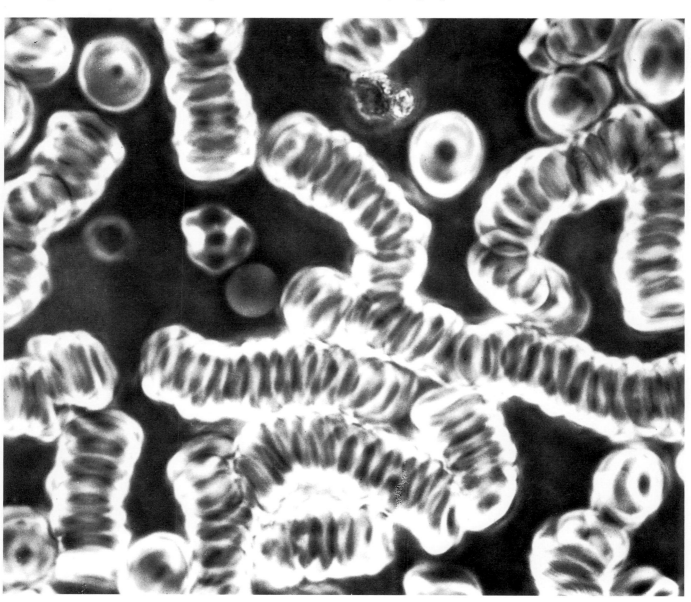

How the Blood Circulates

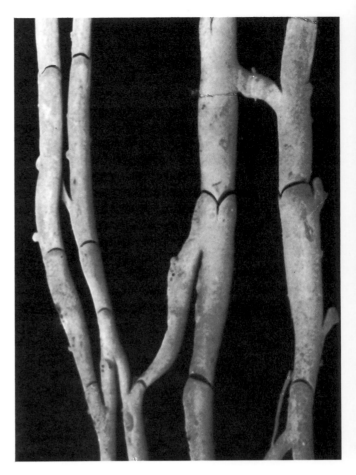

The systemic circulation of blood is a two-way process. The *arterial* system carries blood away from the heart to the tissues, the *venous* system transports blood from the tissues back to the heart. The heart pumps oxygen-rich blood through the aorta, which is the main artery of the whole circulatory system. From the aorta smaller arteries branch off to the various regions of the body, and these in turn divide and subdivide still further. The walls of the arteries contain varying amounts of elastic fibers and smooth muscle. Smooth muscle is found in the walls of tubes that need to contract, and like cardiac muscle it moves involuntarily. The large arteries consist mostly of elastic fibers, which dilate when the heart pumps blood through them and contract after the blood has passed; this has the effect of smoothing out the flow of blood. The smaller arteries, however, contain muscle that contracts rhythmically so that a contractile wave runs along the artery; this helps to speed the blood on its way.

The next stage in this pipeline delivery service takes the form of arterioles, which are branches of small arteries. The walls of arterioles have no elastic tissue, but they are equipped with smooth muscle fibers. Finally each arteriole divides into a number of tubes called capillaries. In the capillaries there is no pulsation; blood passes through them only because of the pressure produced by the pumping of the heart. The capillary walls are one cell thick and consist of an extremely thin layer of lining epithelium. No cell of the body is more than one ten-thousandth of an inch from a capillary tube and it is here that the whole purpose of the circulatory system is fulfilled: the area of exchange, covering in all about 2500 square yards, has been reached.

The blood creeps slowly along the capillaries with the erythrocytes in a single file. This slow movement allows one to two seconds for the exchange of various chemicals with the tissue fluid and thus with the cells. The blood has now completed its mission. It then flows from the capillaries into a collection of pipelines – the venous system. First there are minute venules, the counterparts, we could say, of the arterioles. The venules then join together to form larger and larger veins, which finally deliver blood back to the heart.

Veins have only a small amount of smooth muscle and elastic fibers in their walls and they do not pulsate. Because a human being stands erect, blood on its way back to the heart has to travel uphill

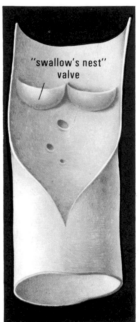

"swallow's nest" valve

Acrylic cast (above) and section (left) of the veins showing the characteristic valves. The pressure in the veins is almost identical to atmospheric, and the walls of the veins have little muscle. The circulation of blood through the veins is actually effected by overall muscular pressure in the body. The valves' function is to prevent a backflow of blood.

against the pull of gravity, and so many of the larger veins have valves to prevent backflow. The veins transport blood at a slower rate than arteries, but they compensate by having a larger caliber. In this way the volume of blood flowing into the heart from the veins is the same as that leaving it in the arteries. The return flow through the veins is assisted by muscular action that compresses the veins lying between the muscles (the so-called muscle pump). It is also assisted by the slight negative pressure

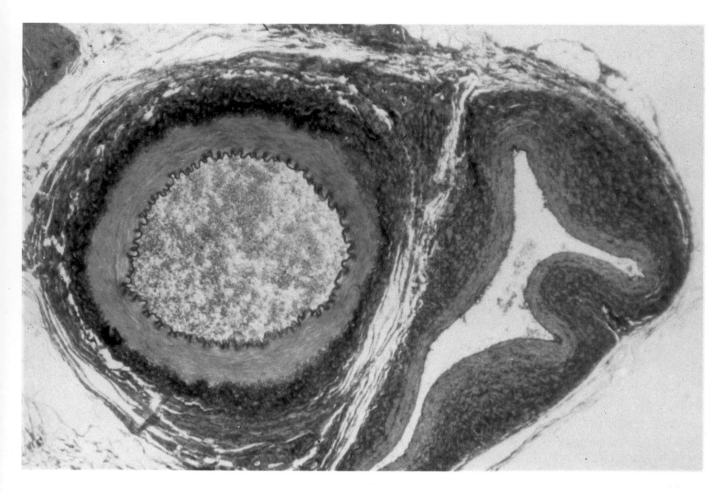

within the chest (the so-called thoracic pump).

Certain blood vessels have the ability to vary their diameter and thus the amount of blood flowing in different parts of the body can be controlled. Although the veins and the large arteries cannot change their diameter, the smaller arteries and arterioles contain muscle that keeps them in a state of tone, that is, a condition of never being completely relaxed, never too constricted. The degree of tone is controlled by two nerves, one of which causes the vessels to dilate and the other to contract. Thus if a gland has to go into action its arterioles dilate so as to ensure a generous supply of blood. Once the gland's task is completed, the vessels constrict and cut down the blood supply. In this way blood can be diverted for a time from a less important to a more important part of the body.

What happens in a runner's body during a hundred yards' sprint? On the starting line the sprinter braces himself for the effort ahead, and his emotions stimulate his brain to send messages to all parts of the body so that his muscles are ready and his blood charged with adrenalin. During the sprint both nerve impulses and adrenalin dilate the smaller arteries and arterioles, and the return of venous blood to the heart is accelerated by the muscle pump. The force as well as the speed of the heart's action also increases. This combined physical and mental striving throughout the sprint enables the athlete to achieve a speed that represents the limit of the body's capability.

Above: section through an artery (left) and vein (right). The arterial walls are regular, thick and muscular, the venous walls thin and irregular.

Below: the arterial system of the lower leg and foot. The arteries were injected with a suspension of lead in paraffin.

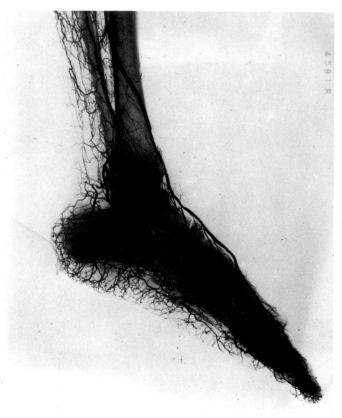

Warning Signs

It is not unusual for a person with a diseased heart to be completely unaware of his or her condition, even when it is advanced. Congenital heart disease is frequently discovered in a child during routine examination by a school doctor, and various heart conditions are sometimes found in a "healthy" adult during a life insurance checkup. This may be because there are genuinely no symptoms, or the patients have automatically learned how to adjust themselves to their disability and are unaware of any limitation to their activity. Many people do not know the symptoms of heart disease. It is easy to associate disturbances in urination with urinary tract disease, but it may not be so easy to attribute such symptoms as shortness of breath, a cough, fatigue, sleeplessness, or sweating to heart disease. On the other hand, with the increased publicity given to heart disease, a great deal of unnecessary fear and suffering may result from symptoms, such

A: the usual pain caused by a heart attack is dull – a feeling of pressure or fullness in the center of the chest (the actual position of the heart). It may radiate, and vary in severity and duration. B: the discomfort may extend into one or both arms, and unlike arthritis, is not aggravated by raising the arms above the head. C: the distress may radiate to the neck and jaws; unlike pain originating in the neck, it is not aggravated by neck movements.

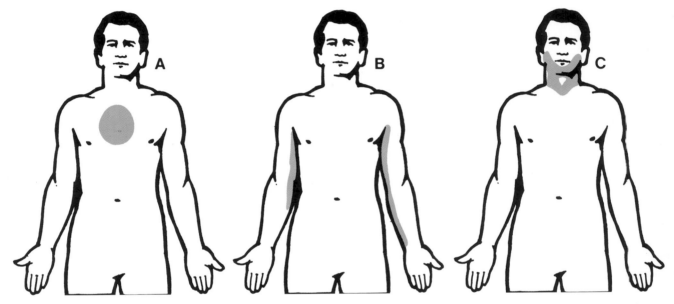

D: another sign is an aching or squeezing pain in the upper abdomen overlapping the lower chest at the fork of the ribs. It is often mistaken for indigestion. E: back pain, often confused with muscular strain, may be the only sign of a heart attack. F: the distress may be a combination of areas sometimes accompanied by nausea, vomiting and shortness of breath. Unexplained heavy sweating associated with pain in this area is usually considered a sign of heart attack.

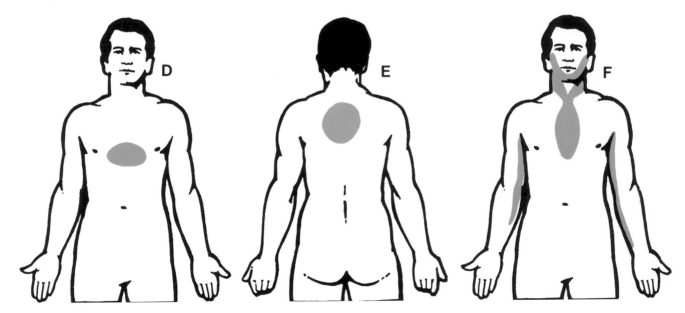

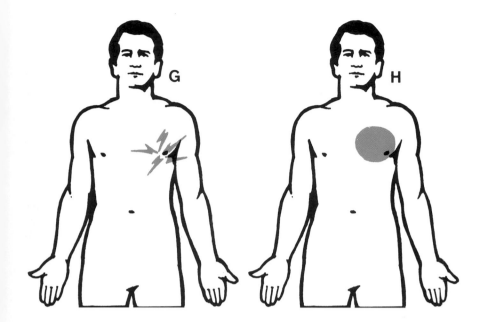

These chest pains are invariably harmless but may often be confused with those preceding heart attacks. Many persons who are by nature tense experience pain in the left chest wall, centering on the nipple. The pain may be sharp, jabbing and last for only a few seconds (G) or it may be a dull soreness lasting minutes or hours (H). Or it may be a combination of both. This is *not* the position of the heart (see A). However, if the pain persists, you should see your doctor.

as pain in the left side of the chest, headache, and fatigue, often wrongly attributed to heart disease.

Shortness of breath can vary in intensity. It can be mild when it occurs only after fairly strenuous effort, such as running for a bus, in a person who until then has been able to do this without distress. Moderate shortness of breath can occur with the ordinary activities of everyday living, such as walking a block or two, shopping, or sexual intercourse. If breathlessness happens with only slight effort, such as minor household activities, walking a few steps, or making beds, then the disability is severe.

Pain from heart muscle is typically pressing, squeezing, or gripping in nature. The duration varies from a few moments to many hours or days, depending on whether ischemia (shortage of blood) is slight and transient, or prolonged and permanent. Commonly it is felt in the center of the chest and it can radiate into the neck, the jaws, down the arms or into the back. Central chest pain on effort, subsequently relieved by rest, is almost always ischemic. Prolonged pain at rest of mounting intensity, associated with restlessness, sweating and anxiety, suggests an infarction – congestion of blood vessels. However, the heart has no monopoly of pain in the chest. Most inner organs can produce similar pain. The most common are the chest wall, bones and nerves in the chest, gullet (esophagus), stomach and gall bladder. Psychoneurotic "left chest pain" is often mistaken for heart disease and is responsible for a great deal of unnecessary mental suffering. Usually it is felt in the region of the left breast, is of short duration, and is stabbing in nature.

Palpitations produce an unpleasant awareness of the heart's action. They may be slow or fast, regular or irregular. They may consist of a thump in the chest, or a throb in the neck. Throbbing in different postures, such as in bed, is often noted, especially in the ears when the head is in a certain position on the pillow. Excitement and nervous anticipation may give rise to slow or fast palpitations.

Since fatigue is such a common complaint in many diseases, it is incautious to attach too much significance to this symptom. There was time when fatigue was thought to be entirely neurotic. Fatigue on effort, however, is now recognized as an important symptom of low cardiac output and of heart failure. Like fatigue, insomnia is a common symptom in all kinds of illnesses. However, it is a very real complaint in heart disease and may be an early symptom. Similarly, loss of consciousness can be an early sign of cardiac malfunction. Any factor preventing oxygen from reaching the brain will produce a faint. One of the main reasons is inadequate filling of the heart, for example in circulatory disturbances associated with sudden dilation of blood vessels, or loss of blood volume as in shock or severe loss of blood. When this happens a return of blood to the heart is interrupted and the result is a failure of venous inflow to the heart. Fainting on effort needs a special mention since a heart malfunction is the usual cause. Obstruction of blood flow from either ventricle, usually the left, prevents an appropriate increase in cardiac output required by exercise.

In heart disease, salt and water retention is of major importance and is associated with a heightened venous pressure. When more fluid leaves the vascular system than is absorbed, the blood volume remains more or less constant, but the extracellular component becomes expanded, causing a swelling called an *edema*. Swelling of the feet is an extremely common complaint when this occurs and is usually not serious. In heart failure the increased fluid gravitates to the dependent parts. When sufficient fluid has collected edema appears and is first seen at the end of the day, disappearing after a night's rest. As more fluid accumulates the hands and feet may become permanently swollen and later this "dropsy" extends to involve serous cavities and the face. The face is often affected early on during kidney inflammation, but the same symptoms may occur in heart disease.

Causes of
Heart Disease

Diseases of the heart and blood vessels have become by far the most common cause of natural death in the world's more advanced communities. Both the incidence of heart disease and resulting deaths have been rising steadily for many years. Ischemic heart disease, particularly, is becoming more frequent. In 1910 there were 137,000 deaths from heart disease in Germany; in 1956 in the German Federal Republic alone, 230,000 people died from heart conditions. There are many reasons for this dramatic increase.

The veins, which carry blood at a lower rate of flow away from the tissues and back to the lungs and heart, are pretty resistant to diseases likely to affect their walls. But the arteries through which the heart pumps newly oxygenized blood at high speed, are subject to more stress. They must be flexible to

Bar diagram showing the percentage of deaths caused by cardiovascular disease, for both sexes, and across all age groups, in the United Kingdom, 1976. In that particular year, cardiovascular disease killed more people in the UK than cancer, respiratory diseases and accidents combined.

handle this high-pressure flow, but as the body ages they have a tendency to harden – a process called *arteriosclerosis*. This degenerative process may begin in the main artery, the aorta, as early as during the first ten years of life, and can be seriously advanced in a man by the time he reaches his twenties. Most often it becomes noticeable in middle age, though some people remain unaffected all their lives. Women of childbearing age appear to be protected against arteriosclerosis, but after 45 they develop it just as frequently and severely as men do.

If ischemic heart disease were confined to the very old and were merely a mode of death in people who had reached the end of a long life, it would not pose a major problem. Unfortunately it often occurs in people who are relatively young, and in the last 30 years it appears to have increased alarmingly in people who are still in their forties and fifties. People who develop heart attacks before the age of 65 are said to suffer from premature coronary heart disease.

Arteriosclerosis and clotting are common causes of "strokes." The damaged vessels cannot supply the brain with enough blood, and depending on what area is deprived of essential nourishment, the parts of the body they control suffer paralysis; often speech and arm movements are impaired. Damage to only a small patch of brain can paralyze one entire side of the body. Sometimes complete recovery is possible when healthy areas take over the work of dead brain tissue. But actual regeneration of dead brain and nerve cells never takes place.

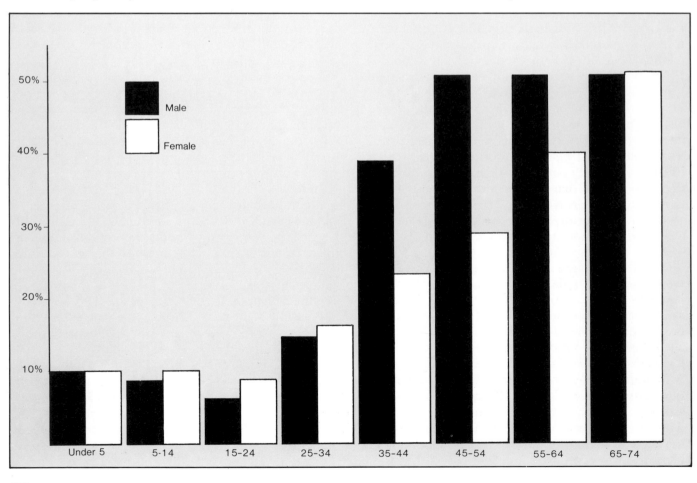

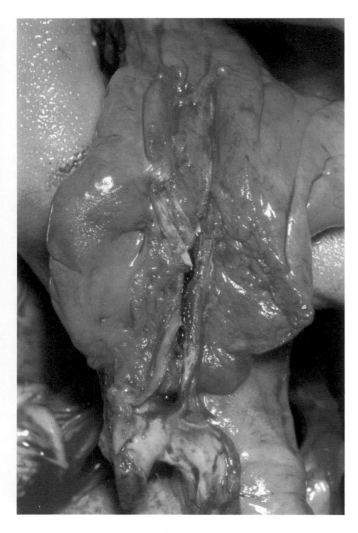

Above: coronary thrombosis. A coronary artery becomes obstructed by a thrombus, or clot, and this blocks the flow of blood to part of the heart muscle. Starved of oxygen and nutrients, the affected area of the muscle dies. Hardened arteries are a major predisposing cause.

Coronary thrombosis is the commonest form of heart attack. A sudden, sharp chest pain that usually lasts a few hours marks a coronary attack. It may be accompanied by faintness and breathlessness. The heart continues to pump, but a portion of its muscle dies. Replacing dead muscle with strong fibrous tissue takes from a few weeks to several months. With care, people who survive such attacks may achieve normal lifespans.

Angina pectoris is not so serious; it results from a less severe reduction of the heart's blood supply, and pain lasts only a few minutes. Most attacks are brought on by physical exertion. With careful avoidance of stress, of overindulgence in eating, and of excessive physical exertion, the outlook is good, even though the heart's arteries remain narrowed or blocked.

Bacterial infections are another important but rare cause of heart disease. Rheumatic fever, which attacks tissues in the joints and muscles, often damages similar tissues in the heart, interfering with the normal rate of heartbeat, and usually some years later, the operation of the valves.

Heart valves that are abnormal, whether through maldevelopment or as result of rheumatic fever, are also liable to attack by bacteria. *Infective endocarditis* is a disease produced by a number of factors including direct infection of the heart valves, certain congenital defects of the heart and aorta, and the presence of foreign material in the heart. The forms of infection have changed considerably since the discovery of antibiotics, the development of drugs that aid in surgery, the widespread use of operations on the heart and the rising incidence of drug addiction. In the past the infective agents were almost always organisms such as streptococci and pneumococci, commonly found in the mouth, respiratory tract, and other parts of the body. Now other organisms are also involved, such as certain bacilli and fungi, the commonest of which are some types of yeast.

In *hypertensive* conditions (high blood pressure), narrowed arterial walls force the heart to work harder to pump blood, and the heart muscles enlarge in order to handle the extra load. The thickened muscle often outgrows its blood supply. Coronary thrombosis and heart failure are common results when blood pressure has been high for a number of years.

Below: an artery in section showing the development of atheroma. This is a deposit of fatty materials, including cholesterol, which causes arteriosclerosis or "hardening" of the arteries. The walls thicken, become less elastic, and more susceptible to the formation of clots (thrombi).

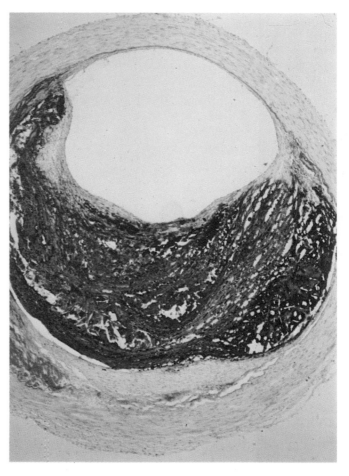

Avoiding the Risk Factors

Because of the increase in the incidence of premature heart disease, much medical research has been focused on its causes. This research has led to the identification of certain characteristics that are found in most heart disease patients under the age of 60. These are called "risk factors" and it is probable that they accelerate arteriosclerosis. If people who possess these risk factors could be identified at an early stage, the probability of their developing coronary heart disease could be reduced by treatment and advice before they suffer a heart attack.

These risk factors include: untreated high blood pressure, high levels of blood fats (cholesterol, a fatty substance derived from animal fats in food, and triglycerides), smoking, lack of physical exercise, emotional stress, and diabetes mellitus. Being overweight and a history of premature deaths in the family also increase the likelihood of heart disease. We do not know whether the removal of these risk factors will reduce the number of people suffering from ischemic heart diseases, but it is likely that the effect will be to delay their occurrence.

Before World War II, heart disease was most common among professional men, such as doctors, lawyers, businessmen, and managers. It was uncommon among unskilled laborers doing heavy manual work. Since the mid-1950s, however, more and more coronaries have occurred among the relatively lower paid sector of the community. The condition now attacks younger men and, increasingly, women.

What can have brought about these changes? Certainly before the 1930s the rich lived – and ate – very differently from the poor. Subsequently, especially in the 1950s, living standards began to rise and have continued upward until the middle of the 1970s. Everyone started consuming more sugar and fats, bought more automobiles and television sets, and smoked more cigarettes. And during this period the incidence of ischemic heart disease began to rise.

In the United States the Metropolitan Life Insurance Company, observing a group of apparently healthy people over a period of years, noted that coronary thrombosis was frequently accompanied by overweight. Their study showed that men whose weight was 40 percent or more above the average for their age, height and body type, were three times more likely to suffer a coronary than other people. Two other important factors have also been recognized: the height of the blood pressure and the level of cholesterol in the blood serum. Could this be due to too much fat in the diet? People who suffer from heart attacks generally have a high cholesterol level in their bloodstream; however, this high level does not mean that the cholesterol has caused the heart attack. The answer may well lie in what happens in the walls of the coronary arteries, and the high level

A diseased coronary artery. The white flecks are deposits of cholesterol, the fat-like steroid implicated in cardiovascular disease.

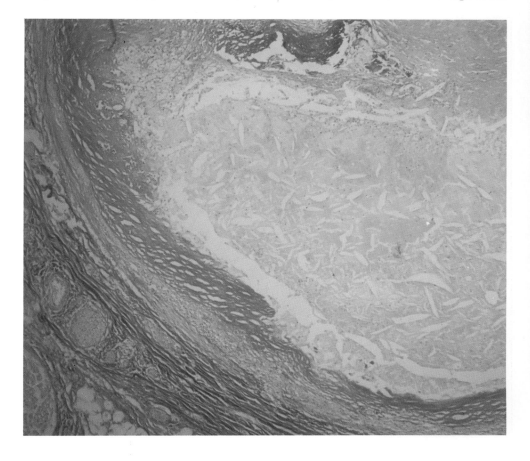

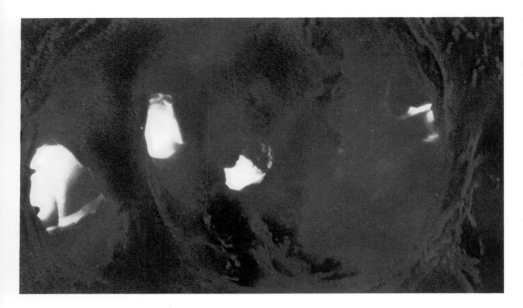

This diseased heart, with its cholesterol deposits, belonged to a smoker. Heavy smokers are more prone to heart disease than moderate or nonsmokers.

of cholesterol may just be a sign that the body is not dealing properly with fat-like substances. It therefore seemed logical to advise people who have suffered a coronary to avoid animal fat, but unfortunately those who have followed such diets do not appear to be less prone to further attacks of coronary thrombosis. However it is a different matter if healthy men of 30 and over adopt such diets: some medical experts believe that animal fat-free diets would prevent them having coronaries in their 40s, 50s, and 60s.

Recently British nutritional experts have pointed out that deaths from coronary thrombosis in various countries has risen step by step with the increase in sugar consumption. It is true that in countries where coronary disease is common, people consume large amounts of tea or coffee, well laced with spoonfuls of refined sugar – as well as a great number of cakes, puddings, and ice cream.

Yet another consequence of affluence is that more people smoke more cigarettes. Studies in both the United States and Britain have shown that cigarette smoking is linked with increased mortality from coronary thrombosis. These studies indicate that the death rate in those smoking up to ten cigarettes a day is about 30 percent higher than in nonsmokers, and for those smoking over 40 cigarettes a day the rate is 250 percent greater.

Two interesting studies, both conducted in London, showed that bus drivers are more likely to die from ischemic heart disease than are conductors on the same buses, and that clerks in post offices suffer a greater mortality from coronaries than do postmen working in the same department. The factor common to both postmen and bus conductors is physical activity. Evidence suggests that lack of exercise may encourage the narrowing of the coronary arteries. Thus affluence, in providing us with more and more sophisticated methods to minimize our physical exertions, would seem to be an enemy of health.

The pressures of modern life would also seem to play a part in the development of heart disease. It is usually the type of stress that one puts on oneself, rather than that caused from outside, that appears to lead to a coronary. It is often the tense, self-driving type, such as the architect described at the beginning of this chapter, of whom people say: "If he doesn't take it easier, he's going to have a heart attack."

So the conclusions are obvious. If you want to avoid the risk factors that could irreparably damage your health, you must: eat lean meats and avoid animal fat, sugar, and other rich foods; give up or cut down on smoking; take more exercise; reduce your bulk if you are overweight; and try to avoid stress.

	High cholesterol foods	Low cholesterol substitutes
Meat, poultry, fish	Pork, mutton, offal, duck, goose, sausages, salamis, bacon, shrimp	Beef, lamb, veal, chicken, turkey (trimmed of fat, boiled, roasted, broiled), fish
Dairy products	Whole milk; cream; whole milk and cream cheeses; eggs, especially yolks, in any form	Fortified skimmed milk and skimmed-milk products; buttermilk; cottage and farmer's cheese, mozarella
Fats and Oils	Butter, lard, hard margarine, peanut and olive oil. Products from coconut oil (non-dairy substitutes); avocado; chocolate	Margarine and liquid shortening made from poly-unsaturated oils such as corn, cottonseed, sunflower, safflower, sesame seed

The Benefits of Exercise

A witty man once said: "Whenever I feel like taking exercise I lie down until the feeling passes away." Sir Winston Churchill, who lived to the age of 91, tended to shun physical exertion whenever possible. But there cannot be any doubt that for most people a certain amount of daily exercise is both necessary for health and helpful in prolonging life.

One of the main functions of exercise is building up cardio-respiratory (heart-lung) efficiency. As already described, the heart is a muscle and breathing is also carried out by muscular activity. Just like other muscles these require regular exercise at more than resting levels to maintain and improve their efficiency. The purpose of controlled exercise is gradually to increase the pulse and respiratory rates

Below: exercise increases the strength, capacity and functioning of the heart and lungs. The key is to start gradually if you are out of condition and to increase your functional capacity slowly. Also, if you are over 50, you should first check with your doctor. Sudden sporadic bursts of activity can do more harm than good.

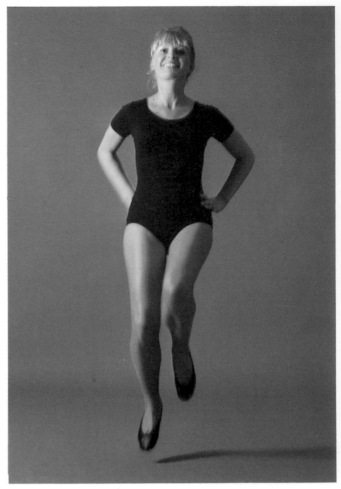

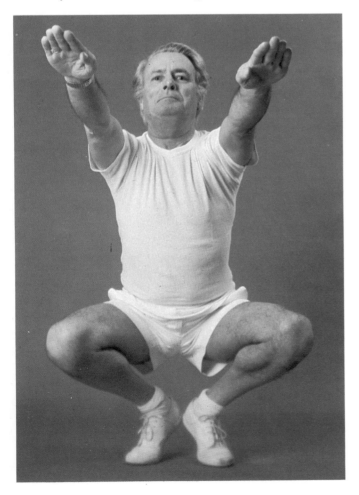

Above: in many cases a good start to fitness can be achieved by dramatically improving the posture. When upright, lift your head and chest, and keep your shoulders back. Pull in the stomach muscles, tuck in the buttocks and tilt your pelvis slightly upward. At the same time relax and breathe deeply.

to levels at which you are comfortably tired and out of breath. In all forms of exercise anything more than a mild discomfort shows that you are driving yourself too hard and this should be avoided.

A program of exercise carried out in the home can, in a few hours spread through the week, maintain adequate physcial fitness for everyday life. But most of us find "physical jerks" rather tedious and have difficulties in sticking to such a program. For this reason it is wise to combine regular participation in games with five to ten minutes most mornings of loosening-up exercises designed to strengthen those muscles that are not used very often. Age is no barrier as long as the exercises are planned carefully. However, the older you are, the longer it will take to get fit after a long period of unfitness, and it is important that you build up gradually after any break of more than a few days.

The key to safe and effective exercise is to introduce a little bit of action into every day. Sudden bouts of strenuous exercise can be dangerous because the body is not prepared for the strain. A person leading a sedentary life working in an office needs an activity that starts out gently but can

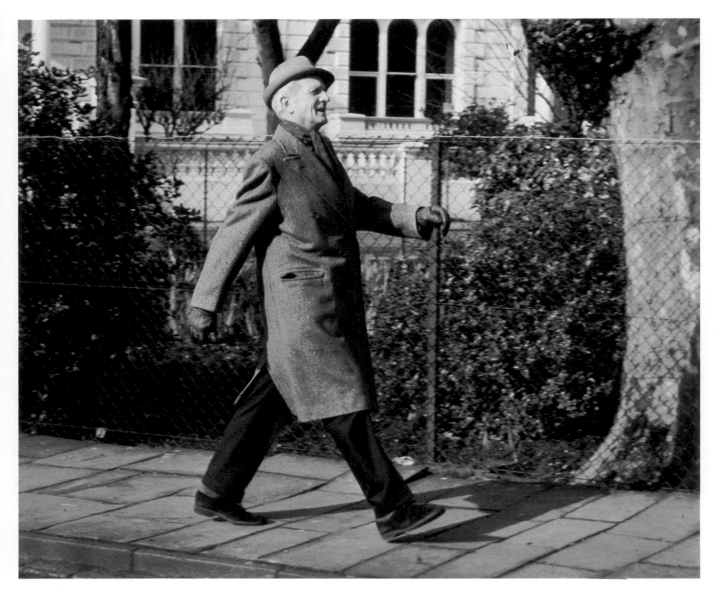

become gradually more demanding as he or she gets fitter. And its needs to be something they can fit into their daily routine – such as walking. A walk to work or to the station is good for you. A walk before bed-time will also help you to sleep better. And a stroll after meals is particularly good, because more food is burned up faster just after eating.

If you can participate in sports, so much the better. Swimming, running, skating, skiing, tennis, squash, table tennis, or bicycling are all excellent activities. Jogging is good too, provided you get your doctor's approval first. Among the exercise routines suitable for the home, the Royal Canadian Air Force program (11 minutes a day exercise plan) is excellent. Or you could join a physical fitness group in your neighborhood.

Physical activity has virtues that are closely related to relaxation. Firstly, the time spent exercis-ing is time taken out of work, and contributes to a more balanced life. Secondly, physical fatigue, particularly in the relatively unfit, promotes sound sleep. An eminent doctor once said that hard exer-cise is the best antidote to anxiety: get physically tired enough and you will sleep through anything.

When embarking on a fitness scheme start gradually. Concentrate on dynamic exercises. These involve large groups of muscles and improve the functions of the lungs, heart and blood circulation. Walking, in particular, is an excellent but neglected form of exercise.

A piece of advice often given by doctors to people with heart conditions is: "Get yourself a dog, and don't let your wife take it out." The third virtue is that many types of exercise involve meeting and participating with an entirely different group of people. This means a change of routine that can lead to relaxation.

To sum up. First you should spend some minutes every day in loosening-up exercise and then a few times a week engage in strength and endurance exercises. In addition two hours should be set aside at the weekend for walking, sports, or games. Use the stairs rather than the elevator if you are going up less than three floors, or get out a couple of floors early and walk the rest of the way. If you already have a heart condition, then certain exercises can be of great benefit – but it is important to remember that strenuous exercise must only be carried out with the permission of your doctor.

The Dangers
of Stress

A certain amount of stress is part of everyday living. Joy and pleasure, for example, are just as much forms of stress as is anger. Watching a football game on television is stressful and so is any sudden excitement. Such emotions cause chemicals to be released into the system to help the body cope with the extra claims being made on it. Normally, once the stress is over, the effect of these chemicals is neutralized. Trouble starts, however, when we undergo too much stress for too long. Unrelieved stress may then play its part in producing a host of physical and mental disturbances, including heart disease, high blood pressure, ulcers, headaches, indigestion, fatigue, anxiety, and general feelings of depression.

It is obvious that we cannot cut stress entirely from our lives. But anyone who feels that their job is making too great and continued demand on their health, should seriously consider whether they might not be better off in a less stressful occupation. This may sound like a pretty drastic solution, but even being ready to discuss it as a possibility can do a

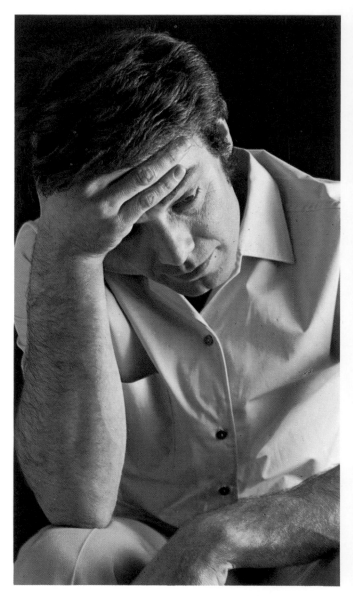

Stress disturbs the natural functioning of the mind and body, and has been implicated as a causative factor in many diseases. High-pressure jobs generate it in their employees, but isolation, loneliness and lack of opportunity to communicate can also cause a build-up of stress.

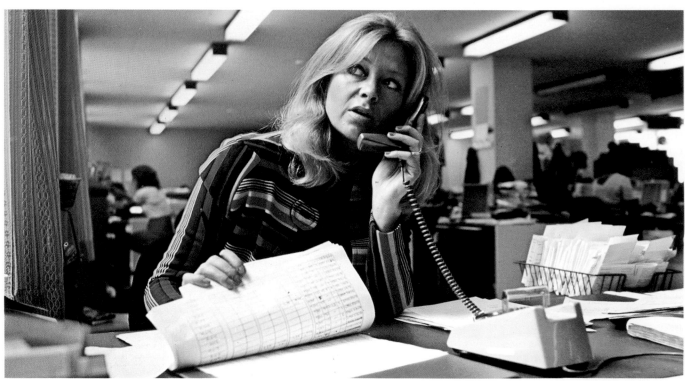

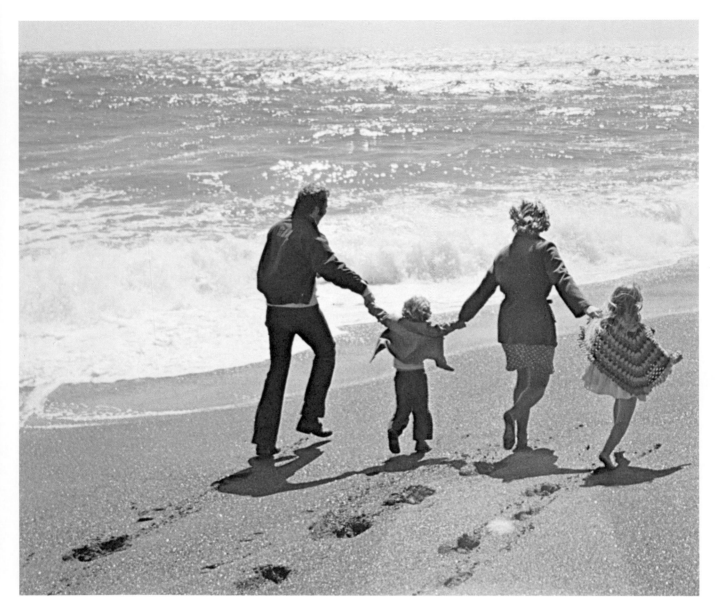

lot to take the pressure off people who feel that they must stick at a job that overtaxes them or make ever increasing efforts to get ahead and earn more money for the sake of the family.

This is what had happened to Philip the architect. Originally he had worked in a small office. But when he joined the urban development project he found that he had twice as much work to do, and lived in constant fear that he might make a mistake. After his heart attack he opted for a less stressful life. In taking this decision he was fortunate in being supported by his wife, because she preferred to have him alive, well and happy, rather than suffering for the sake of a larger pay packet and personal prestige.

But if often happens that husband and wife get so caught up in the frantic scramble of money-earning and budgeting that they lose sight of the facts of life. Naturally a wife worries about having enough money to go around. And naturally parents want to give their children the best possible start in life. But even though few luxuries are desirable, they cannot take the place of a father who is always working, or who is too tired and harassed to play with his

Western civilization has for a long time prized drive, hard work and success at the expense of other values. It is now becoming clearer that the quality of life, including family life, depends on other, nonmaterial factors.

children, or talk to his wife. It takes courage for a husband and wife to step back and reassess their life in these terms, but such a reassessment can sometimes be the key to family health and happiness.

"Moderation in all things," seems to be the most important rule. It sounds rather dull but it may help to be reminded of something Dr Kinsey once wrote about a person's health. "Good health, sufficient exercise and sleep," he said, "still remain one of the most effective aphrodisiacs known to man." And sex is also one of the best ways of relieving tensions left to us in our stress-filled world – as well as being one of the pleasures in life that will not do anything to harm one's health.

The important point to realize is that there is no one way of avoiding stress; there is no universal panacea that will relieve all of the tensions and frustrations of modern living. What is done must be appropriate and satisfying for each individual.

A Return to Normal Life

An acute heart attack is a grave medical emergency. Available statistics suggest that three to five out of every ten people who suffer a major heart attack die during the first two hours, the majority of these patients dying during the first few minutes, before any medical help can reach them. For the remainder the coronary care units in modern hospitals have brought a new hope: hospital death rates from coronaries in the past two decades have been cut to

be treated before heart failure and death occur.

Many of those people who die before medical help can be summoned could be saved if skilled help could be obtained in time. It seems that the majority of the deaths that occur immediately after a heart attack are also due to treatable dysrhythmias. Recognition of this fact has led to the development of mobile coronary care units in many countries, consisting of an ambulance complete with special equipment and a trained team of medical, nursing and ambulance personnel that can be called immediately to a person's house. These units are highly efficient life savers, but for maximum effectiveness it is important to know the main symptoms of an acute heart attack, as every minute counts.

Once in hospital, a patient with a coronary will remain only for a few days in the intensive care unit, after which he or she can be moved to a general

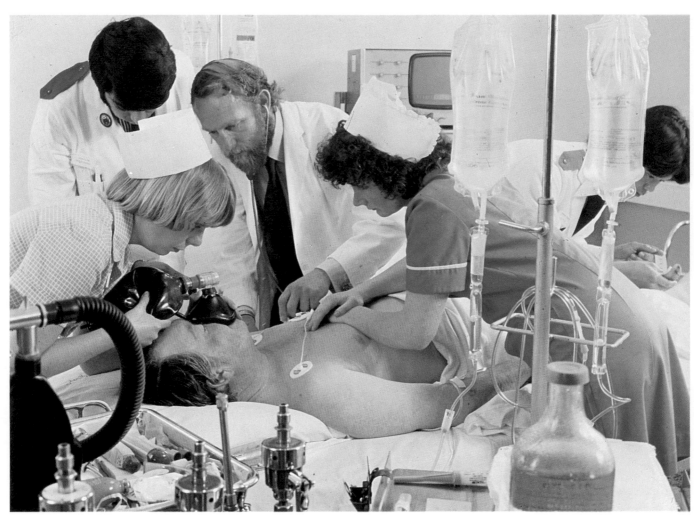

15 percent from over 70 percent before the intensive care units began to operate in the early 1960s. This great improvement was made possible because most deaths that occurred when the patients arrived at the hospital were due to treatable disorders of the rhythm of the heartbeat – *dysrhythmias* – and not because of a severe destruction of the heart muscle. Now, with the use of sophisticated instruments that detect and record changes in the heartbeat, these disorders can

Death from cardiac arrest is usually due to the electrical instability of the heart, and could often have been prevented if help could reach the victim in time. Mobile coronary care units have dramatically reduced deaths from heart attacks.

ward. After three weeks most people are well enough to leave hospital and by this time they are usually free of symptoms. They are given advice and instruction, urged to stop smoking if they are smokers, and to start a reducing diet if they are overweight. If they suffer from hypertension, drugs are usually prescribed to lower blood pressure. If high cholesterol levels are detected in their blood they are advised about a special diet and may be given drugs as well.

Usually a person who has just had a coronary cannot return to work until at least eight weeks after the attack, or take part in any heavy manual work. He or she should not drive an automobile until two months after returning to work. On returning home, he or she should increase his activity gradually, and after a month can start going for short walks, increasing the distance by a few hundred yards every day. At eight weeks they should walk three to four miles each day and they may start playing games which do not demand excessive physical exertion. Many people are encouraged to continue with the walking therapy and walk up to six miles a day for

is still a matter of controversy among experts but in recent years it has been proved that corrective heart surgery can not only help many people but also give hope for those with badly damaged hearts suffering from chronic and severe conditions. Fortunately such severe heart conditions are relatively rare.

As more and more is discovered about the causes of heart disease and as newer and more effective forms of prevention and treatment are found, so the outlook for these people who are likely to suffer an attack – already greatly improved over the last 20 years – will continue to get even better.

Coronary thrombosis does not put an end to a victim's active life. After about 8 weeks the patient can resume light activities such as gardening. He or she will be put on a rehabilitation program, which will include diet and exercise, to restore the body's functional capacity.

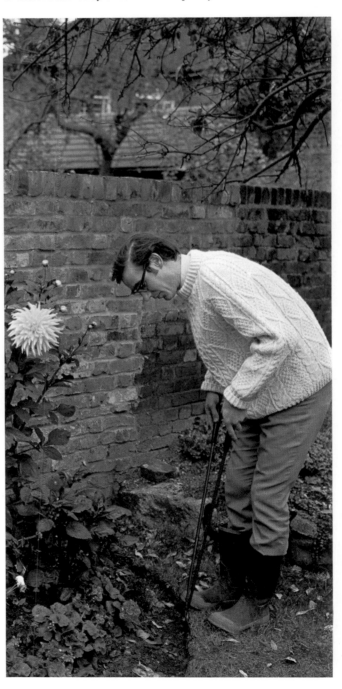

For some days after the heart attack the patient is still in danger and remains in the intensive care unit under constant supervision. His or her electrocardiograph is monitored constantly for irregularities in shape and rate. An alarm system attached to each patient's oscilloscope signals emergencies.

the rest of their lives. This method has given astonishingly good results and most people can resume their professional careers in full after their first heart attack. The risk of these people developing another coronary is only slightly higher than that in people of the same age who have not had a previous attack, and the long-term outlook is good.

Heart surgery can help some people with chronic heart disease. The effectiveness of heart transplants

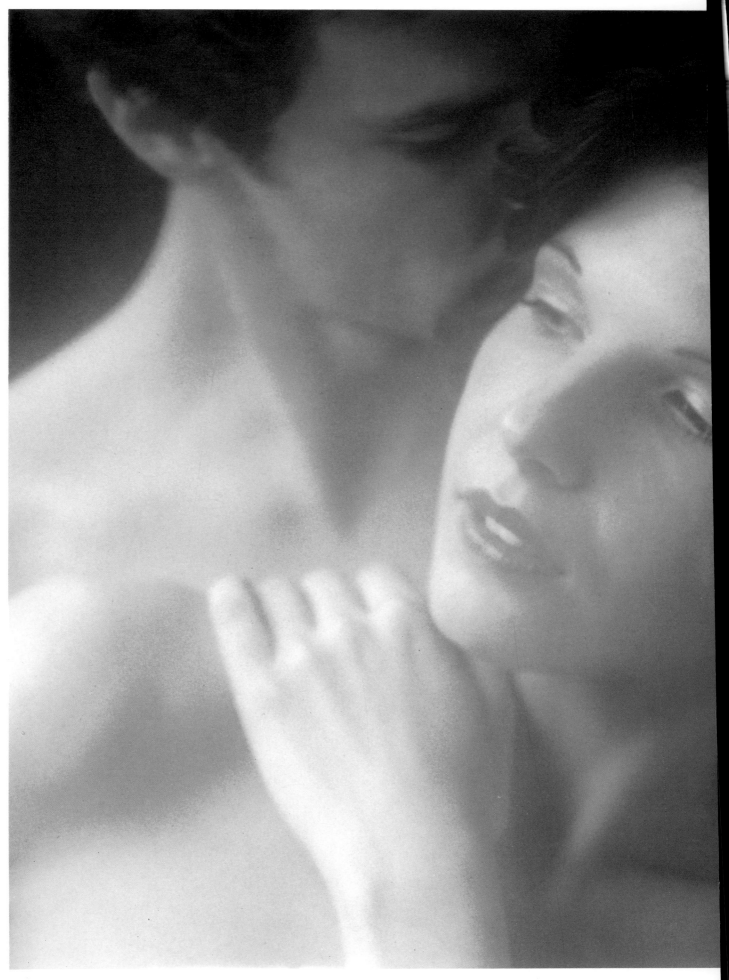

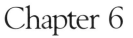

Chapter 6

A Healthy Sex Life

The act of reproduction is not only essential for the survival of the human species, it can also be a healthy and rewarding activity. Sexual function, like the workings of any other organic system, can be described in purely scientific terms. But this will not tell us what "making love" is all about. Sexuality is the basis of primary human relationships. It is fundamental to our acceptance and enjoyment of life and is one of the mainsprings of human motivation. Like the outermost orbitals of an atom's electrons, it shapes the forces of attraction, repulsion, and bonding between people. We need the physical and emotional experiences of sex to live healthy lives.

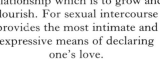

Opposite: sexual compatibility is an essential aspect of a relationship which is to grow and flourish. For sexual intercourse provides the most intimate and expressive means of declaring one's love.

Sex and Loving

Two researchers in the United States, William Masters and Virginia Johnson, have studied men and women during intercourse, and have given us for the first time a detailed knowledge of what our bodies achieve during sexual excitement and satisfaction. Indeed we are all surrounded with so much information about sex that it is often believed that it was discovered in the 20th century. In theory, since the problem of producing unwanted children has almost been solved in the West, we should have reached the ultimate heights of sexual happiness.

Dr William H Masters and Virginia E Johnson. Their laboratory studies of the human sexual response identified the four phases, exploded many sexual myths, and formed the basis for future sexual therapy.

But this has not come about. Sex is too vital, too interesting, and too personal not to arouse continued controversy, and many unnecessary anxieties and inhibitions surrounding sex are still very much with us. Though they might not say so, many women today long to be what "J," author of *The Sensuous Woman* (1970), describes as "that perfect combination of a lady in a living room and a marvelous bitch in bed." This attitude is a remnant of the not-so-recent strongly held male belief that there were "two kinds of women" – those that a man married and those that he could play around with. Though today few women would say, "I'm not that kind of girl," this statement, until very recently, was thought to be a valid way of explaining to a man why a girl would not go to bed with him. In these "enlightened" times, it is more readily accepted that every healthy woman is "that kind of girl" in her sex life. But is this belief totally accepted by everyone?

Though the marriage manuals and the husband,

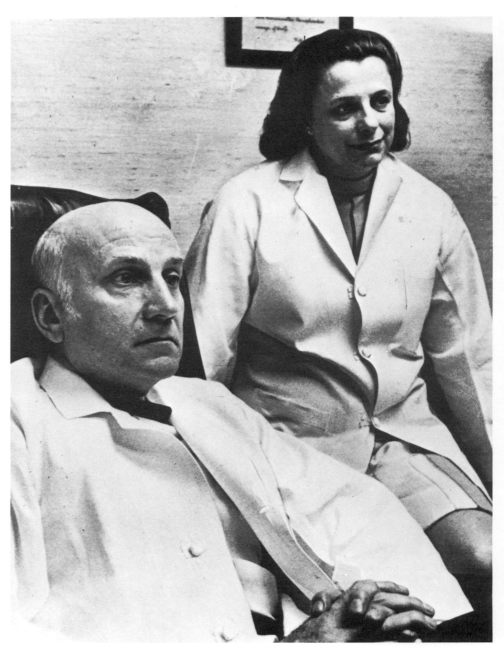

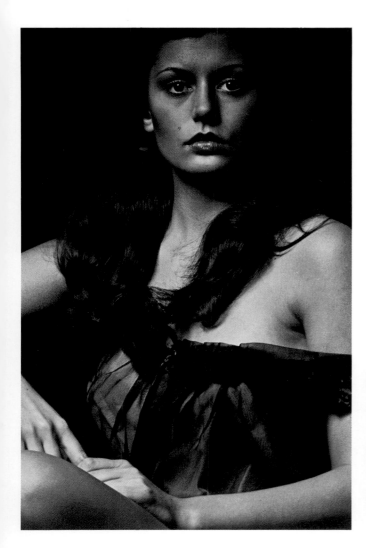

Above: cultural attitudes produce images known as sexual stereotypes. One of the most common is that of the promiscuous or "fallen" woman who could be a whore or a mistress, but never a wife. This stems from a belief, only recently discredited, that a woman should not have sexual feelings.

may encourage her toward "complete abandon in the bedroom," the average woman may question whether a "nice" girl really does act in this way and she may be worried and feel guilty because she finds it impossible to play the part expected of her. There is no easy answer to this problem, but frank honesty and cooperation between partners makes a lot of difference. If two people can cooperate, both bodily and mentally, in their first sexual experiences together, and are able to tell one another about all their sensations and any inhibitions they might have, this will help their relationship to mature and create a strong bond as husband and wife.

May was a chemistry graduate. She and Michael, a salesman, had met at a party, liked each other, and started to go steady. Soon Michael wanted May to make love completely. But May had had a strict upbringing. She was sexually inexperienced, afraid of her own urges and afraid of pregnancy – but could not summon up the courage to be frank with Michael about her fears. So she told him they would have to wait until they had known each other longer.

Michael could not understand May's attitude, and just at that critical time he met Mary Ann, a young secretary. They were immediately attracted to each other and were soon making love. Because they were able to derive great enjoyment from each other's bodies and could talk about sex in an open manner, their relationship – which at first was based purely on a physical attraction – soon matured and they were married a few months later.

Despite the many predictions – usually from men – that the widespread use of the Pill would lead to a totally promiscuous society, it seems that this has not happened. In fact the Pill has had a stabilizing effect and many social workers have commented that "the Pill has replaced the diamond ring as an engagement symbol."

Below: nowadays few would expect that a woman has to be a virgin until marriage. In fact many couples would insist that it is essential for both partners to get to know one another sexually before embarking upon marriage.

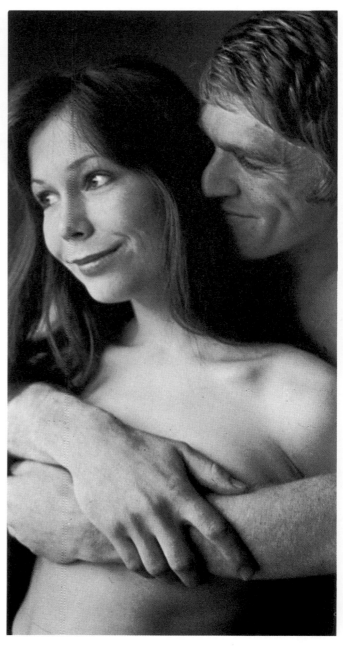

The Human Sex Organs

Although love inspires poets, it is the sex organs themselves that give men and women their greatest sensual pleasure. Yet their primary function is simply to reproduce the species, to insure the survival of man.

The visible parts of the male reproductive organs are the *testes*, which are contained in the *scrotum*, and the *penis*. The testes are responsible for producing millions of sperm cells every day. The penis has two functions: it is the means by which man urinates and by which he has sexual intercourse. When a man becomes sexually aroused, the spongy tissue of his penis fills with blood and stiffens.

During intercourse the sperm travel from the testes to a narrow tube called the *urethra* where they mix with other fluids to form the *semen*. The urethra leads to the outside world and also serves to carry urine from the bladder. At orgasm, ejaculation of semen is brought about by muscle contraction at the base of the penis.

From an early stage in their development the testes produce male sex hormones called *androgens*. These hormones cause the development of the male sex organs. Around the age of 14 or 15, the pituitary gland at the base of the brain starts to produce two hormones that "tell" the testes to start making sperm cells and to produce *testosterone*, the predominant male sex hormone. The testes grow under the influence of pituitary hormones, but it is testosterone that produces the other changes of puberty: the growth of the penis, the deepening of the voice, and the development of hair on the face and body.

Can a man change his sex? Newspapers report from time to time on men undergoing a sex change operation and becoming women. Some of these people are born with a mixture of both male and female organs. The operation simply clears up the

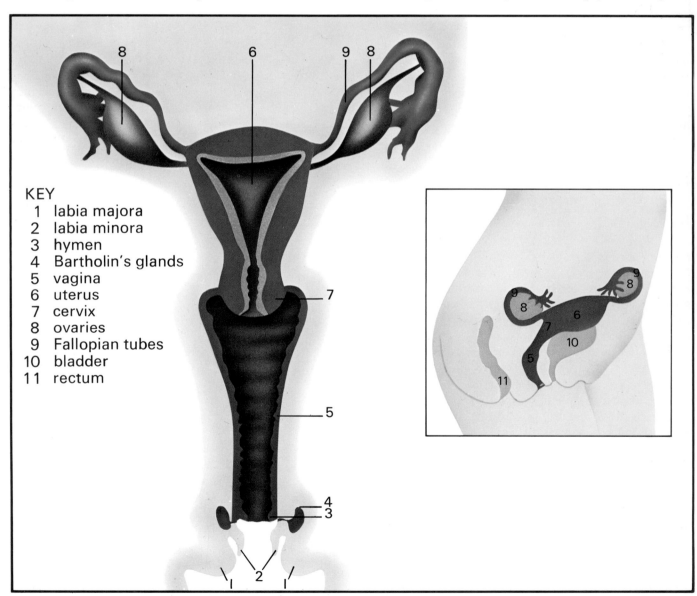

KEY
1 labia majora
2 labia minora
3 hymen
4 Bartholin's glands
5 vagina
6 uterus
7 cervix
8 ovaries
9 Fallopian tubes
10 bladder
11 rectum

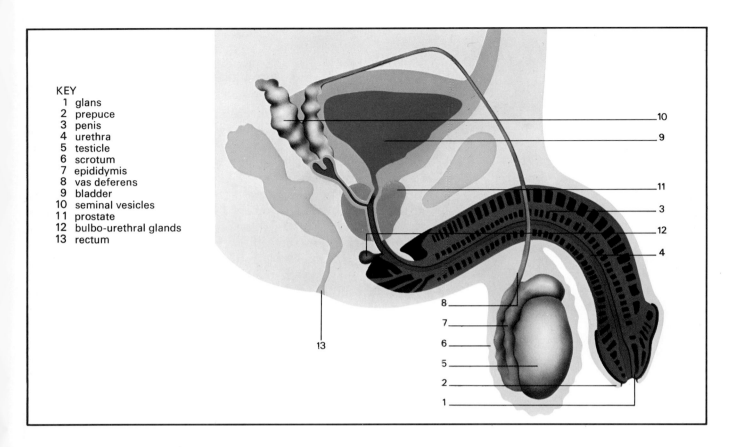

KEY
1 glans
2 prepuce
3 penis
4 urethra
5 testicle
6 scrotum
7 epididymis
8 vas deferens
9 bladder
10 seminal vesicles
11 prostate
12 bulbo-urethral glands
13 rectum

ambiguity, and hormone treatment helps with the transformation. But it is impossible for a normally developed man to be changed into a woman.

The woman's sex organs are designed to conceive and bear children, and therefore it is not surprising that they are far more complicated than those of a man's. The external female sex organs are known as the *vulva* and from puberty are covered with hair. The foremost limit of the vulva is a fleshy mound called the *mons pubis* or *mons Veneris*, and sweeping back from the mons are two folds of skin forming the *labia majora*. Between the labia majora are more delicate skin flaps, the *labia minora*. Almost hidden by the front part of the labia is the *clitoris*. This organ is responsible for the woman's intense physical pleasure during intercourse. The *vagina* itself is a muscular tube about 4 inches long that passes upward and backward and accommodates the penis during intercourse; it is the passage through which a baby is born.

In most girls and women who have never had sexual intercourse, a thin porous membrane called the *hymen* almost closes the vaginal opening. This is torn either by the penis during the first intercourse or quite often by physical exercise, and after childbirth there are only a few remnants of the hymen left. The part of the female sexual reproductive system where the fetus develops is called the *uterus* or womb. It is a hollow organ shaped like a pear, protruding at an angle of 90° into the upper part of the vagina. The womb has a lining which undergoes a cycle of change – the *menstrual* cycle. Two tubes – the *Fallopian tubes* – open into the upper part of the uterus, one on each side. These tubes lead to ovaries,

where *ova* or eggs are produced. Apart from producing eggs, the ovaries also make the female sex hormones *estrogen* and *progesterone*. These complex compounds control all the changes that take place during the menstrual cycle. Estrogen is also responsible for the development of the secondary sexual characteristics at puberty, such as breasts, body hair, and feminine body shape.

Once a month, roughly midway in a woman's menstrual cycle, one or other of the ovaries produces an ovum. The semen ejaculated by the man during sexual intercourse contains millions of sperm cells, and of the few hundred that will swim high up in the Fallopian tube, only one will fuse with the ovum and fertilize it.

Will the scientist ever replace the womb and produce babies in test tubes? Can a system be devised that would be an improvement over the highly efficient one evolved over millions of years? These speculations still lie mainly within the realms of science fiction, but recently British gynecologist Patrick Steptoe and physiologist Robert Edwards made headlines all over the world after their many experiments culminated in success: a healthy child was born from a mother who had a fertilized ovum implanted into her womb.

The mother had been able to produce ova, but her Fallopian tubes did not function normally. An ovum was extracted from the mother and fertilized with her husband's sperm in a laboratory dish. Three days later a developing embryo was implanted in the mother's uterus where it continued to develop normally. Surely the child conceived in this way is one of the wonders of modern medicine?

Phases of Sexual Response

Many individuals, and sometimes whole societies, throughout history have taken up the struggle to satisfy mind and body at the same time — and have then abandoned the attempt. There seems to be a perpetual pendulum in human history between seeing sexual love in terms of the mind on the one side and the body on the other — a swing to and fro between puritanism and promiscuity. But puritanism and promiscuity are in fact two sides of the same coin.

Until comparatively recently, the taboos regarding our attitudes to sexual response, especially in the woman, have been so severe that objective scientific investigation of this important field of human activity has been slow to advance. But the pioneering

There are no rules for lovemaking as long as both partners are willing participants. Even a minor degree of violence has its place in the sexual act.

work of such scientists as Dr Alfred Kinsey and his colleagues in the 1950s, and Masters and Johnson in the sixties and seventies, opened the way to a public awareness of the real meaning and possibilities of sexuality. And now we have a much greater understanding of our sexual urges, and a much more detailed knowledge of what exactly takes place during lovemaking.

The woman's response to sexual arousal is in many ways similar to the man's. Mounting sexual excitement brings about changes in the distribution of blood around the body. The clitoris and labia become engorged with blood. The breasts increase in size and the nipples become erect. The vagina and labia secrete a mucous lubricant that will make it easy for the penis to enter. Almost any area of the body can become sensitive to stimulation during lovemaking, but in the man the penis is the major area of sensation and in the woman it is the clitoris and the area of the sex organs round the vaginal opening. In fact during intercourse the penis does not touch the clitoris directly but massage is maintained indirectly because of the movement of the penis over the labia, which are in contact with the clitoris.

Lovemaking can be divided into four separate phases. The *excitement* phase includes close body

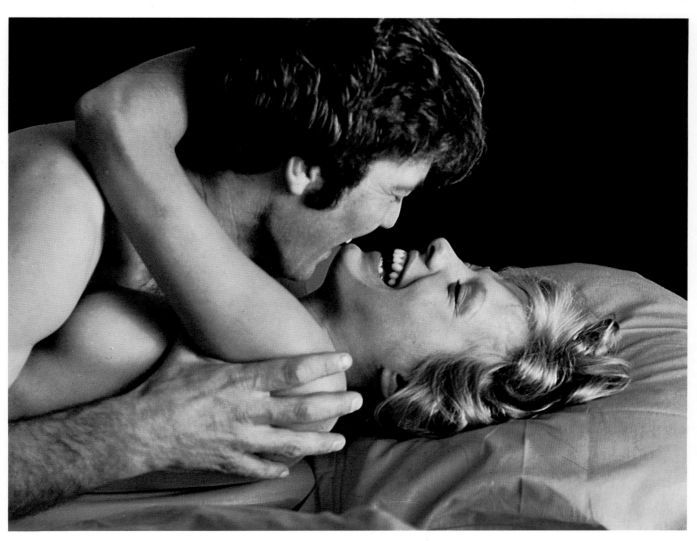

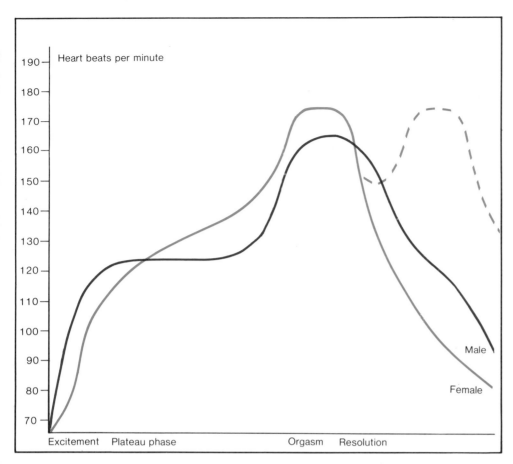

190 — Heart beats per minute
180 —
170 —
160 —
150 —
140 —
130 —
120 —
110 —
100 —
90 —
80 —
70 —

Excitement   Plateau phase   Orgasm   Resolution

Male

Female

Left: a comparison of the heart rates of a man and a woman during the four phases of sexual response. The dotted line represents the pattern of multiple orgasms.

Below left: there are no set rules as to which partner initiates lovemaking.

Below: resolution should be a period of restful tenderness.

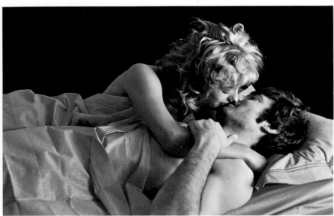

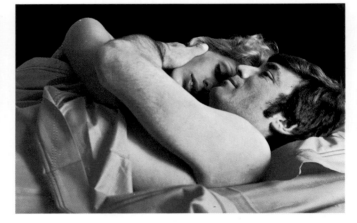

contact – kissing and caressing – but can also include stimulation by sight, smell, or sounds. If these stimulations are maintained and intensified, the next stage, the *plateau* phase, soon follows.

By this time intercourse will be taking place and the man will have put the whole length of his erect penis into the lengthened and distended vagina, moving it in and out to increase sensation.

Passion is unpredictable and the length of the plateau phase varies from couple to couple and from occasion to occasion. Its duration and enjoyment is dependent on many factors, including the position or series of positions used, the concentration of the participants, and how strong the drive is for a release of sexual tension. Depending on the length of time of the plateau phase, there is a swift or gradual buildup to the *orgasmic* phase, when waves of muscular contractions at the base of the penis cause semen

to be ejaculated into the vagina. The climax lasts for a few seconds only and can be shared by both partners – concentrated in the penis in the man, and in the vagina and clitoris in the woman, but affecting the whole body with a series of uncontrollable violent thrusting movements.

Once the tension has been released, the couple enter the *resolution* phase in which all the body organs gradually return to their normal state. Since lovemaking is pleasantly exhausting, this should usually be a time of complete relaxation, sometimes merging into sleep.

Traditionally the man is supposed to assume the dominant role in lovemaking, but really there are no set rules. Either partner can experience the excitement and pleasure of arousing his or her partner and they can both experiment in any way that leads to sexual fulfillment.

119

Which Contraceptive?

During the fertile years of an average marriage, a couple will make love about 3500 times, which makes some form of family planning essential. Yearly pregnancies are an intolerable idea to most women, and thanks to modern methods of birth control millions of couples all over the world are having their children by choice, not by chance.

Today there is a wide choice of contraceptive methods available, but there is not one which is totally troublefree in use and without adverse side-effects to a greater or lesser extent. *Oral contraceptives* – the Pill – are taken regularly by ten million women in Europe and the United States who are able to enjoy lovemaking without fear of pregnancy. Consisting of small regular doses of the female sex hormones estrogen and progesterone, the Pill suppresses the monthly release of the ovum so that

Right: chart of the most important facts about the major methods of birth control. The effectiveness of each method depends not only on the contraceptive or technique itself, but also on whether it is used regularly and correctly. For this reason, effectiveness cannot be measured with total accuracy.

Below: certain contraceptives are more suitable for some women than for others. The same is true for the various birth-control pills available. Your physician will help you decide on the most appropriate method.

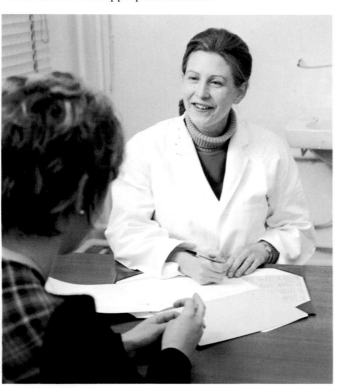

The Methods	What is it?
Pill	Pills containing synthetic estrogen and progesterone hormones
Coil or Loop intrauterine devices (IUD)	Small flexible devices of different sizes and shapes, inserted into the uterus
Diaphragm (together with spermicidal cream or jelly)	Soft rubber cap with flexible metal rim that fits over entrance to the uterus
Condom	Thin, strong rubber covering fitted over the penis
Spermicidal agents (1) Jellies, creams, soluble tablets, vaginal suppositories	Chemicals put into the vagina
(2) Aerosol vaginal foam	Foaming cream in aerosol can
Rhythm method ("safe period")	Finding out time of ovulation by keeping record of period dates and temperature changes
Douche	Syringe filled with water or other special solution
Withdrawal (coitus interruptus)	
Sterilization	Surgical operation

invading sperm find no egg to fertilize. Estrogens alone are effective, but a lower dose of estrogen combined with progesterone is preferred because the progesterone insures regular and normal menstruation. There is also a Pill in use which relies on the effects of progesterone alone.

Unfortunately the Pill can have adverse side-effects, including depression, weight gain, and headaches. Sometimes a change of Pill will alleviate the side effects, but there does appear to be a connection between the Pill and the incidence of such diseases as thrombosis. Therefore doctors do not recommend it for women with high blood pressure, previous blood vessel or blood clotting disorders, diseases of the major organs, or for those over 35 years of age. It should also not be prescribed for women with a family history of thrombosis.

The *diaphragm* or cap is a dome-shaped rubber device. It is placed in the vagina and covers the cervix, thus acting as a sperm barrier. It does have several disadvantages however. It must be fitted initially by a doctor. To be fully effective it must be used with a spermicidal jelly or cream that kills the sperm. Also, many couples are put off by the idea of interupting their lovemaking so that they can insert the device.

The third most widely used contraceptive method

How it works	Advantages	Disadvantages	Effectiveness
Taken daily for a certain number of days each month prevents release of egg	Easy to use. No interference with enjoyment	May cause unpleasant side effects. Prescription required. Unsuitable for some	0.5% pregnancy rate
Prevents fertilized egg from implanting in uterine wall	Usually stays in place indefinitely. Cannot be felt. Does not reduce pleasure	Temporary discomfort after insertion. The woman may expel it unknowingly	With newest types of IUD 1% pregnancy rate
Used in conjunction with cream or jelly, prevents sperm from entering the uterus	No side effects. Cannot be felt by either partner. Can be inserted up to three hours before intercourse	Must also use cream or jelly. Should not be removed for at least six hours after intercourse	With correct fit and good cream, 95-98% effective
Prevents sperm from reaching the uterus	Easy to obtain. Simple to use	Can be felt. May slip off. Interferes with enjoyment	5-6% pregnancy rate. If woman uses spermicidal cream or jelly less than 5% pregnancy rate
Immobilizes or kills sperm	No prescription needed. Usually easy to obtain	Must be applied again before each intercourse. May cause irritation	Not reliable unless used with diaphragm or condom
Forms a chemical barrier against sperm	No prescription needed. More effective than creams or jellies when used on its own	Must be inserted again before each intercourse. May cause irritation	At worst, 20% pregnancy rate. At best, 90-98% effective
Intercourse is limited to woman's infertile period, just before and just after ovulation	No pills or devices involved. Only method approved by Roman Catholic Church	Keeping careful records required. Limits intercourse. Not reliable if periods are irregular	About 20% pregnancy rate
Washes out vagina to remove semen before it enters the uterus	None	Must be done immediately after intercourse. Unreliable. May cause infection	Least effective of all methods
Man withdraws penis before ejaculation	No product required. No cost	Interferes with sexual climax. Unreliable	Poor
In a man, prevents sperm from being released in seminal fluid. In a woman, blocks the passage of eggs from the ovaries to the uterus	Almost always permanently effective. No need for any other birth control method. Does not interfere with sexual desire or enjoyment	Cannot be undone	Virtually 100%

for women is the *intrauterine device* (IUD). This is a plastic loop or coil inserted into the uterus by a doctor. In some way not fully understood, the IUD renders the uterus hostile to the implantation of a fertilized egg. The greatest advantage of the IUD is that once it is in, there is nothing else to remember. New, small devices containing copper have now been developed and these can be used by women who have not had any children, unlike the earlier larger devices. But the IUD can have troublesome side effects, such as intermittent bleeding, heavy periods, abdominal pain, and even infection.

The *condom* or rubber remains the preferred method for many couples, and is particularly useful during the early stages of a sexual relationship while other methods are being considered. It consists of a rubber sheath that is rolled on to the erect penis just before intercourse, and prevents the semen from entering the vagina. Its advantages are that it does not require medical supervision, is inexpensive, easily available, and its distribution does not depend on the medical services. Its main disadvantage is that it reduces the pleasure of intercourse by acting as a sensation barrier.

The *rhythm method* is based on the concept that there is a "safe" or infertile time related to menstrual periods during which a woman is unlikely to conceive. This period of time is determined through keeping a careful record of the dates of the menstrual cycle and of body temperature. The advantages of this method are that it is acceptable to a large number of couples for religious and psychological reasons, and that it involves no contraceptive device or medication. It is, however, the least reliable of the contraceptive methods because menstruation and temperature can be effected by many physical and mental conditions. At the moment doctors are attempting to find new methods of predicting ovulation more accurately, such as the changes in the vaginal mucus that occur just prior to ovulation.

Chemical barriers such as aerosol foams, vaginal foam tablets, creams and jellies are also used. These mechanically block the passage of sperm into the uterus and destroy them chemically. They are not efficient unless used in conjunction with a condom or diaphragm.

Coitus interruptus – the withdrawal of the penis from the vagina just before ejaculation – is widely practiced. It involves no mechanical appliance or chemical product, but is unreliable in so far as it demands a higher degree of control than many men are capable of exercising, and sperm may be released before orgasm. It can also have adverse psychological effects on both men and women.

Methods of Sterilization

Today a relatively new method of birth control is becoming more and more popular because of its near total efficiency: sterilization for both men and women. Female sterilization can be achieved by *hysterectomy* (removal of the uterus), but there is no justification for this major operation simply as a method of contraception, and it is performed only if there is some other reason such as fibroids.

Sterilization for a woman usually involves an operation under general anesthetic in which both Fallopian tubes are cauterized, clipped, or cut. The patient spends only one night in hospital and there is little discomfort. Her sexual life will continue normally, she will have monthly periods, but she will no longer be able to have children.

It is estimated that in the United States alone over one million men are sterilized every year. This operation, called a *vasectomy*, is simple: the sperm-carrying tubes are cut and tied in a minor operation that is performed under local anesthetic and only takes about 15 minutes. It is painless, involves very little discomfort, and the man can leave the hospital or clinic immediately after the operation. A vasectomy does not affect a man's sexual activity; he continues to ejaculate semen at intercourse, but within two or three months of the operation the semen becomes free of sperm.

Sterilization for both men and women is equally effective and involves a small amount of discomfort and risk. But both types should be considered irreversible and therefore should be thought about very carefully by both partners. Only when they are determined that it is the right step for them to take should they go ahead. To help them with their decision, and with any problems of adjustment that might arise after the operation, most health authorities that provide sterilizations also have a counseling service.

Another "birth control" problem that is of importance is infertility. Even if the population explosion may seem to be the world's most pressing problem, to a childless couple a baby is more than just another mouth to feed. And if that longed-for baby does not come, the resulting tensions created can often lead to a breakdown of the marriage. So as soon as a couple begin to get anxious about their inability to start a family, they should seek medical advice.

Initially in most cases the doctor's advice will be to go on trying for a few more months, but first he will make sure that intercourse is taking place. For example the man may be impotent, that is he cannot get an erection or finds it impossible to achieve orgasm. The cause might be physical or psychological, but whatever the reason in most cases it can be treated and cured.

The couple might be sent straight away to an infertility clinic where special tests will be carried out on both partners. The first of a series of tests carried out on the man will be to determine if his sperm cells are normal and whether he has a low "sperm count" – which means that less than the normal level of sperm is present in his semen (at least 100 million sperm should be present in every cubic centimeter). Hormonal and other treatment can sometimes raise a low sperm count. Several other tests can be performed on the man to see if he is functioning normally.

If there is nothing wrong with the man then a series of tests are carried out on the woman to find out if she has some physical abnormality. It will be established whether or not she is ovulating. Cervical secretions removed soon after intercourse will be studied. The entire reproductive tract will be examined in detail using a whole range of highly sophisticated techniques.

Where the clinic can determine that the seat of the trouble is physical, then very often a course of treatment, an operation, or artificial insemination will solve the problem. But if there is nothing wrong with either partner, then a series of in-depth counseling sessions may be needed.

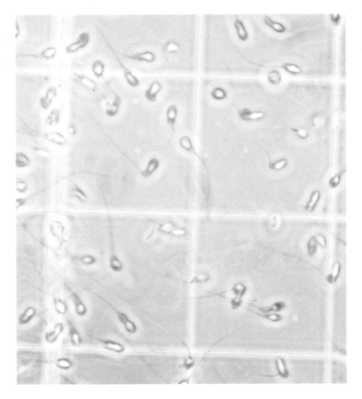

Grid used to determine sperm concentration. A low sperm count is often the reason why a man cannot father a child. In such a case sperm from several ejaculations can be preserved and then artificially injected. If conception follows, the subject is still the true father.

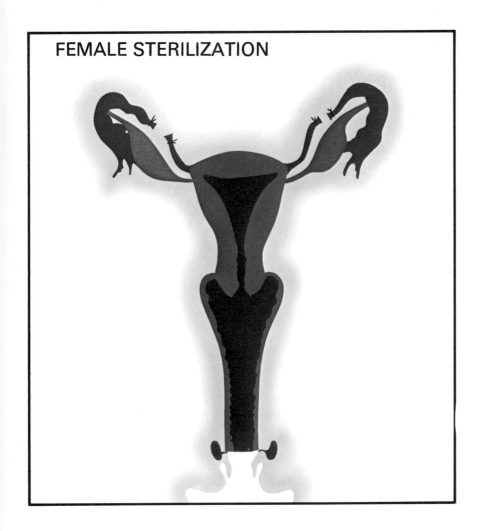

FEMALE STERILIZATION

In tubal ligation the Fallopian tubes, which carry the ova from the ovary to the uterus, are either cut and tied or removed. The operation is performed under general anesthetic.

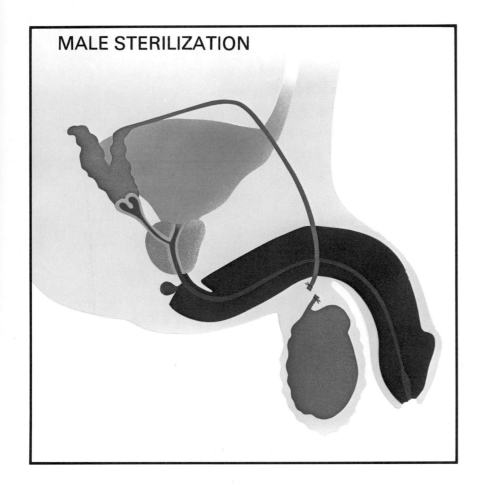

MALE STERILIZATION

A vasectomy involves the cutting and tying up of the vas deferens – the tubes which carry the sperm away from the testicles. The operation is performed under local anesthetic.

Artificial Insemination

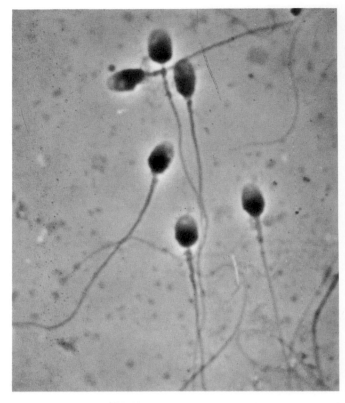

There are several causes of sterility. A man may not produce enough sperm or any at all. Or, in rare cases, his testes may produce sperm but there is a blockage in the tubes by which the sperm travels from the testicles. A woman's vaginal secretions may have a high acid content, and the sperm could in such cases be killed before reaching the womb. This acidity can often be counteracted medically. Sometimes too few sperm reach the egg in the Fallopian tubes and thus the chances of successful fertilization are greatly reduced. However, nature normally provides a great abundance of sperm: a healthy man ejaculates at one orgasm at least 300 million sperm, but only one is needed to fertilize the ovum.

Above right: human sperm. Each ejaculate contains about 300 million, but only one is needed for fertilization.

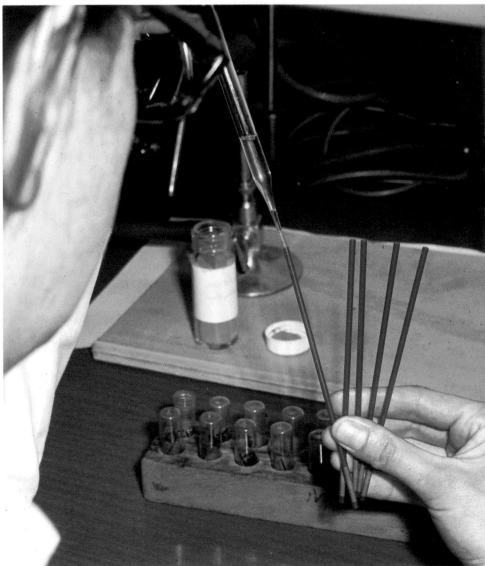

Right: seminal fluid from a donor is transfered to capillary tubes which are then placed in liquid nitrogen for preservation.

124

Provided that a woman is healthy, then a technique which has been used on animals for centuries – artificial insemination – is often the answer to the problem. In artificial insemination semen is injected into the woman, usually by a doctor, using either a glass syringe or a curved tube fitted to a syringe. In order for artificial insemination to succeed, the semen must be deposited in the vagina as soon as possible after the egg has matured. But judging this time exactly is difficult – the most reliable sign is a slight rise in temperature. Despite the difficulties, the success rate is quite high.

There are two categories of artificial insemination. Where the woman produces a chemical barrier to the sperm but her husband's semen is normal his own semen is used. If the husband's sperm count is low, several samples can be collected over a period and freeze stored until there is a sufficient quantity. If the husband's sperm shows a defect, or if he produces no sperm at all, then sperm from an anonymous donor is used.

Artificial insemination by a donor presents many problems – both for doctors and their patients. The donor must enjoy good health and he should resemble the husband as closely as possible. But apart from problems of selection, there are also moral considerations. For some wives contact with the sex cells of a man who is not their husband raises the problem of whether there is any ethical difference between her receiving another man's semen via his penis during intercourse, or via a syringe in a doctor's surgery. Also, considerable psychological difficulties may have to be overcome. The husband knows that the child is not his and this can often create future tension in the family. Many gynecologists suggest that the couple should make love immediately before the injection of the donor's semen; there is then a chance that the husband will be the father.

In spite of the many difficulties associated with the practice of artificial insemination, it has brought personal happiness to a great number of childless couples who would otherwise have felt unfulfilled as human beings.

This couple have had their child through AID (artificial insemination by donor). This method is used if the male partner has no sperm or too little to effect fertilization. The donor's identity is never disclosed.

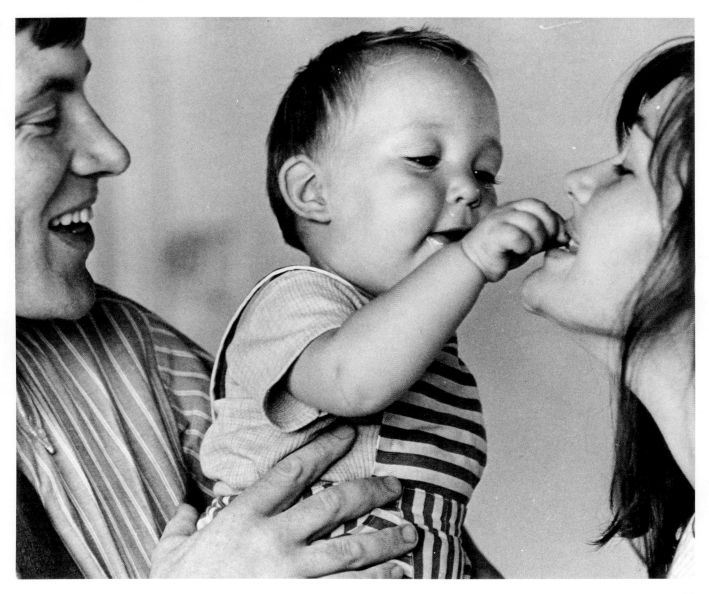

Never too Old

Sometimes after years of successful lovemaking the sexual side of a marriage loses its appeal. One partner no longer enjoys the other's approaches and sex becomes a bore, to be endured simply as a polite ritual. When this happens what is often needed is a change, a rest, a slight if temporary shedding of some of life's burdens, and a chance to feel like a carefree young married couple again.

Couples should try to avoid sliding into sexual inertia. One of the most important findings of modern research into our sex lives has established that men and women can enjoy sensual love well into old age, provided that they keep up a steady, active interest in lovemaking. Contrary to the old myth that a man or woman must not "use themselves up" sexually in their early years, modern science has confirmed that those who keep in practice can best maintain their sexual urges well into old age. In other words, the more you make love, the more chance you will have of enjoying it into middle and old age. As with any other aspect of life, the individual's overall attitude is what determines the outcome – in this case whether sex continues to bring satisfaction into the sixties and seventies or whether it subsides much sooner. Once a man and woman tell themselves that they are too old, they tend to become too old – for anything, not just sex.

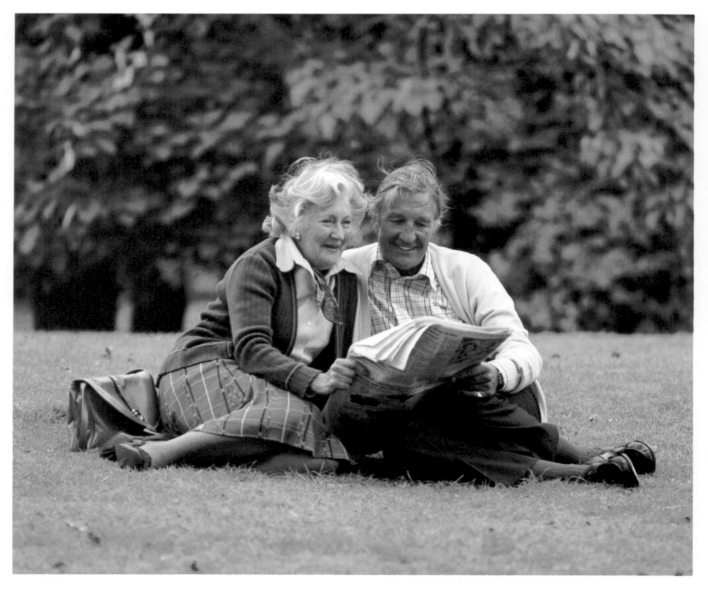

Medical evidence has confirmed that men and women can and should enjoy sex well beyond middle age, provided the couple have maintained a regular and interesting sexual relationship throughout their partnership. In fact, both physically and psychologically, sex would be extremely beneficial for both partners.

A recurring problem that confronts doctors, social workers, and marriage counselors is when either a husband or wife suddenly decides, usually in their mid-fifties, that sex has come to an end for them. Their partners are frustrated and unhappy and the individuals themselves are uncertain whether they should still want sex or not "at their age." This happened to Betty and Henry, but Henry knew what to do. He went to see his doctor to discuss the situation. He told the doctor that Betty had accused him of trying to be "young and foolish," but he was afraid that she had settled for a long wait for death. His doctor told Henry that sexual desire is still as normal, healthy, and essential to a man and woman in middle age as when they were young. The doctor advised Henry to take his wife away for a holiday, and to talk to her in cheerful terms about all the things they could look forward to doing together

Below: with the major pressures of family and business life behind them, a couple approaching middle age will find that they have more time to spend together. They can develop new joint interests, take long vacations and generally rediscover the value of each other's company.

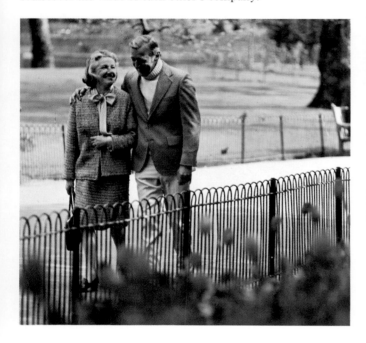

after his retirement. Once her appetite for life itself returned, so would her sexual desire.

A similar problem confronts men. Although it is perfectly normal for people of middle and old age to continue with their lovemaking for as long as they feel like it, the husband's sexual drive sometimes begins to subside a little more rapidly than that of his wife. Often a partnership that had had problems in its early days because the husband wanted to make love more frequently than the wife, may change when they reach their late fifties or early sixties into one which the wife is the more sexually demanding. She has got to learn to be more tolerant and undemanding – just like she wanted her husband to be when they were young. She can also get around the problem by increasing the amount of time spent in sexual foreplay and intercourse not involving ejaculation, and cutting down on the amount of lovemaking that calls for her husband's erect penis to be inside her body. It can be of comfort to know that by the age of seventy, only approximately 25 to 35

percent of men in the United States and Europe have lost their sexual potency – and this figure is decreasing all the time as more and more older people realize that it is perfectly normal for them to make love all their lives.

Even the most problem-free sex lives can be further improved with a little encouragement, and encouragement is the keynote to most of the modern research by experts in the field of sex. Such research has been one of the most daring scientific contributions of the last 20 years in Europe and the United States. Time and again the old myths that once bred anxiety and led people to believe that they could not achieve fulfilment in sensual love have been dispelled. In their place has come the knowledge that sexual performance and pleasure is much easier to attain and to extend into old age than was ever dreamed of.

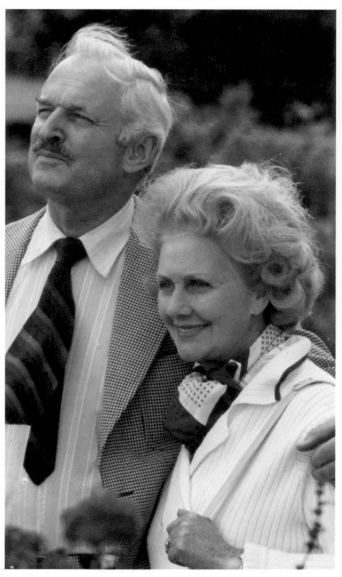

Above: as more elderly people realize that sexual intercourse is perfectly normal for them, and not just the province of the young, there are fewer reports of sexual potency decreasing with age. Sexual capacity may change but this can be more than compensated for by the love and mutual understanding that exists in a longstanding relationship.

127

The Growing Problem of VD

Venereal diseases (VD) are so called because they are usually transmitted during sexual (including homosexual) intercourse. The more casual attitude toward sexual behavior, new methods of contraception, drug resistance, and the greater mobility of people, have all contributed to its spread. Also, the social stigma attached to such infections prevents many sufferers from investigating symptoms and seeking medical treatment. This is a tragedy because if they are caught in their early stages venereal diseases can be cured quickly. On the other hand, if they are neglected they can lead to serious illness and even death.

Gonorrhea in men starts as an inflammation of the

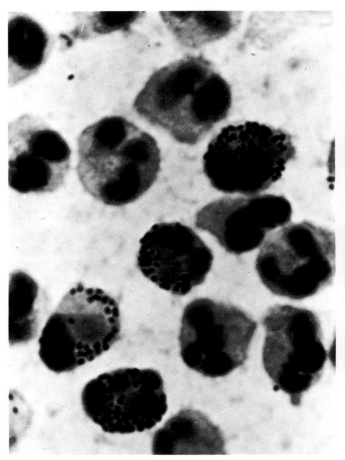

Above: white blood cells in a urethral smear taken from a subject with gonorrhea. The spherical bodies inside the cells are the gonococci bacteria. To survive, the bacterium needs warmth, moisture, darkness, and an oxygen-free atmosphere. After infection it passes to the urethral passage and the cervical canal, where it multiplies.

Below: *trichonomas vaginalis*, the organism responsible for trichonomiasis. It causes inflammation of the bladder, soreness in the genital area and pain during intercourse. In women there may also be a thick, white or greenish discharge. Some carriers have no symptoms.

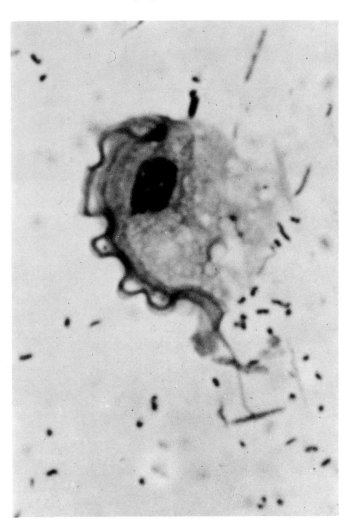

urethra or water passage between two to ten days after the man has had intercourse with an infected woman. The usual symptoms are pain and discomfort when urinating and a greenish-yellow discharge. It not treated promptly the disease can spread to other parts of the body and cause swollen joints and eventually sterility.

In women, gonorrhea is particularly dangerous because often there are no symptoms in its early stages. The reason for this is that the pus and discharge caused by the germs breeding at the opening of the uterus mix with the normal body secretions. Because of this lack of symptoms women are often unwilling to believe that they may be infected and do not seek medical help. Quite often an infected man is the only indication that a woman has the disease. Some early symptoms that do sometimes appear are vaginal discharge, and pain when passing water. If left untreated it can lead to pain in the joints and abdomen, and the woman may become sterile.

Syphilis is the most dangerous form of VD, but fortunately it is not as common as gonorrhea. It begins with a painless sore on the genital organs that is slow to heal. This "primary chancre" may be hidden, and it is easily missed. After a few weeks the sore will heal and if the disease has not been treated, it will enter the secondary stage, in which the germs are being spread by the bloodstream to every part of the body. A few weeks later the person will feel unwell – with a skin rash, sore throat, and sores on the genitals and around the anus. But even these symptoms will disappear eventually without treatment. By this time the disease will have become hidden – "latent" syphilis. The germs can live unnoticed for years in many organs of the body, but eventually may cause insanity, paralysis, blindness, and death. A woman with latent syphilis can pass it on to her unborn baby so that it is born diseased.

Nonspecific urethritis is a disease also transmitted during intercourse. It causes a discharge in men but women – who usually carry the germ – have no symptoms. If neglected it can result in inflammation of the joints, arthritis, and eye disease. Other diseases that can be spread through intercourse, including *trichomoniasis*, which produces a discharge in women, and *candidiasis* (commonly called thrush), which also produces itching and soreness in women. Several other diseases spread in the same way cause discharges, ulcers on the sex organs, and rashes. Like gonorrhea and syphilis, all these diseases can be cured with a minimum amount of treatment if caught in the early stages.

It is obvious from what has been described above that anyone who suspects that they might have VD – or thinks that they have run the risk of catching it – should immediately consult their doctor or attend a special VD clinic. At a clinic a patient will be questioned closely, given an examination, and blood and urine tests will be carried out. Many people who attend a VD clinic turn out to be disease-free, but even when a person has contracted the disease, if it has been discovered early enough it can be cured in a short period of time with suitable drug therapy.

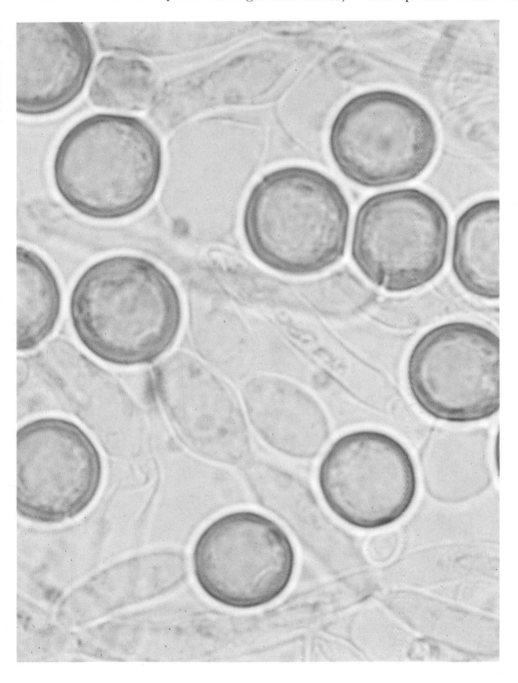

The yeastlike organism *Candida albicans*, responsible for candidiasis. In women it causes vaginal inflammation and a discharge; in men it can live beneath the foreskin, causing inflammation and possibly phimosis.

The New Approach to Sex

After at least a decade of the famous "Sexual Revolution," it is often assumed that most Americans and Europeans have entered a state known as the "New Morality." It is a condition in which pleasure is an important principle, in which more or less anything between consenting adults goes. Yet although some observers have proclaimed the revolution triumphant, new battles keep breaking out.

After an era of revolution, is a counter-revolution underway? Is it even possible that the revolution never really happened, that much of civilized world watched the New Morality – voyeristically – without abandoning the Old Morality? Undeniably recent years have seen major changes in social patterns, most notably a greater openness about sex, homosexuality and birth control. But young people who favor the new standards are still paying a high price in family conflicts, and conservative protesters are increasingly vociferous. It is not too difficult to show with a few typical examples that on all sides there are doubts and misgivings.

Kathy, a 27-year-old teacher, has been living with her boyfriend for over a year: "When I first told my parents I had a new roommate, they immediately knew what was going on. My mother's first words were: 'Don't do all the cooking and cleaning. With your brains you should be using your college education.' But I'm sure that what she really wants is for me to get married and have children."

Henry knows that his daughter has had several affairs: "I know what is going on with my daughter, but I don't want to see it, and I don't want to discuss it with her. This generation has no qualms about sharing a bedroom before marriage. I accept the right of young women to make that decision, but I don't see that they are much happier. And it's very difficult for me. I have a lot of personal feelings about it."

Kathryn, 25, a graduate, lived with her husband for a year before marrying him two years ago: "Intellectually, I think it's fine to sleep around. But emotionally I'd be very upset if my husband slept with other women. I wish I could be more liberated about this. I always felt I had conquered this until I started living with my husband and got dependent on him."

Wilma was married to a psychologist who often advocated "open marriage." She took him at his word and had an affair. When he found out, it broke up the marriage: "A lot of people accept intellectually that their partner will probably have an extra-

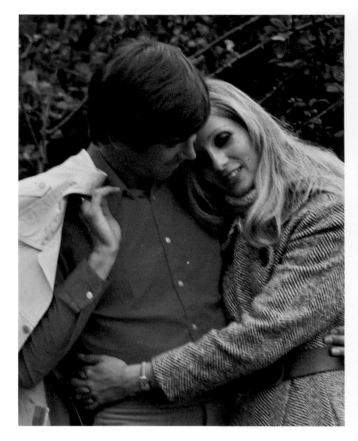

Many couples will now live together without even considering eventual marriage. However, the love element has retained its central importance to the relationship.

marital affair. But it's easy to be glib about it when it's not happening to you."

Sociologist Wayne Youngquist thinks that most people today are in a state of what he calls "betweenity": "They are caught between the new morality and the old. As long as they are not asked to make a statement, they'll ignore what's been going on." Youngquist also feels that while people are freer about private morality, they are becoming more conservative about the public and commercial exploitation of sex. But parents apparently suffer few illusions about how much effect any proposed clampdown would have on the young. The majority approve of classroom sex education, even before high school, and more than three quarters think that parents are correct in instructing their own teenage children about the use of contraceptives.

At a time when sex is being widely commercialized, when people's emotional needs are often manipulated and exploited, it is interesting to record that a substantial majority of Europeans and Americans cling to a belief in many of the values of family life that they learned in their homes. Yet even those who are critical of the Sexual Revolution admit that it has brought many good things: greater frankness, greater tolerance, greater willingness to experiment, and less guilt. And many also point out that the time has come to stop equating morality with sexual morality, to separate it from cheating, betrayal and cruelty.

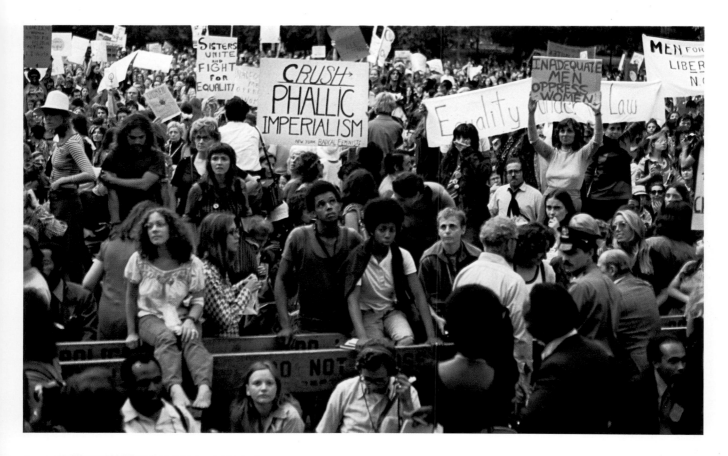

Above: the so-called "sexual revolution" did not actually bring sexual equality, and the women's liberation movement was born out of this pressing need.

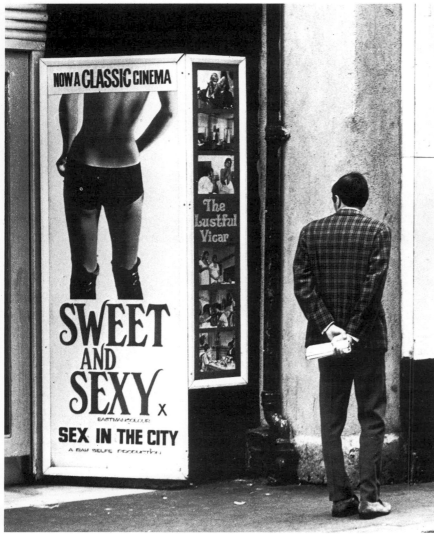

Left: the increase in pornographic films and publications has made many wonder whether the trend toward sexual permissiveness has gone too far.

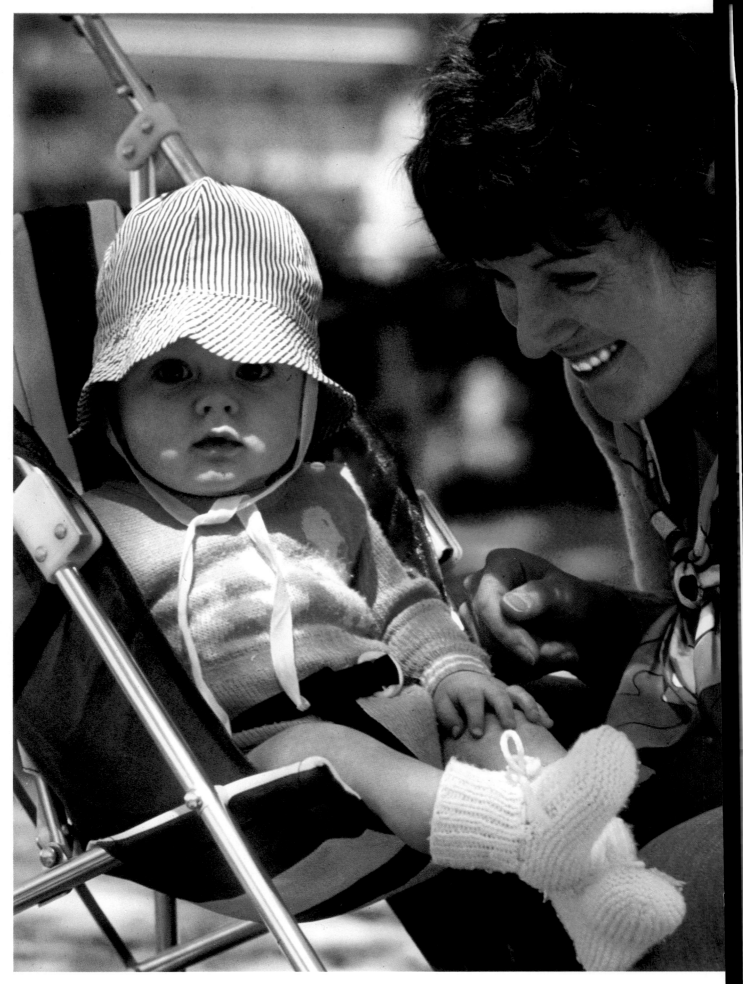

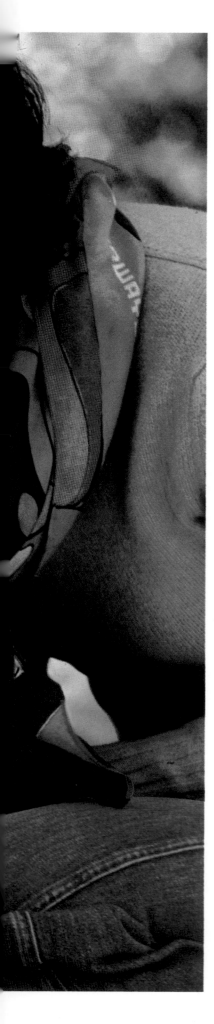

Chapter 7

Having a Baby

Parenthood is an ongoing experience that starts nine months before a child is born and from that moment never really comes to an end. Having a baby is not just a matter of insuring your child's physical health and wellbeing: it is also a state of mind. If an expectant and nursing mother has the confidence to know that she can make sensible decisions that are right for her child and – equally important – right for herself, then all the other members of the family are sure to benefit. The key to this confidence lies in the mother's realization that she is a changed person – emotionally as well as physically – and that this change can lead to a newfound maturity.

Opposite: from a very early age infants have an insatiable curiosity. Their eyes follow moving objects and people. Taking your child out regularly exposes him or her to new and interesting stimuli.

Receiving the News

Motherhood is supposed to be a woman's ideal state. She should be overjoyed when she finds out she is pregnant and spend the whole time in a continual state of happy anticipation – dreaming about the new baby. When it arrives she should slip into the maternal role with care and delight. This is all true to a certain extent, but it is only one side of the picture. Medical studies have discovered that there are normal *negative* feelings connected with pregnancy, especially when it is the first.

For Christine, the first pregnancy meant the end of a carefree existence. From a girl she was gradually turning into a mother, and this was accompanied by a decline in her exuberant femininity and natural grace. Both eclipses were very real. She was fully aware that after the baby arrived there would be distinct limitations on her social life and many other pleasures. There would be financial restrictions too, the same budget would have to be spread thinner. Also she knew that her husband's attention would soon be split in two, between her and the new arrival.

The changes to be expected because of the arrival of the first child do not usually look so drastic after you have had two or three children. But every pregnancy will probably arouse different feelings, often associated with problems within the family. Perhaps the pregnancy was not planned or expected, or the father is having work problems, or there is a serious illness in the family, or there is much tension between mother and father. These problems occur in the very best of households, but in the great majority of cases they are temporary. The child, when he or she arrives, usually proves to be less of a challenge than the parents had anticipated.

Christine was proud and pleased to be pregnant, but she found it hard to feel a personal love for a baby she had never seen. But its first move inside her stirred her profoundly and she realized that it was a real person. Her thoughts from that point became more positive and she began to think about and plan the baby's care.

A great majority of mothers who admit that their first reaction to pregnancy was predominantly one of dismay are reassured as they come to accept the pregnancy and become fond of the baby well before the birth. However, there is often a letdown for the inexperienced mother when the baby actually arrives. She may find that the intense love she was expecting to feel for the baby when it arrived just does not show itself when the time comes. But she will find that after caring for the baby at home for some time, her true feelings will emerge.

Sometimes parents get off on the wrong foot with

During the first few weeks of pregnancy there are no visible outward signs. Then the uterus elongates and the upper part becomes spherical. As the pregnancy progresses the uterus rises out of the pelvis and into the abdominal cavity, and becomes top-heavy. Toward the end it may descend again.

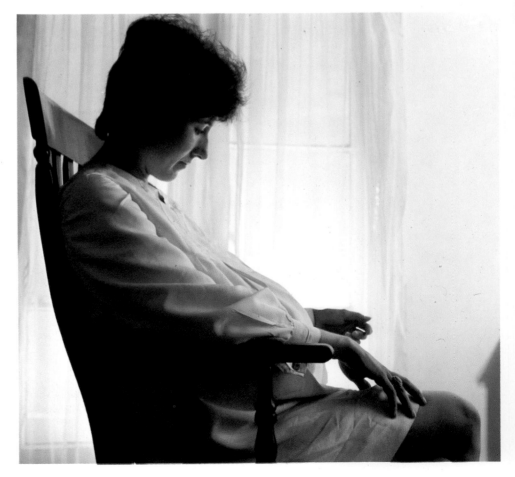

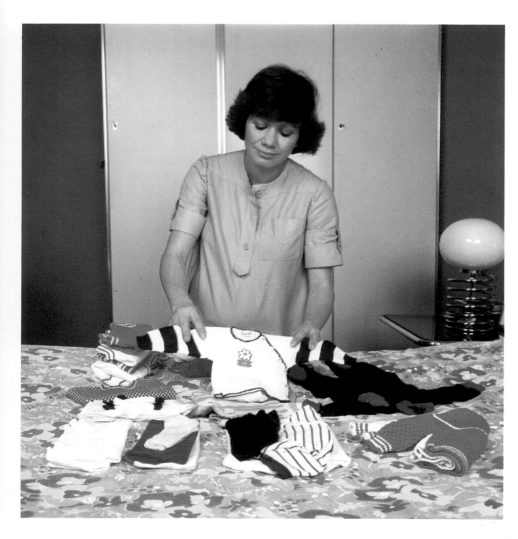

Left: by the end of your pregnancy you will probably be inundated with clothes for your baby by enthusiastic friends and relations.

a child. This may be because they did not feel ready for another pregnancy, or there may have been unexpected family tensions just at that time, or the baby is completely different from what they expected – a boy when they wanted a girl, an ordinary girl when they anticipated a beauty, or a frail infant compared to the other robust children. The baby may cry for several months with colic and seem to spurn the parents' efforts to comfort it. Whatever the problem, comfort can be derived from the wise words of Dr Spock: "So it's human and normal, and inevitable that we should feel quite differently about each of our children, that we should be impatient with certain characteristics in certain ones of them and proud of others. All these mixed attitudes are only different aspects of our deep feelings of obligation to bring up our children properly."

Most mothers find that they are more anxious than usual during the first few weeks at home with the baby. They worry about every sneeze and every spot or rash. But usually there is a sudden change of mood. At first, in hospital, a woman may feel very dependent on the nurses and grateful for the care they give the baby. Then comes a quick change of heart: she becomes confident she can take care of the baby herself and secretly resents the fact that the nurses do not let her take over. If she has a nurse or other help at home, she may go through these two

Below: in most Western countries at least the first confinement occurs in a hospital, and the newborn child is cared for initially by nurses.

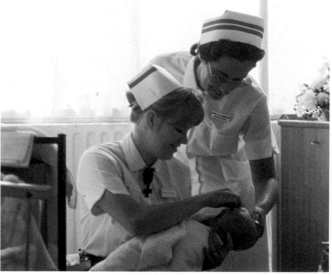

stages again. It certainly is normal for a mother to want to take care of her own baby by herself. The main reason she may not have this feeling at the start is because she is convinced she is inadequate. The stronger the sense of inferiority, the stronger will be the determination to assert her competence when she gains the courage. As the mother's confidence increases, she soon realizes that most of her initial fears were without foundation, and she is ready to face the future with a new-found confidence.

Health during Pregnancy

Do you know that mothers who smoke frequently bear smaller babies than nonsmokers? Smoking may be more harmful to the unborn babies of women who have already experienced childbirth difficulties or who live in poor communities. It is interesting that the smaller babies of women who smoke grow faster during the six months after the birth than do babies of nonsmokers. This is thought to be a response to the removal of the infant from an "inhibiting and toxic" influence in the womb. There is also evidence of a relationship between mothers who smoke excessively at home and the incidence of pneumonia and bronchitis in their babies from six to nine months of age. The lessons are obvious: pregnant women should either decrease or break the smoking habit completely.

Alcoholic drinks, taken in moderation, have not been associated with any known detrimental effects on the course of pregnancy or the health of the unborn child, but some new studies at the University of Washington indicate that pregnant women who are severe alcoholics may give birth to malformed babies. With drugs the position is much clearer: no drugs should be taken during pregnancy without the approval of your doctor. Certain drugs are known to cause malformation and drugs such as heroin and methadone taken during pregnancy may produce newborne drug addicts.

Sometimes aspects of general behavior and hygiene may puzzle expectant mothers. For example, how much rest, relaxation, and exercise do you need? Pregnant women should conserve their energy resources by getting adequate rest. They may not want to nap in the morning or afternoon, but at least they should sit down and put their feet up! Walking outdoors is wonderful exercise, available to most, but often neglected. Golfing, bowling, dancing, and swimming, when not done to the point of fatigue, are all good forms of exercise. Which sports may be beneficial during pregnancy depends largely on the health, exercise habits, and medical history of the individual. Curtailing the exercise of a previously active woman can be a negative factor in her physical emotional, and mental health. Prenatal exercises are extremely beneficial and these can be learnt at special clinics.

A woman may perspire profusely during pregnancy, and frequent baths and showers are needed. Bathing may become a problem in late pregnancy

Right: maternity clothes are designed to accommodate the increase in size of the abdomen, thighs and breasts. They should be loose and comfortable, but need not be unfashionable.

Below: there is no reason why you should not continue your favorite sport during the early stages of pregnancy. Your doctor will advise you when to stop.

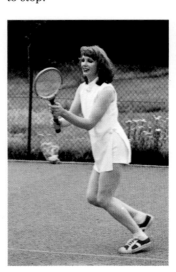

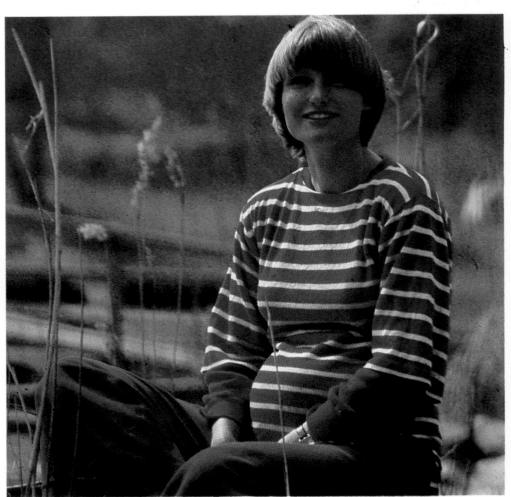

because of the woman's awkwardness, and she must take great care not to fall. The hair may need extra washing because of the increased activity of scalp oil glands. It is a good plan for the pregnant woman to have a dental checkup around the end of the third month so that plenty of time is available for any treatment to be carried out.

Maternity clothes should be lightweight, non-constrictive, adjustable, and absorbent and should also provide a morale booster. Never before has a mother-to-be had the opportunity to take advantage of such an attractive and versatile maternity wardrobe as is available today. Probably more important are adequate supportive underclothes. It is especially important that the pregnant woman have a good breast support to prevent fatigue and maintain a good figure. A maternity corset is rarely advised. However, a light maternity girdle may be worn.

Most women wonder whether they should douche or not. Normal vaginal secretions are usually intensified during pregnancy. Most doctors believe that douching should not be carried out during pregnancy – or at any other time for that matter.

Nowadays many pregnant women have a job. Whether they continue their employment and for how long depends on several factors, one of which is the type of work they do. As long as there is no danger to the expectant mother, she may safely continue working until four to six weeks before the birth.

Sometimes the question of travel arises. If a trip is arranged, it is best to travel during the middle three months of pregnancy, since the expectant mother is more comfortable, the danger of abortion can be discounted, and the threat of premature or unprepared for delivery is at a minimum. If trips are made by car, adequate rest stops should be made. Commercial airline travel in pressurized airplanes is now considered as safe as other methods of transportation until very late in pregnancy.

Doctors' advice regarding sexual intercourse during pregnancy is now much more sensible than it used to be. Many doctors say that most couples can have sexual intercourse until full term is reached, unless the bag of waters has ruptured, or there is discomfort. Others, believing that orgasm may initiate painful uterine contractions or premature labor, advise that intercourse should stop in the last few weeks before birth. If a woman has had a previous problem with abortion, premature birth, or bleeding during pregnancy, additional modifications in sexual life are advised. If in doubt – consult your doctor.

For your own sake, as well as the baby's, you should take care of your body during your pregnancy. Relaxation is important, and so is some form of exercise. It improves your circulation and prevents cramp in the legs. Walking and swimming are ideal because you are less likely to overexert and strain yourself.

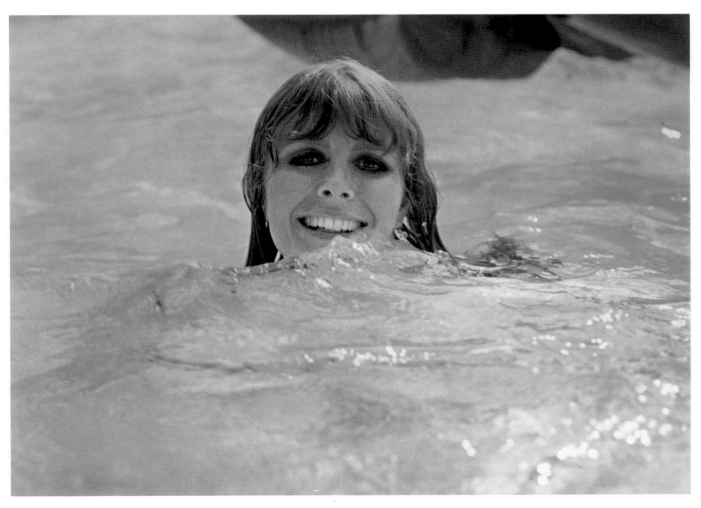

Prospective Parenthood

How do you know that you are pregnant? The most consistent symptoms of pregnancy are:

A missed menstrual period.

Enlargement of breasts and tenderness of nipples, occurring for a few weeks.

Increased frequency of urination.

Nausea and vomiting – "morning sickness." This may not begin until the second month of pregnancy. Actually, these symptoms are not limited to the morning, but may happen at any time. By the third or fourth month, abdominal enlargement becomes apparent and the first movements of the baby in the womb, known as "quickening," are felt, usually between the fourth and fifth months of pregnancy.

As soon as a woman thinks she is pregnant, she should consult a doctor so as to gain proper care, even during the early months. The doctor will arrange for regular checkups to be made and discuss the baby's arrival.

In nearly every community classes are available for prospective mothers – and fathers too. In these

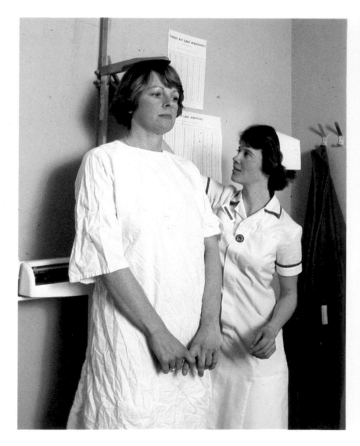

Above: measuring is part of regular antenatal checkups.

Below: pregnant woman undergoing an ultrasonic scan. In this painless technique ultra-high frequency sound waves are reflected from the fetus onto a screen for examination.

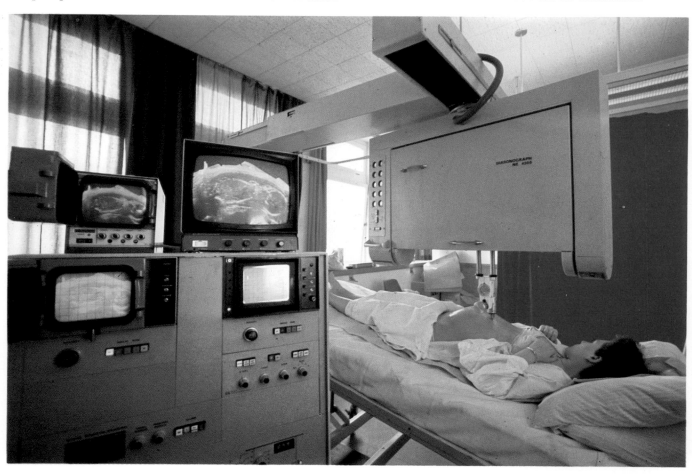

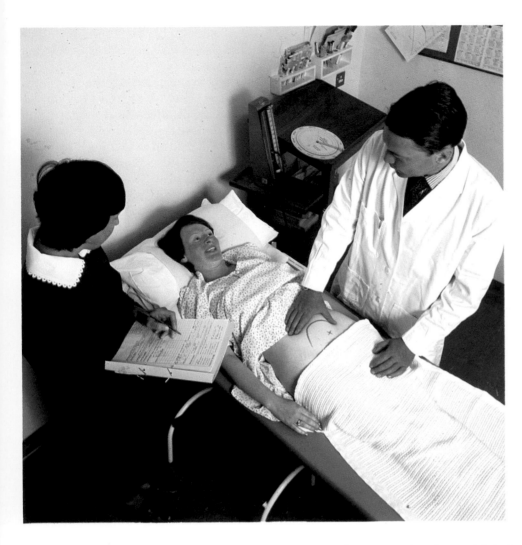

Various tests are performed in antenatal visits to insure that the fetus is developing normally. These include hormone tests, amniocentesis (analyzing the amniotic fluid), and possibly X-rays.

classes, prospective parents will be given a thorough understanding of what to expect during pregnancy and childbirth, and many helpful hints about child care. Such classes are extremely useful and will help to relieve some of the fears that young people have about the experience of becoming parents. The aims of *prenatal* (before birth) care are to help a woman through pregnancy with a minimum of mental and physical discomfort and a maximum of gratification; and to make sure that the delivery will be accomplished under the best circumstances and that the baby will be born healthy.

The psychological needs of the pregnant woman will also receive attention from the doctor and his staff. Indeed the physical and psychological needs of the entire family unit – mother, father, and other children – will be considered. This modern approach is often called "family centered maternity care."

Usually prenatal care is begun shortly after a woman misses her second menstrual period and the most lengthy visit the future mother makes to her doctor is often the first time she attends. She is given a complete physical examination. She is weighed and her temperature, pulse, blood pressure, and respiration are checked. The histories of any previous pregnancies and their outcome are noted. This will determine whether special treatment is necessary.

The visit usually includes an internal, or pelvic,

examination, which is completely painless and can indicate to the doctor that the patient is definitely pregnant. At the conclusion of the visit arrangements are made for the necessary laboratory tests to discover possible hazards, either to mother or baby, such as anemia, syphilis, and German measles.

During most of the pregnancy, expectant mothers should visit their doctors or prenatal clinics every four weeks routinely. In the last months, checkups will be made more often. At each visit the mother is weighed and her blood pressure recorded. A urine specimen is checked. Then the doctor estimates the height of the uterus to see if the pregnancy is progressing at the expected rate. After about four months he or she may listen for the baby's heartbeat, and after eight months the doctor feels the abdomen carefully to determine which way the baby is lying in the womb.

Toward the time of giving birth the expectant mother will be making weekly visits to her doctor. By this time a feeling of trust should have been built up between the two. This will make it easier for the doctor and staff to identify areas in which the expectant mother may need special help, information, or reassurance. They may possibly be able to advise in organizing her household so as to give her more rest and peace of mind. They also act as interested human listeners.

139

Prenatal Exercises

Many women in prenatal classes are taught exercises to prepare themselves for the demands of labor, delivery, and adjustments after the birth. The exercises will vary from group to group. Here three basic exercises are described that are of positive help to expectant mothers.

Pelvic rock

This is a great aid to comfort during pregnancy. It increases the flexibility of the lower back, strengthens the abdominal muscles, and shifts your center of gravity back toward your spine. It relieves backache, improves posture, and improves your appearance in late pregnancy. It should be practiced daily as an exercise, and in addition, once you have learnt it, you should always walk and stand with the pelvis tilted forward, thus providing your baby with a cradle of bone in which to lie. This prevents the baby from being supported by your abdominal wall so much,

which always results in increased stretching. The pelvic rock minimizes the tendency toward a sagging stomach and a tired back.

You can perform this exercise in three positions. First lie on your back, knees bent, feet flat on the floor. You may put a small pillow under your head.
1. Tighten lower abdominal muscles and muscles of the buttocks. This will cause your lower spine to lift, so press the small of your back into the floor. Do not lift buttocks off floor.
2. Relax abdominal and buttock muscles. As you do this, arch your back as high as you can.
3. Again tighten abdominal and buttock muscles, making sure that the small of your back presses tightly into the floor, your back becoming a straight line.
4. Do this five or six times daily. Do it before getting out of bed in the morning if your back feels stiff when you wake up.
Then do the same exercise on your hands and knees, hands directly under the shoulders, knees under the hips.
1. Contract abdominal and buttock muscles and at the same time hump your back up as far as possible. Bend head down.
2. Slowly relax abdominal and buttock muscles and let yourself sag through the middle as you lift your head.

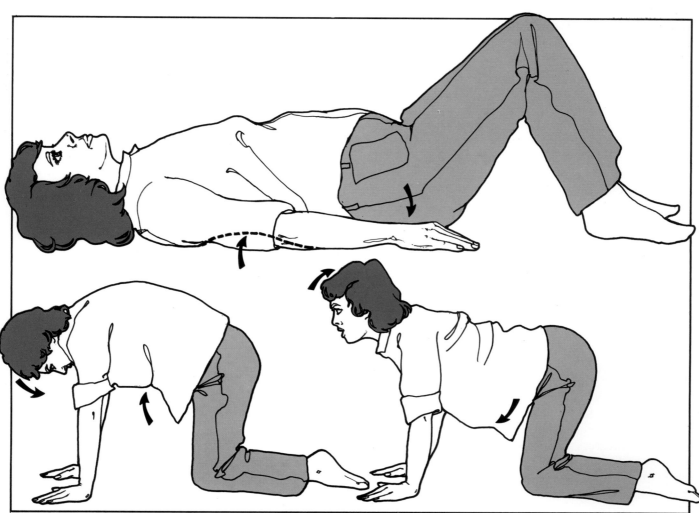

The third position is performed standing up.

1. Stand about 2 feet away from the back of a chair or other prop that is level with your hips.

2. Bend slightly forward from the hips, placing hands on chair back, elbows straight.

3. Rotate hips backward and sag with your abdominal muscles creating a real "sway back."

4. Unlock your knees, flexing them ever so slightly,

5. Slowly rotate hips forward, tucking the buttocks under as if someone were pushing your buttocks from behind. In this position your pelvic cradle will be parallel to the floor.

6. After doing this three times, stand erect with buttocks tucked in, knees slightly flexed, arms at side, chest high. This is the ideal position for standing and walking, especially during the later part of pregnancy.

Abdominal breathing

This type of breathing utilizes the diaphragm (the arch of muscle separating the chest from the abdomen) as opposed to the chest muscles. It is the type of breathing singers use to achieve perfect control and will be very helpful during the first half of your labor. When you breath with your diaphragm the abdominal muscles automatically relax, thus allowing the womb to rise during contractions without tension against the tight abdominal wall. You can practice lying down, standing, or sitting.

1. Place hands on abdomen.

2. As you inhale, allow the abdominal muscle to go down slowly.

3. Inhalation and exhalation should be of the same length. The chest should be completely still during abdominal breathing.

4. Work toward breathing as slowly as possible – a slow, rhythmic inhalation and exhalation.

5. As you become more adept at this type of breathing, it will require less effort for you to expand your abdomen during inhalation.

Panting

You will be asked to pant during the final stages of actual delivery of your baby, letting the womb do the work. This will prevent you from injuring yourself and is better for your baby too. Furthermore, if the baby's head is very low during the late first stage of labor, sometimes your urge to push prematurely becomes very great. In these circumstances only by panting can you stop yourself from pushing. Your doctor will of course instruct you as to when it is time to push, and when it is best to pant. As simple as panting may seem to be, you should actually practice it.

1. Place hands on breastbone.

2. Open mouth, allowing jaw to hang loosely.

3. Pant, making the breastbone move up and down. Pant slowly, deeply, and rhythmically.

4. Practice for 45 seconds at a time, at least once a day.

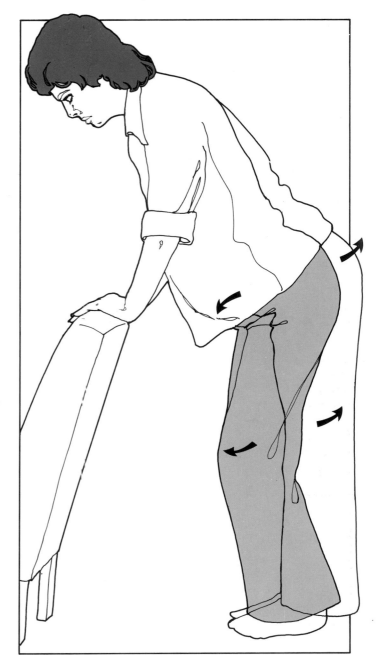

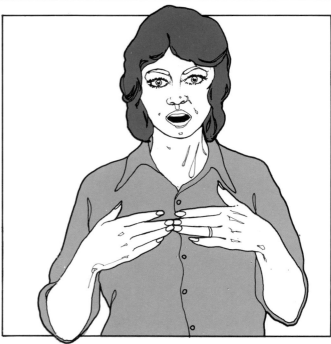

The Importance of Diet

Correct diet has long been considered important in prenatal care. However, it is now becoming apparent to doctors that nutrition is not simply important but crucial in determining the health of the mother, her offspring, and perhaps even that of future generations. A normal healthy woman needs greater amounts of calories and nutrients when she is expecting a baby – but only during the latter six months of pregnancy. She needs plenty of protein, increased amounts of folic acid, calcium, phosphorus, iodine, magnesium, and zinc, and vitamins B_6, B_{12} and C. But remember that excessive vitamins may be dangerous as well as wasteful, and routine multivitamin supplementation should not be necessary. As long as the mother is eating adequate amounts of milk, meat, vegetables, fruit, bread, and cereals, then she has nothing to worry about. Many expectant mothers do not realize the importance of weight control. "Eating for two" is overeating; it results in excess fat which apart from being difficult to shift, is dangerous to the pregnant mother and her baby.

Milk, and the calcium and protein it provides, are considered an important constituent of the expectant mother's diet. However, if she does not like milk then cheese provides an adequate substitute. Meat and offal are recommended, particularly for iron. Sources of high-grade protein, such as lean meat, eggs, fish, and poultry contribute other nutrients as well.

Whole grain or enriched breads and cereals provide sources of the B vitamins, thiamine and niacin, as well as some iodine, iron, and roughage. Fruit and properly cooked vegetables are important sources

A good diet, rich in vitamins, is especially important during pregnancy. Many women worry about the extra fat gained at this time. This is designed to provide the extra reserves needed during breast feeding and there should not be any attempt to lose it until after the birth.

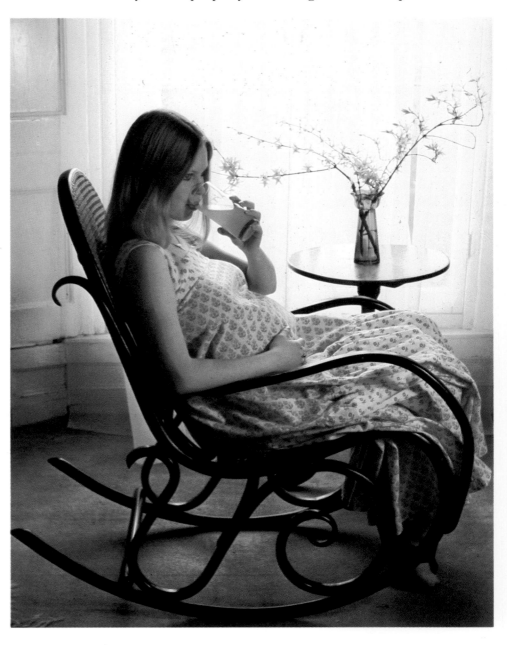

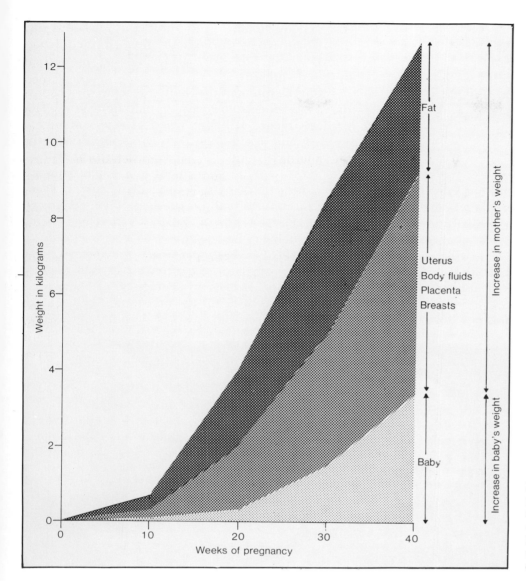

The graph y-axis: Weight in kilograms (12, 10, 8, 6, 4, 2, 0). The x-axis: Weeks of pregnancy (0, 10, 20, 30, 40). Labels on chart: Fat, Uterus, Body fluids, Placenta, Breasts, Baby, Increase in mother's weight, Increase in baby's weight.

Left: the average increase in weight of the baby and the mother during pregnancy. In addition to fat reserves, the weight of the mother is increased by the greater size of the womb and breasts, and by the fluids in which the baby develops.

Below: the increased demands of pregnancy mean that you will need extra supplies of the essential salts and vitamins. At least one pint of milk, drunk or used in cooking, will supply the extra calcium needed.

of vitamins, minerals, and roughage. The use of bulk-producing foods, including whole grain bread and cereals, and an increase in fluid intake, help to solve the problem of constipation during pregnancy. A high vitamin-C intake is advised for tissue building, so two servings a day of fruit – raw, cooked, or as juice – are recommended.

High-carbohydrate foods that contribute little or no nutrient value other than calories are called "empty calorie" foods. These include sugar, candy, most breakfast cereals, cakes, pies, soft drinks, doughnuts, and cookies. Taken in excess they add unwanted pounds but, apart from potential energy, contribute nothing that would assist the expectant or nursing mother.

Sometimes women during pregnancy experience cravings for unusual foods or food combinations. These desires are trivial and may be indulged if they do not threaten good diet. The important consideration is that anything that has an adverse affect on good nutritional intake, whether it be nausea or vomiting, food fads, lack of finances, alcoholism, or other social and personal problems, should be evaluated and treated so that the expectant mother is receiving a well-balanced, healthy diet.

The Pregnant Woman's Guide to Balanced Eating

Here is a guide to balanced eating in pregnancy. Each day, eat something from each food group set out below: the quantities are a rough guide only. Remember that the ideal is to eat all things in moderation, and not to have too much of any one food, which can be harmful; you may, for example, put on unnecessary weight.

Foods rich in protein	Meat/fish 4oz. 2 eggs, liver, beans, nuts, cheese 3 oz
Foods containing Vitamin D	Kippers, sardines, mackerel, eggs, margarine
Foods containing B-group vitamins	Wholemeal bread (4 slices), eggs, meat, liver, green vegetables
Foods containing iron	Bread, cereals, meat, apricots, figs, peaches, most nuts, beans, green vegetables
Useful sources of energy	Bread, cereals, biscuits, beans, cheese/dairy products, fish
Foods containing Vitamin C	Citrus fruits, potatoes, green vegetables
Foods containing Vitamin A	Kippers, sardines, mackerel, liver, eggs, butter
What you crave	Food cravings are mainly psychological. Indulge them a little. When you are pregnant, "a little of what you fancy does you good" is especially true

Labor and Delivery

Childbirth and the *puerperium*, the weeks immediately following it, should be a time of great happiness for a woman. If it is not, then something is seriously wrong. All too often a mother understands little of the emotional and physical changes taking place within her at this critical time. She should be psychologically prepared for what will happen, since a woman's emotions exert a great influence on the course her labor will take.

The climax to all the preparations during preg-

way. Today an increasing number of husbands stay with their wives throughout most of their labor. Some wives, however, prefer not to have their husbands present.

From the moment the mother reaches the hospital the professionals are very much in charge. Her prenatal record will be looked at, she will be examined, and asked about her symptoms during the previous few hours. The baby's heartbeat will be listened to with an instrument like an ear trumpet. The contractions, by now probably occurring every 15 to 20 minutes, will be checked. Then comes the routine: bath or shower, possibly a shave and enema to make delivery easier.

Once she has been prepared, for the next few hours the mother-to-be has to wait – this is the first stage of labor. It lasts an average of 14 hours for a woman giving birth for the first time. At the end of this stage the contractions will become more severe

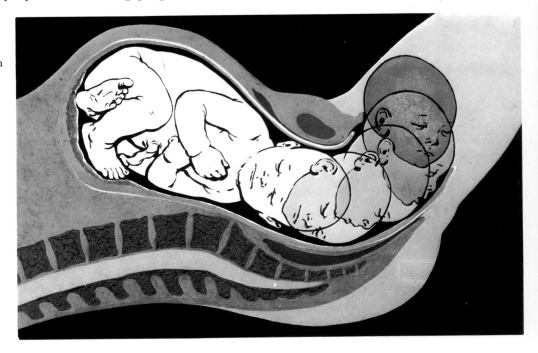

Descent of the fetus. The muscular walls of the womb contract (first stage) and the head of the baby presses down on the cervix, causing it to dilate, so that the head can pass down the vagina.

nancy comes approximately in the fortieth week. The woman starts to feel the first symptoms of labor, sometimes experienced as backache. This is known as "false labor" and may be mistaken for actual labor, except that the contractions diminish in intensity after a short time and usually disappear completely. True labor starts with regular contractions which produce some pain; they last 30 to 60 seconds, with intervals of 20 to 30 minutes. Another symptom of true labor is a slight loss of mixed blood and mucus from the vagina. Sometimes the first sign is the "breaking of the waters." This happens when the membranes which surround the baby and which bulge down into the neck of the womb have broken and the baby's protective fluid rushes or trickles out of the vagina.

If the mother is to give birth in hospital, now is the time for her to be taken there – and the whole process of birth, on average a 16-hour affair, is under

and frequent and some women may need an injection to reduce the pain or discomfort.

The second stage begins when the contractions occur every two or three minutes and the neck of the mother's womb has been fully opened by the pressure of the baby forcing it downward. This stage can last a few minutes, but also as long as two hours. The average for a woman having her first child is about one hour. Normally the baby's head is the first part to appear.

In the meantime, the womb's contractions get stronger still, forcing the baby's head through the vagina and out into the world. Sometimes the doctor may help with a procedure known as *episiotomy*: a small cut is made with surgical scissors at the lower end of the vulva to increase slightly the opening available for the baby's head to get through and to prevent minor accidental tears. Once the baby's head has appeared, the rest of the baby follows fairly

144

quickly – usually within two to three minutes. As the baby is taking its first breaths its umbilical cord is tied and cut. The baby is handed to the mother and the second stage of labor is over.

The third and final stage, which lasts about 20 minutes, involves the expelling of the "afterbirth" (the remains of the placenta and umbilical cord), by the uterus.

In most developed countries a mother who has her baby in hospital will remain there for about five to ten days, sometimes a little less. While she is there her whole physical condition – as well as that of her child – will be watched and any stitches will be examined regularly for signs of infection. During this time the uterus will be shrinking back ot its normal size, producing a fluid discharge called the *lochia*. Each day the color and nature of the lochia is checked for infection, so that this can be treated promptly.

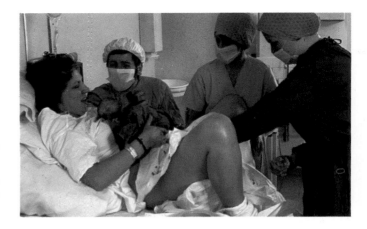

Above: a first pregnancy is always more difficult and labor is slower than in subsequent pregnancies. A hospital delivery, doctors and midwives at hand, is advisable.

Below: the delivery of the fetal head. The rest of the body slips out relatively easily, followed by the placenta.

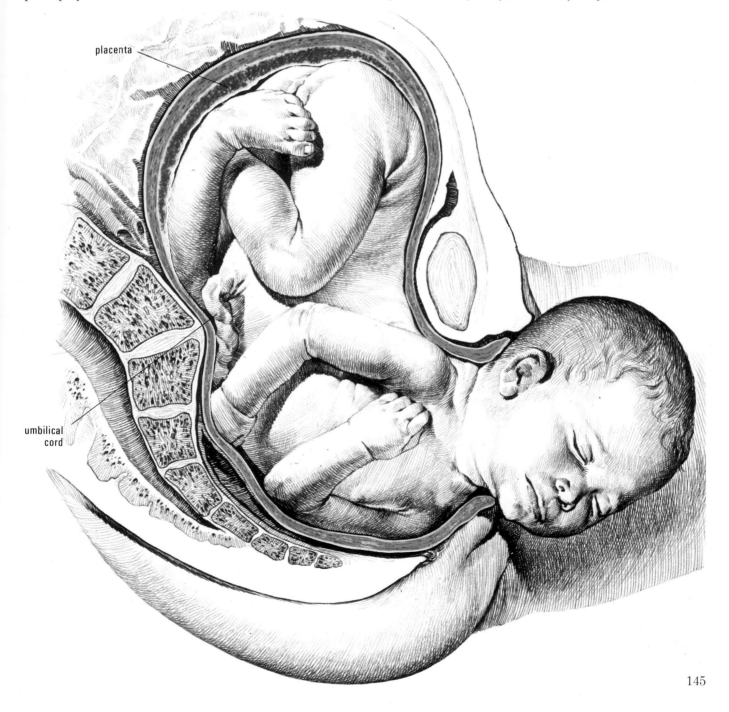

placenta

umbilical cord

Prenatal Problems

During most of the nine months a baby spends in its mother's womb, it is safer from injury and disease than it is likely to be for the rest of its life. But on rare occasions things can go wrong and the baby may develop so abnormally that he or she cannot live or is severely handicapped perhaps by a malformed heart, or blindness, or a limb deformity. One type of heart malformation causes blood from the arteries and veins to mix, giving children with this defect a bluish tinge. These are the "blue babies" and this condition used to be fatal; today it can be remedied by surgery. Sometimes a maldeveloped heart is only mildly affected; despite a "murmur" that indicates some structural abnormality, the child can, with care, lead a normal life.

Doctors call defects like these *congenital* – they are there from birth. No one knows what causes most of them. But maldevelopment sometimes happen because a woman takes a harmful drug while she is pregnant, or suffers an illness that affects her child too. Among the diseases that may endanger unborn children, the best known is *rubella* (German measles). Minute infective particles – rubella viruses – pass from the mother's bloodstream into the baby's where they can cause serious defects. To combat

It's all over! After the hours of labor and exertion, the baby has been delivered safe and well. The most anxious question that the mother and father will have: "Is the baby healthy and normal?" has been answered positively.

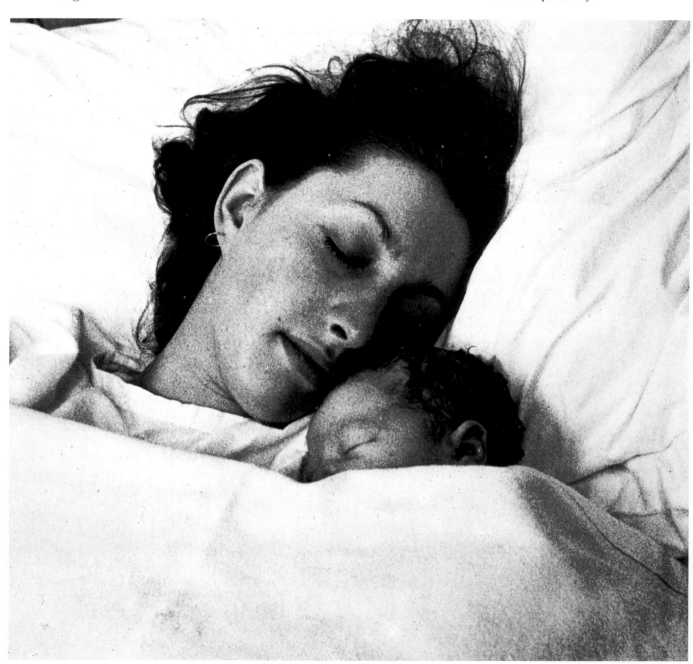

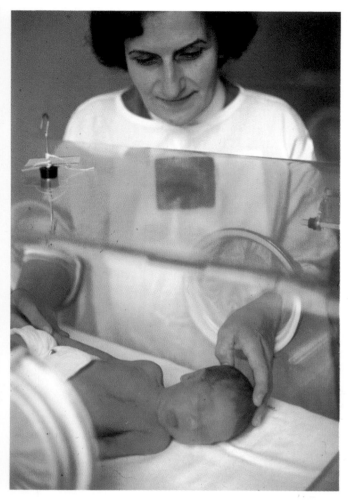

Above: premature babies experiences several problems, including digestive trouble, breathing difficulties and the inability to maintain their body temperature. They may have to be kept in an incubator.

this danger a vaccine has been developed which is given to girls between the ages of 12 and 14 and which insures that they will be resistant to German measles at the time they may be pregnant.

From 1961 to 1963 there occurred in Europe a surprising increase in the number of deformities among newly born babies. It was traced to the drug thalidomide, which doctors at first believed was a harmless sedative; it had been given to women who were nervous or upset, or who vomited excessively in the early days of pregnancy. But the drug turned out to have serious consequences for their unborn children. Doctors exercise the utmost caution when they administer medicines to pregnant women, and the thalidomide tragedies have helped to increase this vigilance and bring about the development of more sophisticated screening techniques. The United States escaped the thalidomide tragedy because the Food and Drug Administration objected to the drug being sold – with the sole argument that it was "not proven that the drug was beneficial."

Maldevelopments usually originate in the first eight or nine weeks of life in the womb. Just at that time the nervous system and such organs as heart, eyes, and ears show a fast rate of development. After

that the child is reasonably safe until the tremendous upheaval at birth. Never having breathed, and then suddenly being separated from the lifegiving umbilical cord, the child must adapt within a few minutes to a new environment. In normal childbirth, as a baby passes through the mother's pelvic region the skull bones are squeezed together. There is sometimes a danger that delicate brain tissues may be damaged, with the risk of disabilities such as spastic paralysis, so called because the child's limbs suffer from stiffness and involuntary spasms, or cerebral palsy, whose victims have difficulty speaking and coordinating their movements. Usually in these cases intelligence is not affected.

A few diseases – producing congenital defects –

Below: despite the traumas of labor and birth, and the possibilities of congenital defects and other problems, the majority of babies are born healthy. Even premature babies have a very high chance of survival.

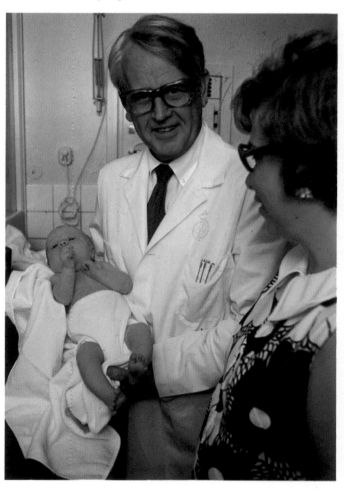

run in families according to the laws of heredity. Such a rare disease is *hemophilia*, passed on from mother to son, even though she has no symptoms of the disease. With this condition the blood does not clot and sufferers have difficulty in stopping bleeding, even from minor injuries.

It must be remembered that despite all the dangers of pregnancy and birth, the vast majority of mothers leave hospital with perfectly healthy and happy babies.

147

The Newborn Baby

Helpless and tiny, a newborn baby can inspire its parents with love and tenderness, often pride. The infant's needs are not many: the right food, warmth, feelings of protection, security, and love. It should sleep most of the time – especially after meals. If the baby seems to find this difficult then the right kind of help is needed. It may take the form of rocking the crib, wheeling the baby up and down, patting its bottom, or placing a ticking clock near the cot. Rhythmic sound, lullabies, or music can be comforting to a young baby.

A young baby's distress may be caused by wrong feeding. Breast milk provides a store of perfect food and does not usually upset or constipate the baby. But some substitute formulas may cause tummy upsets, abdominal cramp and pain, or vomiting, and if this happens the doctor may suggest an alternative food.

A newborn baby is often irritated by uncomfortable clothing. He or she should be dressed according to the weather – but never overdressed. Clothes should be light in weight and should not restrict movements. A newborn baby's hands and feet need to be kept warm, as the heat regulative mechanisms are not yet functioning properly.

Both parents should be able to react to the baby with confidence. This is important, as the baby is highly sensitive to atmosphere and will be influenced instinctively and automatically by the mood of the people around. The best way to gain the baby's confidence is through gentle but firm handling, and even when it is only a few days old, by speaking comforting words quietly and soothingly.

The baby must also learn the customs of the society in which it is born, which will include bathing. The water should be warm, never hot, and so should the room in which the baby is bathed. Test the temperature of the water with the elbow, not the hand. The baby's clothes should be removed only when all the preparations have been completed. When the baby is placed in the water, its head and back should be supported firmly with one hand and arm all the time. The head and face should be washed first, to insure that the water used for this is clean. Do not attempt any excessive cleaning of the

When you bathe your baby first insure that the water is warm by testing it with your elbow. Support the head and talk softly to keep the baby reassured.

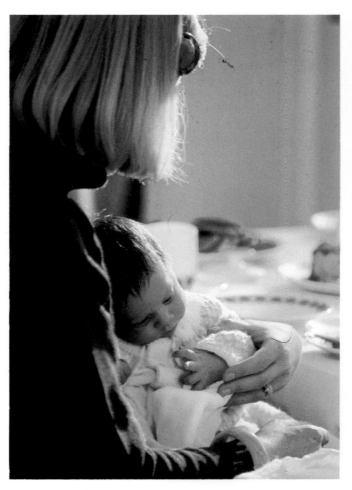

Many mothers feel that too much fussing will result in a spoilt child. But a baby is totally dependent and needs all the love, warmth and reassurance that you can give.

148

baby's nose, ears, or mouth, or the baby girl's vagina as these are delicate tissues and do not require special cleaning. The baby should be dried with a soft towel.

Overbathing is unnecessary. If the baby is fed and cared for correctly, he or she will not get too dirty and a bath three times a week is usually quite adequate. There is no need to wash the baby's

with no side ventilation could result in the baby breathing in a poisonous accumulation of carbon dioxide.

Before you buy a crib check that it is secure and that it has no gaps in which the baby can get stuck. There have been many fatal accidents due to babies slipping through the gap between the side and base of the frame, getting stuck by the head and being

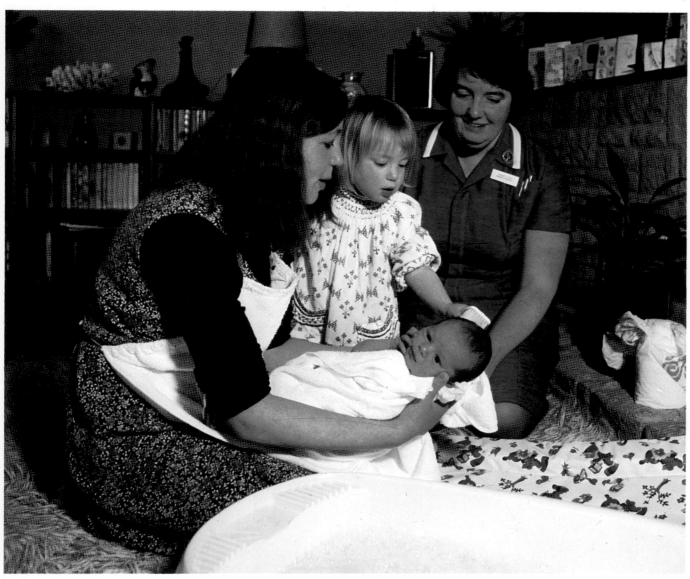

bottom every time the diaper is changed as constant wetting would only produce tenderness and a rash. Creams are only necessary if the skin has been damaged.

Parents often buy expensive baby equipment. However, couples should not feel that they are depriving their child by improvizing and using the kitchen sink as a baby bath and a shallow drawer as a crib. Nevertheless a few safeguards have to be considered. A baby should sleep on a firm mattress. This will be good for its back, but a more important reason is that it will avoid any risk of suffocation. For this same reason any form of pillow should be avoided. The crib mattress should be encased in cotton and not in plastic, and a crib which is too deep

The correct way to handle, feed and bathe a baby does not come naturally, but neither is it very difficult. A nurse or experienced relative will show you what you have to do.

strangled. Ornamental knobs which can catch clothing and painted interiors which can flake should be avoided. Safety should be placed above every other consideration where the baby's equipment is concerned.

With love and understanding and some creative effort, caring for your new baby can be a most joyful experience. As well as supplying its simple, basic needs – five or six feeds a day and a bath three times a week – it can be guided and taught to behave in a way which will help to make it happy, secure, and confident and a source of pride and joy to its parents.

149

The Baby's Weight

A baby that begins to wake earlier and earlier before each feeding and complains with a cry that the mother recognizes as one of hunger, is usually saying that it needs more food. Such a child will finish all its bottles to the last drop and look around for more, maybe even trying to eat its own hands. When the baby is weighed the mother will notice that it is gaining less than before. If the child is getting really hungry, it will show its discontent by crying at the end of some of the feedings.

If a baby on a formula shows such signs of dissatisfaction, it is necessary to get in touch with the doctor to talk about an increase or change of formula. According to some child experts it is reasonable to increase the formula just as soon as a baby is regularly finishing all its bottles, even before signs of dissatisfaction appear. There is one caution: if the child is given an increase on the slightest provocation, he or she probably will not be ready to take it all. There is also a danger of overfeeding the baby, so be careful not to urge it.

Some breast-fed babies start to wake up early. In this case he or she can be nursed early, even if this might mean an extra feeding a day. The more frequent feedings will be more satisfying, and the more frequent emptying of the breasts will stimulate them to produce a larger supply if that is possible. Incidentally a nursing mother should always give both breasts when feeding the baby.

There is no easy answer to the question of how much weight a baby should gain, and at what rate. It may seem too simple, but the best answer is that the baby should gain at the rate that it seems to want to increase. If a baby is offered more food than it needs, it will usually refuse it. On the other hand a hungry baby will wake early before a feeding, and demonstrate its hunger by screaming and eating its fists.

Always remember that when a doctor talks about an "average" baby, it refers to the weight taken of fast, slow and medium gainers, added together and averaged out. One baby is meant to be a slow gainer, another fast. There is nothing to worry about if your baby is a slow gainer provided it is happy and healthy, and receiving its regular checkups.

The "average" baby doubles its birth weight at about five months. But in practice babies that are small at birth probably grow faster, as if trying to catch up. The average baby gains about 2 pounds a month during the first three months. It is obvious that some healthy ones gain less, and others more.

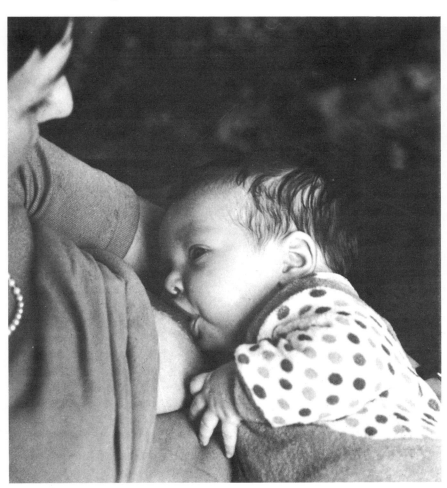

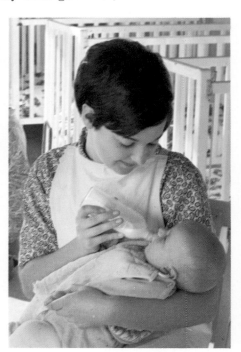

Above: for bottle feeding use a specially prepared formula. When feeding, keep the teat filled with milk so that the baby does not swallow air.

Left: the mother's milk production itself is stimulated by suckling, so you should start offering your baby the breast as soon as possible.

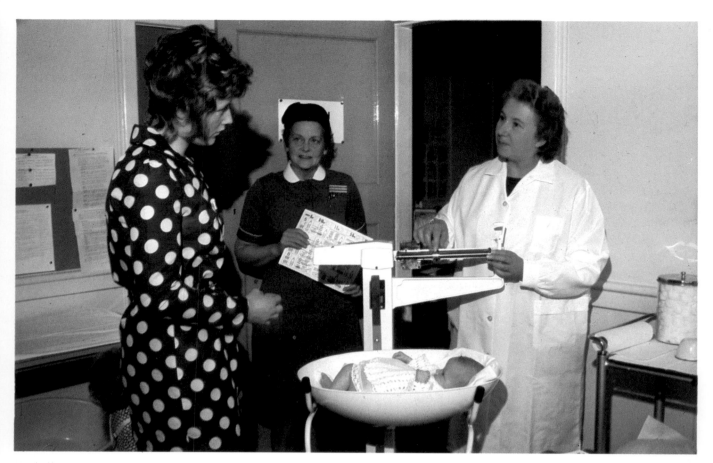

Above: at the postnatal clinic your baby will be weighed to check that it is gaining sufficiently without becoming fat. You will also be advised when to change its diet.

Below: regular medical checkups insure that everything is progressing smoothly with both the baby and mother. This is the time to discuss any anxieties you may have.

Then the baby's growth slows down. By six months the average gain is down to 1 pound a month, and during the second year to about half a pound a month.

As the baby grows older, you can see that the gain in weight is slower, and less regular. Teething, for instance, may somewhat depress the baby's appetite for a few days, and he or she may hardly gain at all. When the baby feels more comfortable, the appetite revives and the body weight catches up with a rush.

Do not get too wrapped up in the fluctuations in your baby's weight. A number of factors affect the weight, including how recently it has urinated, how recently it has moved its bowels, and how recently it has eaten. If you find one morning that your baby has gained only 5 ounces in the past week, whereas in previous weeks it has always gained 7 or 8 ounces, do not jump to the conclusion that the baby is starving or that something else is wrong. If it seems happy and satisfied, wait another week to see what happens. The baby may make an extra large gain to make up for the small one. Always remember, though, that the older the baby, the slower it's gain.

Most mothers do not have scales, and most babies get weighed only when they go for their checkup. When a baby is happy and doing well, weighing more frequently than once a month serves no purpose but to satisfy curiosity. If you have scales, do not weigh more frequently than once every two weeks. On the

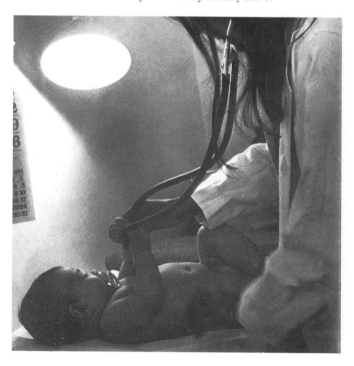

other hand, if the baby is crying a lot, or having indigestion, or vomiting a great deal, frequent weighing may help you and your doctor to decide what the matter is. For instance, if he or she is crying excessively but gaining rapidly, the cause of distress is not hunger but probably colic — intermittent internal pain.

The Father's Role

Men react to their wives' pregnancies with a variety of emotions: protectiveness, increased pride in the marriage, pride about their virility, anticipatory enjoyment of the child. But quite often unexpected feelings can arise.

Stephen and Ann were happy, but when Ann discovered she was pregnant, Stephen felt rejected (small boys often have similar feelings when they find that their mother is pregnant). This feeling he expressed by grumpiness toward Ann, seeking the company of friends outside the home, and flirting with other women. This behavior came just at the time when his wife needed Stephen's support and help the most: this stage of life was as new to her as it was to him.

He felt particularly left out when Ann went into hospital to have the baby. He had done all he could possibly think of to get his wife safely to the hospital. Then suddenly he was quite alone, with nothing to do outside of working hours. He would hang around the hospital, sit in a waiting room with some old magazines, and worry about how the labor was going.

He discovered that his home has become utterly empty and unbelievably lonely. So he tried to hide in the first bar he came across to get some "support." He got some attention from work colleagues, but even some of his best friends were making jokes at his expense. When he went to see his wife and the new baby, he had to stop the car and vomit from the inner tension. The hospital made him feel even more dejected and inadequate. When he finally came to take the baby and Ann home, the concern of everybody (grandparents and other people at hand to help) was all for the baby and Ann. He was literally treated as a chauffeur. At this time he felt less important than usual and despite himself he blamed the newborn baby for his unhappiness.

Stephen's story is not unusual. At a time like this most fathers are often surprised to discover that they have mixed feelings toward their wives and babies. But it might have helped Stephen a lot if he had considered his wife's feelings: she had really been through the equivalent of an operation. Her whole hormonal system was suddenly switched to an entirely new situation. She was feeling anxious – not unusual with a first baby – and had to find new reserves of strength and spirit. And that is why most women need as much support from their husbands as possible at this time. To be able to give so much to the baby, they must receive more than the usual assistance from their husbands. The help needed may be quite practical – with the care of the baby, with the housework.

While the mother rests after the pregnancy, the father can begin to take an active role in caring for the child. This will enable him to establish a direct relationship with his son or daughter.

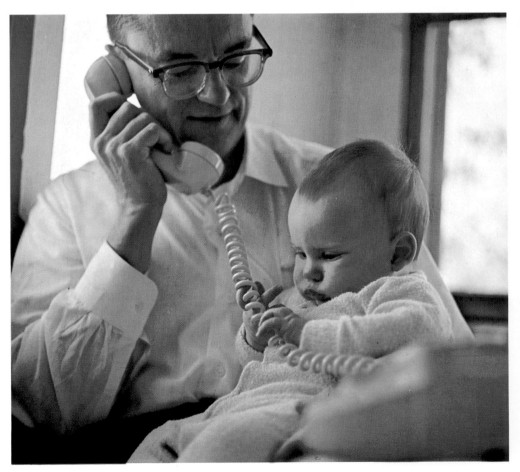

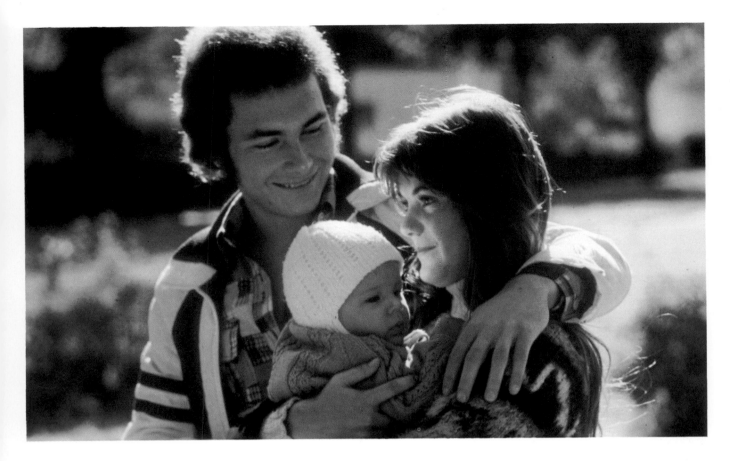

But a husband's moral support is also of great importance. The new mother needs considerable understanding, appreciation and affection. And it is often the case that at this time she is so pre-occupied with real and imaginary worries, that she has no time to be charming, appreciative, and lovable. Quite often she might be depressed, irritable, and complaining, but every husband should realize that this is a crucial time for his wife and he should give her all the support and love she needs.

Many men have been brought up to believe that the care of babies and children is the mother's job. But it is obvious that a man can also share many of the responsibilities of bringing up the baby and yet lose none of his manliness. This is why lectures and classes on baby care should also be attended by fathers. If the wife is expected to take sole charge of the children, then the father will have difficulties later on in becoming a real part of the family unit.

Any help that a father can give in feeding the baby, bathing it and changing the diapers, will be greatly welcomed by the wife. This is especially so in the early weeks when she will still tire very easily. Also, if the mother suddenly became ill the father would be able to cope. Fathers who show repugnance at having to change a baby's soiled diaper should realize that it is no less so for a mother and a little practice will soon cure this feeling. The father could also take the baby on some of the early visits to the doctor's office. This would be an opportunity for him to clear up any problems that are bothering him and would enable him to participate actively in his child's welfare.

Above: the newcomer should be treated as part of a family unit and not usurp the mother's feelings for the father.

Below: when a baby is on frequent bottle feeds, the father can take turns with the mother.

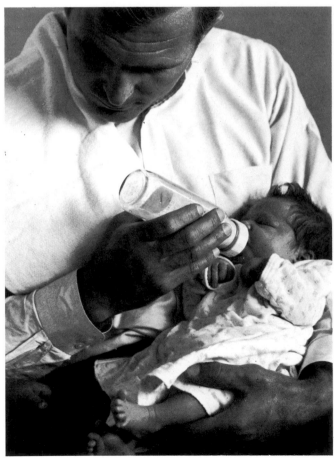

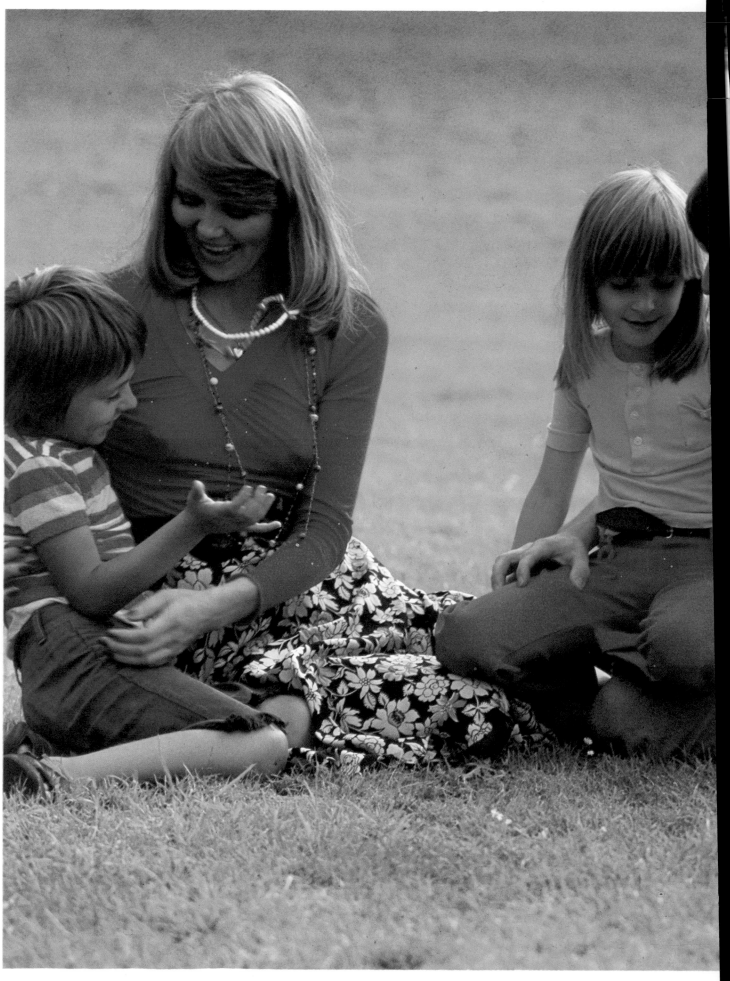

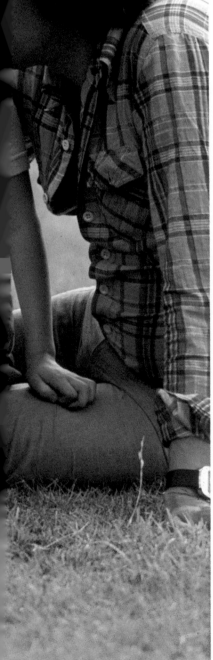

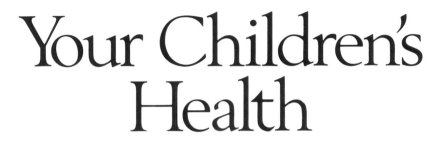

Chapter 8

Your Children's Health

It is true to say that healthy children almost always grow up into healthy adults. Laying the foundations for physical health in the early years is not too difficult a task, despite the many illnesses that children are prone to at these early stages in their development. Most childhood diseases can be avoided by preventive measures, such as vaccination; the others are rarely serious and with adequate nursing are soon over. Emotional stability – just as important as physical health – is also established at this time, and although parents can never be absolutely sure they are bringing up their children in the right way, a plentiful supply of love and understanding will insure that they do not make too many mistakes.

Opposite: not every family is lucky enough to live in or near the countryside. But family outings provide the opportunity for the the adults, as well as the children, to get plenty of fresh air and exercise.

Understanding your Baby

It is often said that babies demand attention to such an extent that they are determined to dominate their parents by any means possible. This is just not true. Babies are born to be reasonable, friendly human beings.

Do not be afraid to love and enjoy your baby: it is its basic necessity. Every baby needs to be smiled at, needs to be talked to, played with, fondled, gently and lovingly – just as much as it needs proper feeding. The parent's love will make the baby into a person with a positive atttitude who will be able to enjoy life to the utmost. The baby who is not loved

house and treating you as a slave. In the early weeks the baby will cry because of hunger, indigestion, fatigue, or tension; sometimes, in order to be satisfied, the baby just needs to be held, rocked, or walked. If you are responding to your child's desires, it does not mean you are spoiling him or her. Spoiling does not happen when a baby is being treated in a sensible way, but comes on gradually when a mother is too afraid to use her common sense in dealing with everyday matters of baby or child care and is inconsistent in her behavior.

It is important to remember that although parents always want their children to conform and be easy to live with, their bowels will move according to their

A child is dependent emotionally, as well as physically, on its parents, and must not be deprived of these basic needs. Even before your child can speak, you should communicate with him or her by singing, cooing, kissing and cuddling, and playing hand games. But do not forget to also use adult speech. Children are highly imitative and pick up their vocabulary in this way.

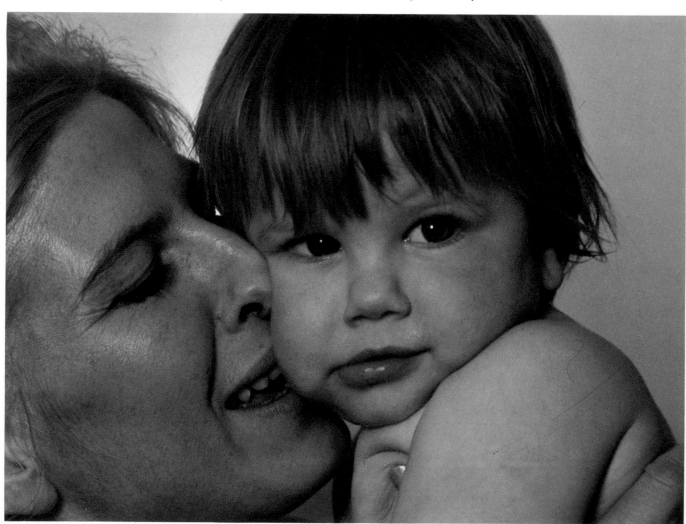

by its parents will grow up unresponsive and will find it difficult to relate properly to other people.

It is wrong not to give your baby what it wants, as long as these needs seem sensible to you and as long as this newcomer is not becoming a tyrant in the

own pattern, which may or may not be regular. Also children will develop their own pattern of sleep according to their own needs. In these and other habits the child will sooner or later fit into the family's way of life, with only a minimum of guidance – but it will take time and sometimes a lot of patience from the parents.

It is also wise to remember that every baby's pattern of development is different. One must never forget from what a mixture of different qualities and patterns of growth each individual person is made of. One child may be very advanced in general bodily strength and coordination, and yet is slow learning how to be manually skillful. A child who turns out later to be clever at school work may have learned to talk relatively late. One baby is born robust, while another is more delicate. Sometimes an individual seems destined to be fat. Other individuals remain slim, no matter what they eat.

Below: one of the problems of a new baby is its effect on the other children in the family, particularly if there is only one. The older child may resent the baby for taking up the parents' attention and become aggressive toward it. It is important that the baby becomes part of the total family unit, and the older child is given some part, however minor, in its upbringing.

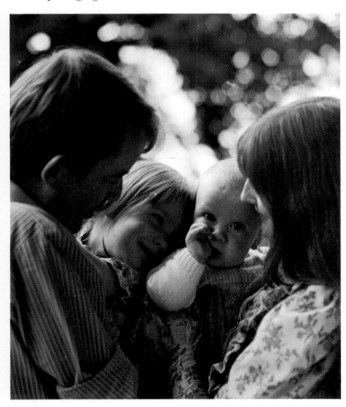

Parents should try and love their children for what they are, for what they look like, for what they do, not for what they would like their child to be. The child who is appreciated for what he or she is, despite being clumsy or slow, will grow up self-confident and happy. But the child who never had parental acceptance, and who is made to feel a failure will start life with a handicap and grow up lacking confidence.

Mothers naturally worry about a "frail" baby. But babies are really rather more tough than you think. If its head drops back by mistake, the baby will not be hurt. The soft spots on the baby's skull are covered by a tough membrane. The system controlling a baby's body temperature works efficiently by the time the body weight is about 8 pounds. The baby has some resistance to germs and gradually builds up immunity to others. If there is a cold spreading among a family, the baby's will probably be the mildest case. The baby knows how much sleep it needs and takes it. For a person who cannot say a word and knows nothing about the world, it can take care of itself pretty well.

A consistent mother-child relationship allows the child to learn gradually about the world outside his or her own demands and needs. At first the mother represents the whole world to the child. Then she widens the child's horizon, showing him or her, in stages, places partly of her own making – such as the rooms of their home – and people of her own choosing, so that the child can learn to accept these first. Then she shows the child the stranger realities of the big wide world that lie beyond the limitations, the strength and intimacy of their close relationship.

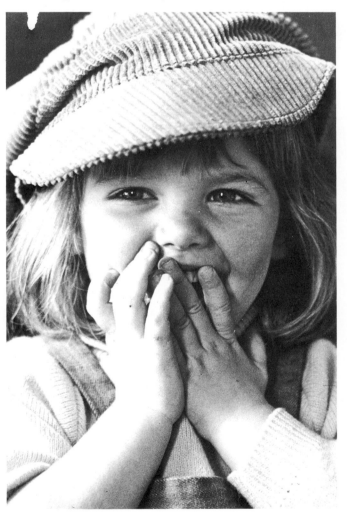

Above: parents want their child to grow up happy and selfconfident. But children, like adults, have different moods and personalities. Parents who try to change their child's character or mold it along preconceived ideas do more harm than good. The child will feel resentful, unwanted or a failure, and its selfconfidence may be completely destroyed. Serious behavioral problems may also develop.

The Young Child

A child's first two years are the most exciting and the most fascinating period in a mother's life. Many mothers would say that they never before or later enjoyed life more. A woman can attain enormous self-fulfillment and satisfaction from caring for her young child, and if she can share this excitement and fascination with her husband, then the success of the marriage is as certain as anything can be in this imperfect world of ours.

For the child this is the most crucial part of life as well. The way the child is handled, loved, and introduced to the rules and regulations which form the basis of family life, all determine whether he or she will grow up a healthy, happy, and contented child. This is one occasion when the seemingly tremendous responsibility thrust upon mother and father becomes a pleasure and a joy.

The secret of success in handling a baby or young child is not to be afraid. Just as nothing is more likely to produce a painful labor than fear, so nothing is more likely to produce a fretful baby than a frightened mother. A baby will soon appreciate whether the mother loves it and wants it. It will also notice at once if mother is afraid for it, and whether she is unsure of herself. Confident mothers are a boon and blessing to their baby in its first year of life.

This influence will continue to have a beneficial effect when the baby becomes a toddler.

It should not be forgotten that both mother and father must be firm with their child. A toddler can be spoiled very quickly. The sooner regular habits are gently instilled the better. A good lusty crying period or temper tantrum does not harm, provided the child is well and not suffering any discomfort. But if there is no apparent reason for the crying, a little exercise of the child's lungs will do no harm, and it will avoid the assumption at a dangerously early age that mother and father will come running the moment the child starts making a noise.

Nothing will keep the healthy child out of mischief. There is usually something wrong with the child who is never annoying or who never gets into trouble. But it is the mother's and father's responsibility to keep their children out of serious danger. It is little short of tragic the number of very young children who are hospitalized as a result of the many different types of accident, including falls, burns, or swallowing medicines. Some of these accidents are inevitable, however vigilant the parents are; but many are avoidable and are due simply to carelessness. A toddler should never be left alone in a room full of dangerous temptations, such as shiny glass ornaments in the living room, or interesting pots and pans bubbling away on the stove. All small swallowable objects and poisonous liquids should be kept well out of reach.

Parents should not, however, veer to the other extreme and overprotect their child. Once a toddler gets to the crawling stage he or she must be allowed to take reasonable risks. The sooner the child starts learning that there are certain things you do not do

Children are very sensitive to their parent's moods and apprehensions, but they will not at this point understand the reasons. By handling your child with confidence you will dispel any fears that it may have.

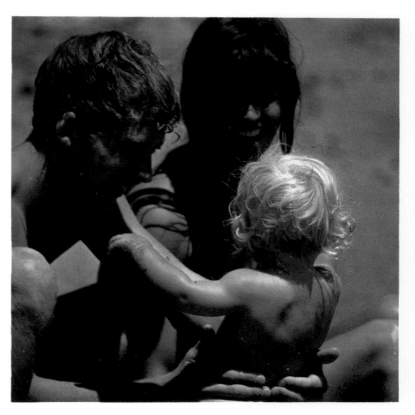

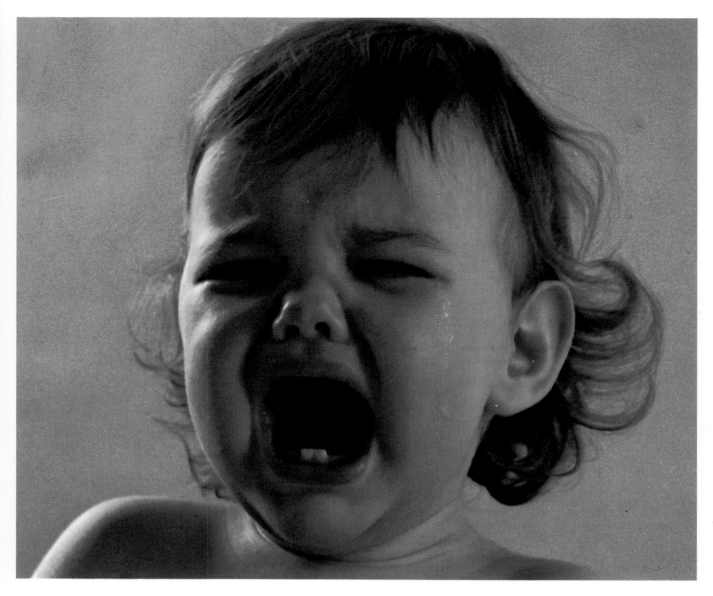

Above: your child may be crying out of fear, distress or frustration. You should always investigate the cause.

Right: a child's indefatigable curiosity can lead it into dangerous situations. Electrical sockets tempt a child to stick its fingers in, and should always be covered.

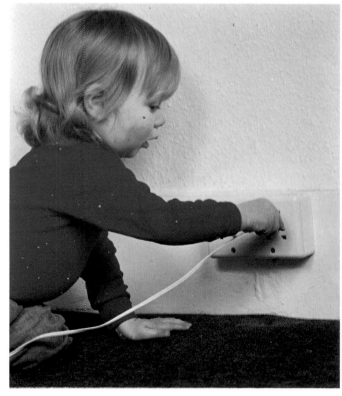

– or, at least, if you do them the consequences may be unpleasant, or even painful – the better. Children learn this just as they must learn that there is a time for eating and a time for sleeping, and, even more important, that when they are awake they must learn to amuse themselves. This is probably the most important lesson to be learned, whether as a young baby lying crooning contentedly in the cot, or as a toddler amusing itself in the bedroom. Young children who are never left on their own will be troublesome both to themselves and to their parents in the years to come.

A mother will be much less tired at the end of a long and strenuous day if she can accept motherhood as a privilege. The more she can enter into the life of her child in an understanding way, the more she will achieve that satisfaction that makes life really worth living.

The Common Illnesses

In their early years children usually suffer from a variety of minor illnesses. Children are naturally healthy, their strong young bodies resistant to most infections. But health problems may occur. For example the diseases which at one time almost every child had – and mothers had to contend with – were chickenpox, measles, whooping cough and mumps. Despite the widespread use of vaccination to prevent some of these diseases, they still occur occasionally.

Colds are produced by viruses, unfortunately by a great many different ones, and some colds can be aggravated by secondary bacterial infections of the upper respiratory tract. Even tiny babies can catch a cold. Also one of humanity's greatest plagues, influenza, can make a child severely ill, even if this illness is usually milder in children than in adults. Muscle pain, sore throat, cough, and some fever are the main symptoms of influenza in children. Some viruses produce only chills and fever and others a "running nose" in toddlers and young children, but very little fever. Unfortunately these kinds of colds can only be treated according to their symptoms, which usually means keeping the child in the house and well cared for until the cold is over.

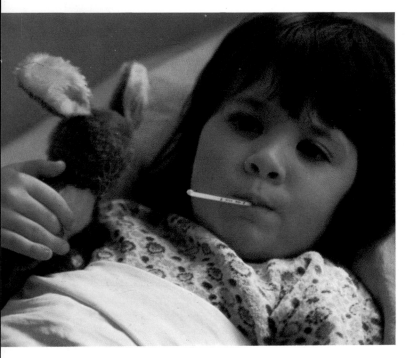

The normal body temperature is about 98.6°F, varying throughout the day, and a sharp rise often indicates an illness. If the fever is mild (100°F), give your child cool drinks and sponge him or her down. If the fever is high (101°F or more) call the doctor immediately.

Young children are prone to skin disorders. Diaper rash is a familiar part of baby care. Ringworm (a fungus infection) and impetigo (hard crusts and blisters, especially on the face, which are yellow and later form scabs) can spread rapidly, particularly when little fingers pick at them. They should be treated early by your doctor in order to avoid discomfort. Eczema, which is characterized by rough, red and often scaly patches, is caused by an allergy and aggravated by rough clothing and cold weather. Eczema in babies is often due to an allergy to cow's milk; breast fed babies rarely suffer from it. Ointments and other preparations prescribed by the doctor usually get rid of the majority of these skin troubles very quickly.

Ear infections occur quite frequently among young children, and they can be a painful experience. Most of the inflammations are not serious but should be watched carefully under the advice of a doctor because of the damaging complications that can develop.

A baby's teeth need periodic attention from the dentist just as permanent teeth do. A three-year-old should have his or her teeth examined twice a year. Then decay can be checked to insure that the baby's teeth stay healthy and the dentist can also follow the development of the permanent teeth and the condition of the gums. This will enable the dentist to treat special problems which might otherwise have a damaging effect on the growth of the teeth and jaw.

When children first start kindergarten or school they seem to get infection after infection. Gradually they become less susceptible to them and while at school most children have good health. Serious disease is rare and death from disease virtually unheard of. The main cause of death among schoolchildren are accidents – road accidents being the most common. Cancer, including leukemia, is the next most common – but is rare. Deaths from congenital defects such as severe heart defects do occur occasionally. A few children die each year from pneumonia and other respiratory troubles. But although common most respiratory troubles are extremely mild.

Young children often complain about tummy aches or headaches. The likely cause is a hidden worry or stress. It may be a child's way of saying "Why does my mummy spend all her time with the new baby?"

Perhaps the most important point to remember about most of these complaints is that while they may be of no importance to the child's health in later years, they may be desperately worrying at the time – both to the child and parents. Doctors should never say, "It does not matter," for in most cases it clearly does matter to the child. In an effort to show understanding of the problem, the doctor may ask to talk to the child alone – to show the child that he or she is looked upon as an important person whose worries matter.

Disease	Incubation period*	Prevention	Symptoms	Length of contagion	What you can do
Chickenpox	12-20 days, usually	None. Immune after one attack	Mild fever followed in a day or two by rash. Successive crops of pimples appear and fill with clear fluid. Scabs form later	7 days after rash appears, or until all scabs are dry	Rest. Ease itching with a paste of baking soda and water, alcohol, or calamine. Dress child in loose clothes, keep him or her cool and trim fingernails to avoid scratching. Usually better in 2 weeks
Diphtheria	2-5 days	Immunization	Sore throat, swollen neck glands, pains in limbs, foul breath. Possibly hoarseness and sharp cough. Child obviously ill	Until laboratory tests clear	Rest. *Call doctor urgently.* Follow his or her advice
German measles	10-21 days, usually 18 days	Immunization	Mild fever, mild cold symptoms, rash of tiny, flat, pink spots. Glands at back of neck and behind ears may be tender and swollen	Until rash has faded. About 4-7 days	Moderate rest and general good care. Usually better in 4 days
Measles	7-21 days, usually 10 days	Immunization. Gamma globulin given shortly after exposure may lessen or prevent the disease in an unvaccinated child	Mounting fever, runny nose, sore, red eyes, barking cough, followed in 3 to 5 days by blotchy rash starting behind ears and spreading downward	Until rash disappears. About 10 days	In bed for about a week on fever regime. Darkened room. Eye washes. No reading while eyes sore. Measles may be mild or severe; follow doctor's advice. Child usually feels better in 4-5 days
Mumps	12-28 days, usually 17 days	Immunization	Sometimes mild fever and headache or sore throat one day before main symptoms: swelling and ache of glands in front of ear, one side only at first. Painful to open mouth. Other parts of the body may be affected too	Until all swelling disappears	Moderate rest. Hot water bottle to relieve pain. Plenty of fluids. Mouth washes usually mild, especially in a young child
Roseola	4-5 days	None. Usually affects children under 3 years, commonest under 12 months	Sudden high fever which drops before rash, or large pink blotches appear over whole body	Until temperature returns to normal and rash fades	Rest and general good care
Strep throat (septic sore throat) and **scarlet fever**	1-7 days, usually 2-5 days	Doctor may advise antibiotics to lessen or prevent an attack	Possibly vomiting and fever before severe sore throat. If followed (usually in 1-4 days) by rash of tiny red spots on body and limbs, it is called scarlet fever	Until all symptoms disappear and laboratory tests clear, or doctor agrees	Rest and general good care. Usually cured by 10-day course of penicillin. Child will probably feel better in a week
Whooping cough	7-21 days, usually 7-10 days	Immunization. For an unvaccinated child, protective serum may be given shortly after exposure	Cold symptoms and cough which changes at end of second week to bouts of coughing accompanied by a noisy gasp for air (the "whoop"). Coughing often brings on vomiting. "Whoop" does not occur in babies who have the disease	At least 4 weeks	Rest. Soft, non-irritating foods; frequent small meals. Fresh air when doctor will allow. Breathing exercises may help. Child needs careful supervision of doctor throughout illness. Cough may continue for eight weeks

Usual time between exposure to disease and first symptoms.

Recognizing the Symptoms

New parents often ask for a list of symptoms that might indicate when something is wrong with their child. This is hardly practical – you cannot consult your doctor about every little cough or cold – but child experts agree that it is by far the most important rule to consult your doctor promptly if a child appears changed in general appearance or acts abnormally. These symptoms include unusual paleness, tiredness and drowsiness, lack of interest, unusual irritability, anxiousness, restlessness, or even prostration. Many other common signs and symptoms are described below, all of which need attention from your doctor. However, after you have had the experience of raising your first child, you will have a good idea of which symptoms require prompt contact with your doctor and which can wait till tomorrow or till the next visit to the health center.

Pain in the ear, particularly when it follows a cold or is associated with fever, may be due to a middle-ear disease. Such pain usually responds rapidly to early treatment. Do not waste time putting warm drops into the ear.

If hoarseness and noise in the throat on breathing in and out follow a cold, the most likely cause is *laryngotracheitis*, which can be serious if neglected. This can sometimes happen at night and parents should call a doctor as soon as possible.

Enlarged glands in the neck can be caused by a number of diseases, such as tonsillitis or glandular fever. Also any septic area, however small, on the skin of the face, scalp or neck, can result in painfully enlarged glands in the neck. As there are many possible causes of this symptom, you should consult your doctor. You should do likewise with a persistently bleeding nose, or any other bleeding that does not stop within an hour or so.

Any type of convulsions should be reported to your doctor. Convulsions are not due to teething. In many small children they are caused by simple infections such as tonsilitis, but you cannot be sure. If your child is having a fit, slapping or a hot bath are not the answer. Just let the fit abate naturally and make sure the child does not hurt itself. If the child is feverish sponge him or her down with tepid water.

If there is no obvious simple cause for a fever, such as cold, that you can treat without medical advice, it is best to consult your doctor. The most likely cause is a sore throat or an infectious disease,

Left: you can examine your child's throat by pressing gently on the tongue with the handle of a warm tablespoon. A complaint of a sore throat should always be investigated. The throat does not become sore of its own accord, but indicates that there is an infection present.

Below: subacute tonsilitis. The tonsils, a mass of lymphoid tissue which usually disappears by late childhood, becomes inflamed usually as a result of a streptococal infection. The symptoms include muscular aching and stomachache, but rarely a sore throat.

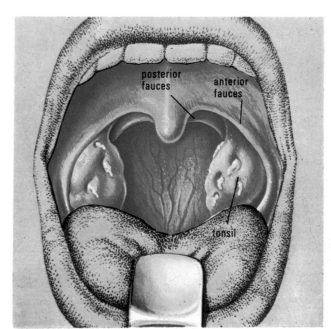

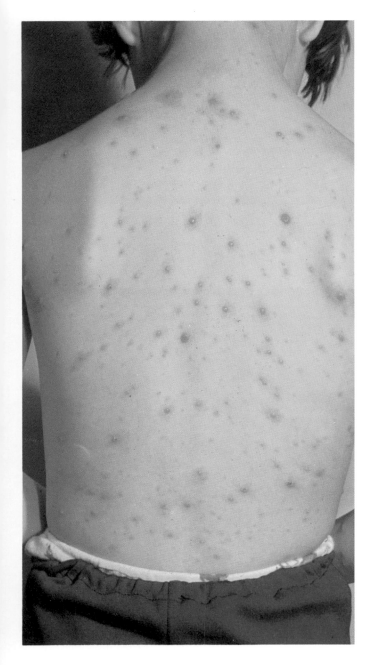

Above: the rash produced by chickenpox (varicella). This highly infectious viral disease has an incubation period of about two weeks, after which the temperature rises sharply and a rash appears. The rash spreads from the trunk to the rest of the body and may blister. Recovery is rapid – within a few days, but the patient is considered infectious until all the blisters disappear. One attack of the disease usually confers lifelong immunity.

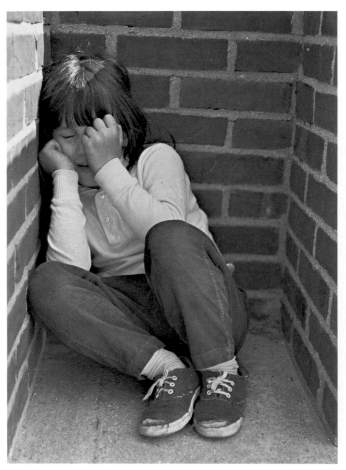

Above: sometimes your child may not display any obvious physical signs of illness. Instead there may be emotional distress, depression or lassitude. You should not let these symptoms go by uninvestigated.

but it may be due to something more serious. If in addition to fever there is some pain or stiffness in the back on bending the neck forward, a prompt examination is called for.

You will obviously not consult your doctor every time your child gets a cold accompanied by a cough. But if he or she is also feverish, breathes quickly and makes a grunting noise on breathing, and you see the side of the nose being drawn in and out on breathing, or if there is a pain in the chest or abdomen, your child may have pneumonia, which calls for prompt treatment by the doctor. A chronic and persistent cough may be due to a variety of causes and should be investigated.

The vast majority of cases of "vomiting" in small children are due to infections, such as a sore throat. Sometimes vomiting in babies may be due to congenital *pyloric stenosis* (an obstruction at the lower end of the stomach). Vomiting with diarrhea could be due to some form of food poisoning, and the child should be seen by the doctor.

Children often complain about pain in the abdomen. However, you should consult your doctor if there is vomiting and pain, especially if, when you gently press the abdomen where it hurts, there is also tenderness. You should also call the doctor if the child is also feverish or vomiting. There are several causes for this, but it may be an attack of appendicitis, which requires early treatment. On no account give a child with an abdominal pain a dose of castor oil or any other laxative.

A change in personality can be a matter for concern. When a child who has previously been happy becomes different, bad tempered, irritable and cries easily, you should discuss the situation with your doctor. It is most likely due to some sort of fear or insecurity at home or at school, but it may be a sign of disease.

The Role
of the Doctor

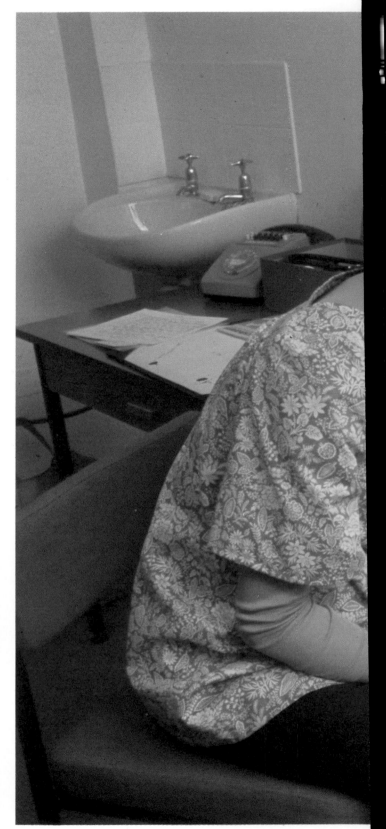

You can always be sure that your baby is making good progress if you have it checked periodically, by a doctor. In the first year your child should be taken to the doctor monthly at three-monthly intervals until the second year, and whenever vaccinations are advised.

Many people take their children to a child-health center. The doctors and nurses on a child health team have specialized in pediatrics (child medicine) and provide a particularly comprehensive service in dealing with your child's health and many other practical child care matters.

Of course for some people who live in isolated communities these visits to the doctor may have to be rare and it must be admitted that few babies get into trouble just because they do not see a doctor regularly.

Some parents prefer a doctor who is casual and

Below: when your child is obviously ill and weak, then it is imperative that you call the doctor. During his or her visit, stay with the child and discuss the problems openly: the child is already worried, and you must not generate further unnecessary fear.

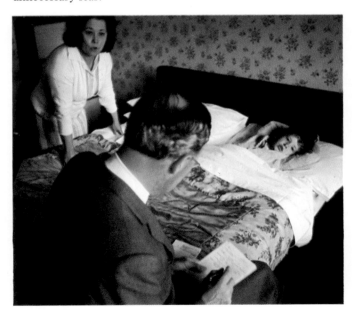

not too fussy about details. Others feel confident only if the doctor gives them explicit instructions down to the last detail. Some may have more confidence in an older man or prefer a woman doctor. Whatever the preference, the important factor is that the parents should be able to communicate easily with the doctor.

Most parents are initially bashful with their first

Above: many parents feel inhibited about bothering their doctor with what they think may be malingering or a trivial illness in their child. But many children do not have a vocabulary adequate enough to describe their pains and symptoms, and only a doctor's thorough examination can discover the underlying causes.

child about asking questions about baby care that may seem too simple, ignorant or silly. It is foolish

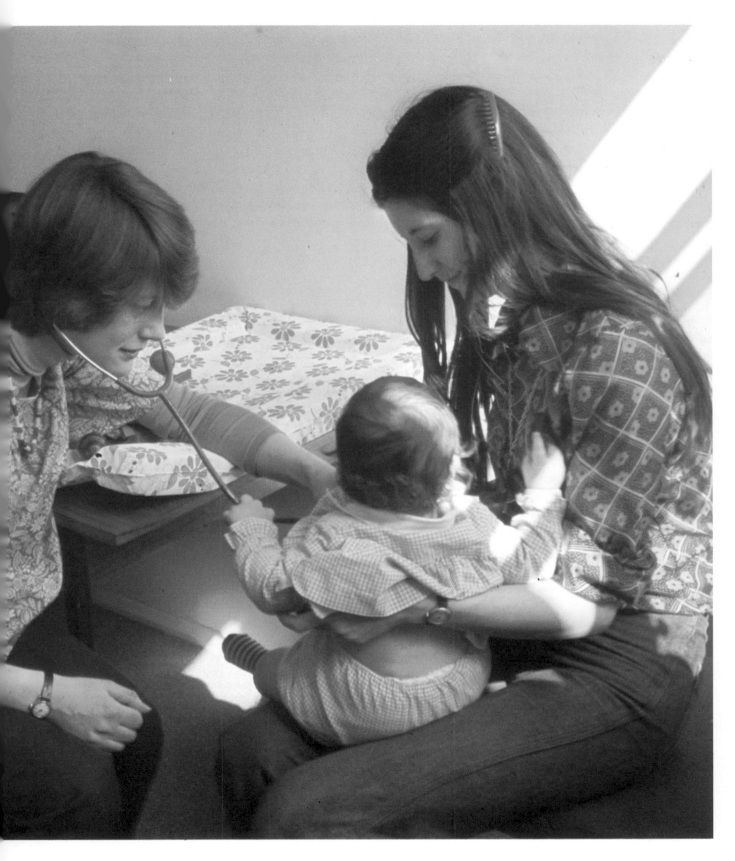

to worry about it. All good doctors are only too pleased to answer any questions they can. Even if you feel sure that your doctor will be grumpy about something that is probably not serious, but that you are very much concerned about, it will do no harm to be on the safe side and contact him or her. Your child's health is more important than the doctor's mood or your own reluctance or shyness. If your child has an illness or a condition that worries you intensely, it is always your right to ask for a specialist's opinion. Many parents are hesitant about doing so, fearing that this would express a lack of confidence in their own doctor. But most doctors will be more than ready to call in an expert if they cannot cure an illness, and very often suggest this course of action themselves.

The Value of Immunization

Immunization is vital in protecting children from potential serious illness. Various vaccinations are given from about the age of three months to about six years. The routines by which these vaccines are administered vary enormously from country to country and from area to area. But all children should receive their basic inoculations at some time.

At birth many babies receive a vaccine to protect them against tuberculosis. At the age of three months children are often given a first shot of a combined vaccine against diphtheria, tetanus (lockjaw) and whooping cough, and also one against poliomyelitis.

Three injections are usually administered over a period of about six weeks. These combined vaccinations often produce a reaction (caused mostly by the whooping cough antigen), consisting of fever, loss of appetite, and soreness around the injected area. These difficulties usually disappear within a day or so, but if a fever persists, it may be due to a new infection and it is wise to call your doctor. Booster vaccinations against diphtheria and tetanus are often given when the child is about four years old and again at about age seven.

Polio vaccine is one of the greatest achievements of modern preventive medicine. Since its introduction, the polio viruses causing infantile paralysis

Preparing an influenza vaccine. A vaccine induces active immunity against a bacterium or virus in the body, in the same way as if the body had actually been infected by that disease. There are three types. Toxoids (diptheria, tetanus), are nonpoisonous modifications of bacterial toxins. Bacterial vaccines (typhoid) are dead strains of bacteria, viral vaccines (polio), weakened viruses.

	Immunization
2-3 months	DTP, Sabin Type 1 or Trivalent
3-4 months	DTP, Sabin Type 3 or Trivalent
4-5 months	DTP, Sabin Type 2 or Trivalent
9-11 months	Tuberculin Test
12 months	Measles Vaccine
12-24 months	Smallpox Vaccination, Mumps Vaccine, German Measles Vaccine
15-18 months	DTP, Trivalent Sabin
2 years	Tuberculin Test
3 years	DTP, Tuberculin Test
4 years	Tuberculin Test
6 years	TD, Smallpox Vaccination, Tuberculin Test, Trivalent Sabin
8 years	TuberculinTest, Mumps Vaccine (if not given earlier or if child did not have mumps)
12 years	TD, Smallpox Vaccine, Tuberculin Test
12-14 years (girls)	German Measles
14 years	Tuberculin Test
16 years	Tuberculin Test

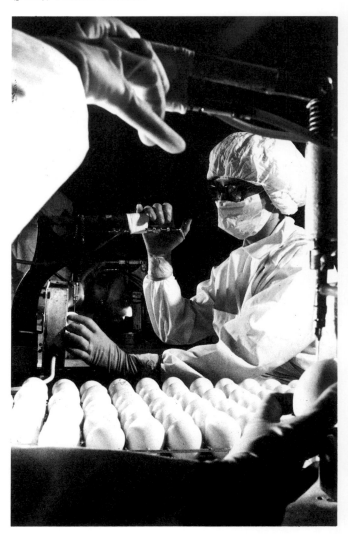

have been virtually eliminated and the illness itself has become an anachronism: many countries have been free from the disease for the last 15 years, but will only remain free if vaccination levels are maintained in the population. Three injections of polio vaccine are given, or the child may receive an oral variety of vaccine on a lump of sugar.

Smallpox has been virtually wiped off the face of the earth. Because of this, in Western countries it is rarely necessary to give children antismallpox vaccinations. Its administration is not recommended if the child has a severe cold or any other upset. The reaction is usually worst on about the eight or ninth day. In moderate cases, the child feels sick, and there is loss of appetite and a fever. After the height of the reaction, the vaccination site dries up and turns into a tough, brown scab, which falls off on the fifteenth day after vaccination.

Within recent years two new vaccines have been added to the armory of public health. One is the measles vaccine which is given to children at about 12 months. The other is an antirubella (German measles) vaccine given to 12- to 14-year-old girls to insure that they will not contract the disease at the time they may be pregnant. Rubella virus can cause serious malformations in the developing fetus.

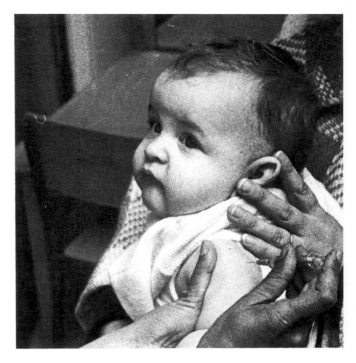

Above: if your child displays marked symptoms after an immunization, you should consult your doctor immediately.

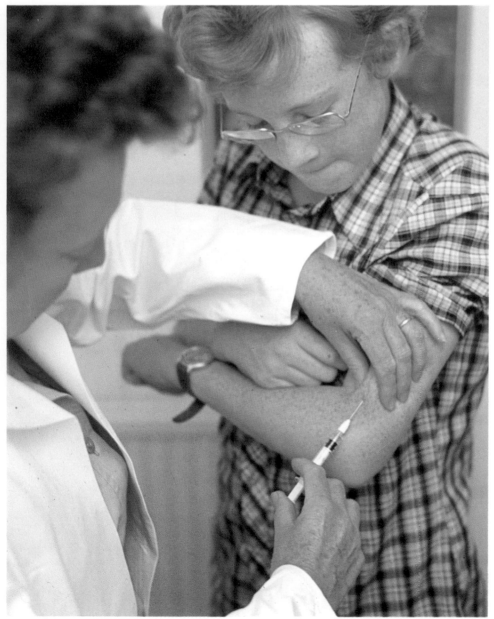

Left: your older child may be vaccinated at school.

167

Caring for a Sick Child

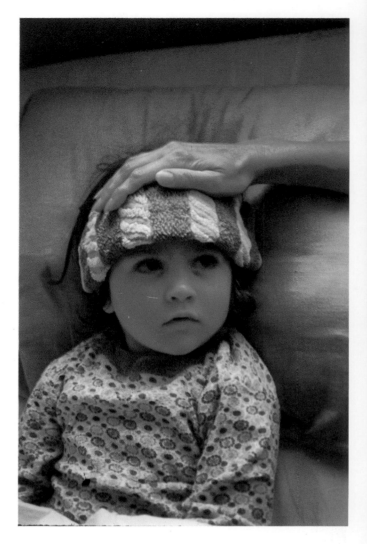

Caring for a sick child is inevitably bound to be a strain for the mother, with all the extra duties involved as well as the natural concern. But children make a fast recovery from most illnesses, so there is every reason to look on the bright side and share your optimism with your child. The medical care is taken care of by your doctor who will give you advice on any required treatment. All that remains is for you to keep your sick child cheerful and comfortable.

Bed is not a very comfortable place when you have to stay there for many days. For sitting up in bed, bolsters, or a slanting wooden board attached to the bedhead, can provide a firm foundation for pillows that would otherwise slide down. An adjustable table that can be swung across the bed is ideal for mealtimes and toys. Your child will probably feel more comfortable wearing ordinary clothes during the day, and a change of clothes before sleep will be refreshing.

Provided your doctor agrees, it is better to let your child get up, at least for part of the day, rather than stay miserably cooped up in bed. A makeshift bed can be made up on the living room sofa so that he or she can feel part of the general household activity. Sick people feel better, and recover sooner, if they can participate even a little in normal day-to-day life. But make sure that the invalid does not get overtired. When your child has to stay in bed then try and make sure that there are plenty of visitors — unless, of course, the illness is contagious.

Above: a sick child will be uncomfortable and distressed, particularly if the illness is accompanied by a fever. You can reduce the discomfort with cool compresses or by sponging the patient down with tepid water, until the body temperature drops to 102°F. Insure that a feverish child has plenty of fluids to drink.

Age	Companionship	Useful toys	Occupations	Games
1—4+	Soft toys, doll to dress and undress, toy telephone	Bricks, large, simple jigsaws, fitting pictures, plastic cups and other fitting-together toys, doll's house, toy cars	Picture books, cutting out, drawing, coloring, large beads and buttons for threading	Nursery rhymes, stories, fantasy games
4—8+	Soft toys, small mobile toys, hand puppets, pets, bird, aquarium, radio, record player	Bricks, jigsaws, model-making, mosaics, easy constructional toys, miniature garages, farms, zoos, toy cars	Reading, drawing, painting, stenciling, modeling clay, sewing, weaving, knitting, cutting out, making scrapbooks	Guessing games, simple card games, playing out the illness, doctor and nurse sets
8—11+	Soft toys, pets, bird, hamster, fish, puppets, Solitaire, card games,. radio, record player	Jigsaws, model-making, constructional sets	reading, writing, painting, sewing, weaving, soft-toy making, basket-making, theater	Doctor and nurse sets, board games
11 and upward	Pets, puppets, Solitaire, card games, radio, record player	Jigsaws, model-, toy-, and jewelry-making, complicated construction sets	Reading, painting, carving, sewing, and other crafts, making a miniature garden, collecting stamps, badges, photos, etc	Play-reading, word games, crosswords, board and card games

A sick child will thrive best on a regular routine for washing, eating, playing and resting, and this can be a boon when a mother is planning her day. The child should start the morning with a cool drink and a refreshing wash before breakfast. Your doctor will have advised you if a special diet is required. Otherwise, light foods, such as toast, cereal, crackers, cookies, soup, custards, junket, stewed fruit, and ice cream, will probably satisfy a sick child. If he or she does not feel like eating at all during the early stages of an illness, do not let this worry you, but continue to offer plenty of fruit juice and sweetened drinks throughout the day. Later, as the child begins to get better, you can start gradually reintroducing easily digestible foods, such as eggs, fish, ground meat, fruit and vegetables.

Even when children are convalescing, they may still not show much interest in food. This is not only as a result of the illness, but because they are still not getting much exercise and therefore are using up less energy than usual. Overencouraging the child to eat could cause feeding problems that last long after the illness is over. It will be easier if you stick to the foods that you know appeal to the child and try to make the meals look as attractive as possible.

Once your child is over the worst phase of the illness, he or she is likely to become demanding and bored. This is trying for the mother, but it is a good sign because it signifies that the child is getting better. This is when a plentiful supply of toys or pastimes should be made available – but only one or two things should be given at a time. A sick or convalescent child tires easily and cannot concentrate for long.

Doctors say that a child who is sick becomes at least a year younger mentally than when well. The child is likely to revert to more babyish habits, to be more dependent and to need more direct signs of affection. However, once the child starts to improve, it is wise to encourage gently but firmly a return to ordinary routine, so that there will not be an excessive attachment to the privileges of being pampered.

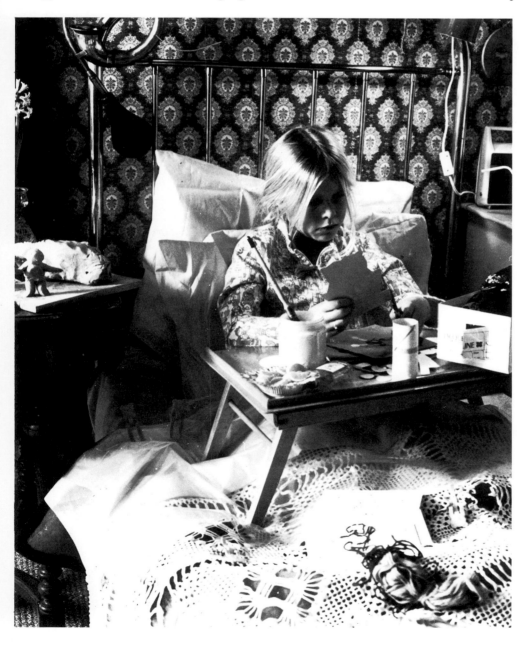

Many convalescing children complain of boredom. A tray or bed table will enable your child to indulge in a variety of play activities.

Understanding Your Child

How do we know whether we are bringing up our children in the right way? This is one of the most fascinating of life's questions, but one that unfortunately has no precise answer. The difficulty is that all children are different and methods most suitable for the bringing up of one child may be wrong for a younger brother or sister. Children differ in their personalities, aptitudes, rate of development, and intelligence. Some are far more active than others; some are happy from the first days of life; others take life much more seriously and hardly ever smile. Some prefer toys to people, others prefer people to toys. This usually happens in the same family in children growing up under the same circumstances and enjoying the same care. At the age of 12 months some children would rather starve than have to feed themselves, while others would rather starve than be fed by their mothers. Some require much more sleep than others.

It is obvious that rigid methods of child care are not suitable for most children. It would make matters much easier if parents could always have the really difficult child first, so that they could face any crisis after that experience, instead of having the placid easygoing child first, after which they think that they know everything about child management, but become seriously disillusioned when the next one has a thoroughly difficult character.

Some aggressive, restless children are very difficult to manage. Other, placid children are very little trouble at all. Some are shy, some are timid, some are fearless. They are all different, and they all differ in their rate of development. Some learn new skills sooner than others of the same level of intelligence. Some learn to sit, walk, dress themselves or control their bladder sooner than others of equal intelligence. Children of the same age often differ widely in intelligence. It would be clearly unreasonable to teach discipline in exactly the same way to a three-year-old with a mental age of four, as you would to a four-year-old with a mental age of two.

We can only finally judge the lasting influence our care has had when our children grow up and we can see how they cope with life's problems, and especially how they handle their own children. And even though we may think that our adult son is perfect, his wife or employers might have different views. We may think that our parents made many mistakes in our upbringing, but how can we tell that we would

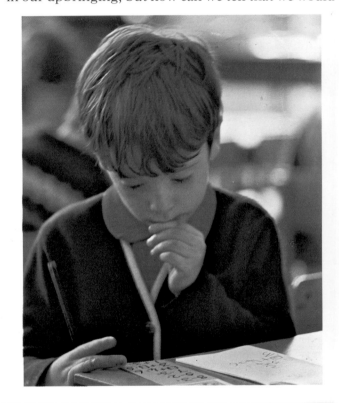

Some children are quiet, pensive, and retiring; others laugh a lot and are sociable. Each child is a unique individual, its individuality determined by heredity, its relationship to the family, and its surroundings.

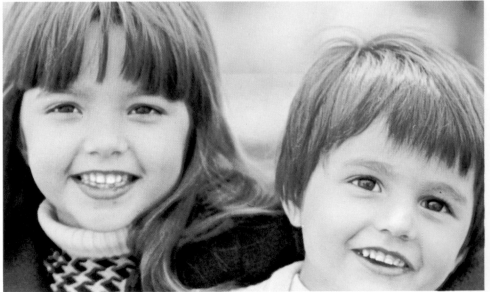

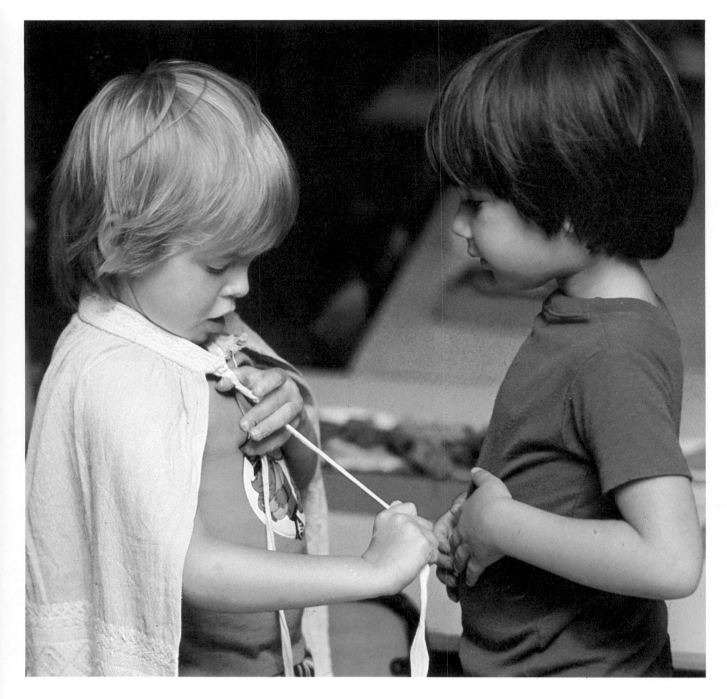

have been better and happier if they had treated us differently? They made mistakes which we are determined to avoid, but we make mistakes which they successfully avoided.

We can never always be sure that what we are doing is right. But we should strive to learn as much as we can about how children develop, discover how they respond to love, teaching, overprotection, insecurity, punishment, jealousy, play, separation from parents, rivalry, puberty, and illness. By our own observations, and by learning from the observations of experts who have made children their life study, such as Arnold Gesell, Jean Piaget and Benjamin Spock, we can learn about children's thoughts, life and development. As well as learning about the common problems of childhood development and behavior, we can come to realize that children are not the only ones with behavioral problems – parents

Most children settle down very well at school but some do have serious problems. They may find it difficult to make friends, and become either very aggressive or susceptible to bullying.

and teachers have them too! We can then begin to know when our own children are responding normally and predictably to our methods of managing them; and we can observe the clash of their own developing personality with their own personality and attitudes.

Being fully aware of the problems involved will not help parents to make their children perfect, because no one is perfect or ever will be. But perhaps it will help parents to accept their children for what they are (and children cannot be blamed for taking after their parents), instead of demanding perfection and then being disappointed when perfection is not achieved.

171

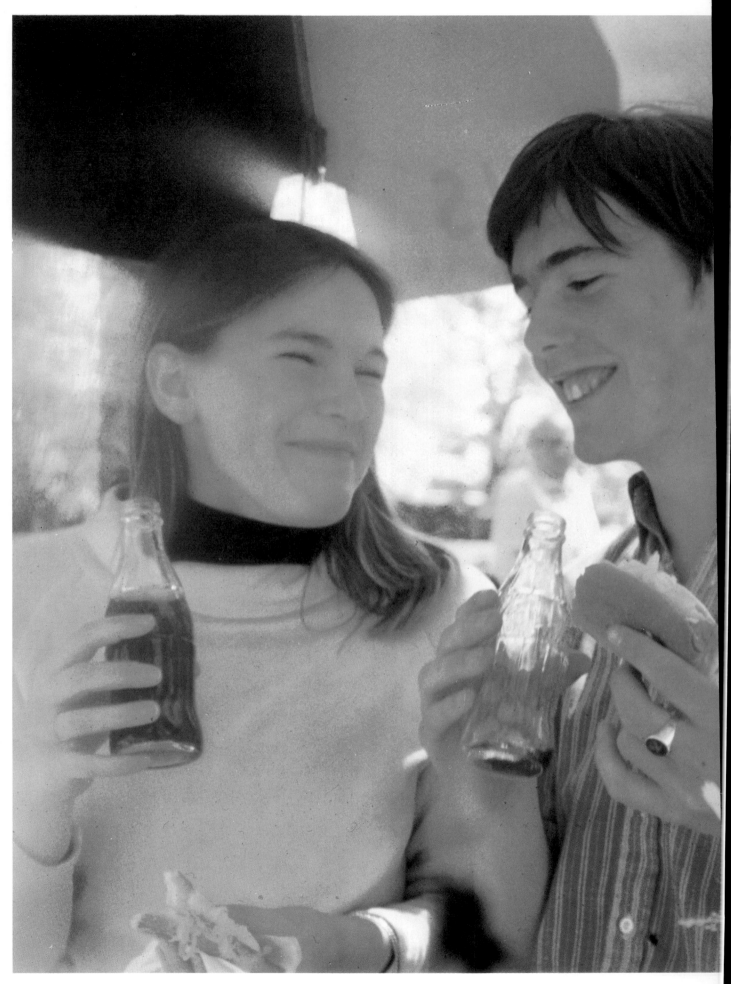

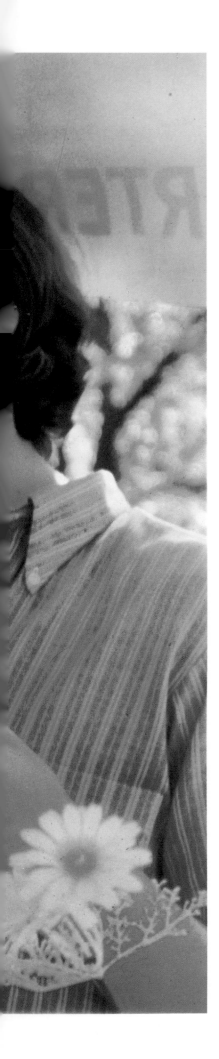

Chapter 9

The Adolescent Years

Medical problems during adolescence are few. A teenage boy may run the risk of a motorcar or motorcycle accident more than the other members of his family; the teenage girl may have a real or imaginary weight problem – and they both may suffer from the teenager's curse: acne. However, to the young person these minor problems can assume monstrous proportions and come to dominate their lives. This is because the real problems that all young people face are psychological: those of adjusting to the demands of their changing bodies, and striving toward their new identities as adults in a sophisticated society. During this vital stage, teenagers need their parents' love and understanding more than ever before.

Opposite: adolescents soon become aware of their sexuality and of the attractions of the opposite sex. It is also important, however, that boys and girls learn how to develop friendships with each other.

Neither Child nor Adult

Headlines such as "Promiscuity among teenagers is soaring, says doctor," "Parents didn't know their son was a junkie," "10 wounded in student riots," are enough to alarm the parents of any teenager today. A common attitude toward adolescents is that a dreadful disease takes hold of normal, happy youngsters and transforms them overnight into alien beings with whom communication is impossible.

Of course everyone knows that the teenage years are a critical period. Boys and girls alike may go through a period of some physical and emotional awkwardness as they try to gain control of their developing bodies and new feelings. A boy's changing voice shows how he is both part man and boy, and yet not wholly either. Adolescence, however, does not change the character of your child, and it need not destroy happy family relationships. It is simply another stage in your child's development, and by

understanding what is happening to your teenage children, you can help them pass through this period with the minimum of pain. For your children need you now as much as ever – often despite appearances to the contrary – and with your continued love, understanding and guidance, their teenage years will not prove too much to handle.

Children do not explode into adolescence overnight. The changes are gradual, beginning at around age 11 for girls and 13 for boys, although they may begin a couple of years earlier or several years later. Biologically, a child may become a teenager as early as age 9 or as late as age 16, and the teenage years will span the whole period from the first signs of puberty to the age when your child is mature enough to leave home and start an independent existence.

The social and educational activities that adolescents take part in tend to be set at levels determined by school achievement, by their social peers or simply by age, rather than by physical and emotional maturity. The peak of physical difference between the sexes is reached when most girls are larger than their male classmates.

The psychologist Erik Erikson refers to the most marked stage of adolescence as an *identity crisis*, a crisis because the increasing emotional tension and pressure of natural bodily drives must meet and be

Rather than lose your temper with your child, you should try and persuade him to tell you what the problem is. A rational discussion produces better results.

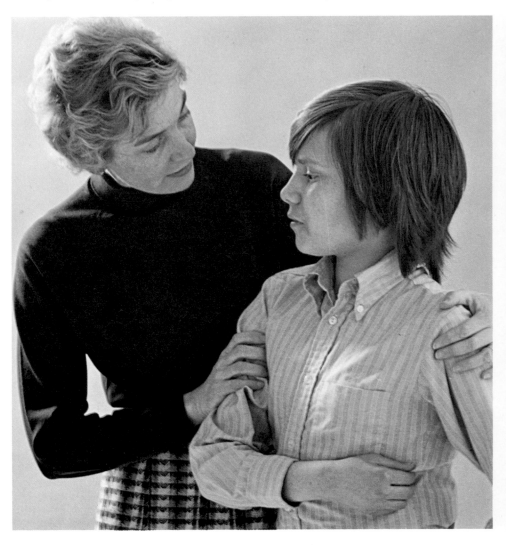

balanced so that the teenager can cope with the increased demands and expectations of society. The process of attaining one's own identity, of "finding oneself," in adolescence and early adulthood has become prolonged in Western culture as the duration of formal education and dependency on the parents increases, and has become complicated by the breakdown of traditional patterns of family life and social class. The quest for one's own set of values involves a search for sexual awareness, social class identity, identity with a job or career, and identity with activities outside the spheres of home or employment.

A further stage in adolescence, which Erikson calls *intimacy*, is the ability to avoid emotional isolation, or an inability to relate to others, by seeking comfort in shared, close experiences. Intimacy involves facing the fear of rejection by taking part in shared physical activities such as sports, in close friendships and in sexual experiences. Intimacy is private and not usually shared with parents. Intimacy implies the sharing of feelings, which is the essential quality of *empathy*, the ability to know how others feel and to respond understandingly.

Erikson describes the next stage as *generativity*, which involves the strong commitment of young people to each other in love affairs, courtship or

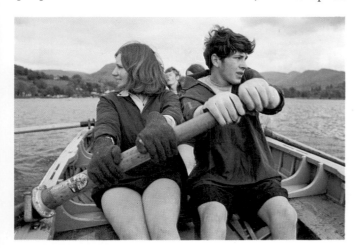

Above: for many teenagers sport provides the ideal means of combining exercise and communal activity. Belonging to a team is also a way of establishing social identity.

marriage, and the acceptance of adult responsibilities and behavior.

The final stage of growth Erikson calls *ego integrity*. He visualizes this as the ability "to accept one's individual life cycle and the people who have become significant to it as meaningful within the segment of history in which one loves. . . . Integrity thus means a new and different love of one's parents, free of the wish that they should have been different and an acceptance of the fact that one's life is one's own responsibility. It is a sense of comradeship with men and women of distant times and of different pursuits, who have created orders and objects and sayings conveying human dignity and love."

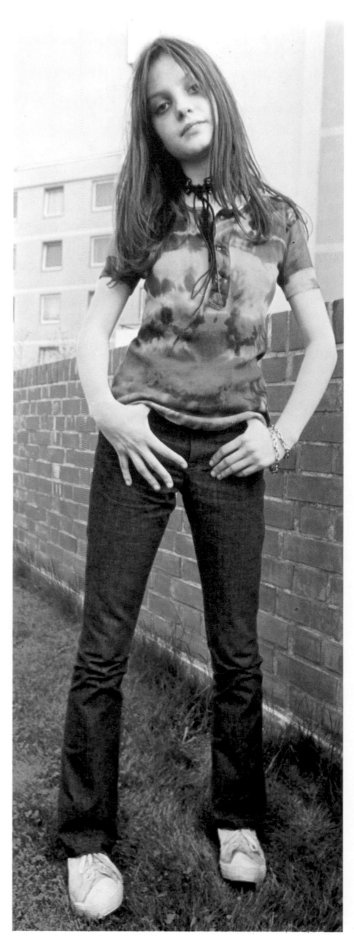

Above: one of the problems that parents face with adolescents is that of discipline. This is a period when your child will be desperately trying to assert her independence.

175

The Impact of Puberty

What are the changes that transform a child into a teenager? For a girl, the arrival of puberty is firmly established by her first menstrual period. This will probably happen soon after her twelfth birthday, although it is perfectly normal for a girl to have her first period as early as age 9 or as late as age 16.

Well before the girl's first period, however, the hormones responsible for puberty will have brought about other changes in a young girl's body. The breasts begin to develop. First the dark area round the nipple (the areola) enlarges and becomes slightly puffy. Then the whole breast begins to take shape. The pubic hair starts to grow, the hips widen, the skin changes in texture, and her height increases considerably.

It is important to realize that there is no regular age at which puberty begins. The largest number of girls begin their development at around the age of 11. But lately an increasing number begin their development at an even younger age, as young as nine in some cases. Late developers may not start before the age of 13. Early and late developers have nothing wrong with their glands. The timetable in these cases, which seems to be an inborn trait, is just faster or slower. Parents who were late developers are more likely to have children who are late developers and vice versa.

By the age of 13 the average girl has almost developed a woman's body. She has acquired most of the weight and height she will ever have. At this point her growing slows down and for the first year ot two the periods tend to be irregular and infrequent, as if the body still lacked experience of its new status. Sometimes it is difficult for a girl who is not aware of what is happening to her body not to feel awkward and self-conscious when she finds herself the only one in her class shooting upward and acquiring a woman's shape. But the girl who has a good relationship with her mother and wants to be like her is inevitably pleased with her newly acquired height and figure.

It is not unusual for the late developing girl to feel out of step with her friends. She may be convinced that she is abnormal and at this time she needs her parents' reassurance that when her time comes she will develop a woman's body just like her friends.

When you notice the first signs of puberty in your daughter, it is time to prepare her for the onset of menstruation if you have not done so already. You should explain simply but accurately why periods happen, pointing out that they are a normal, healthy part of growing up and reaching womanhood. It is

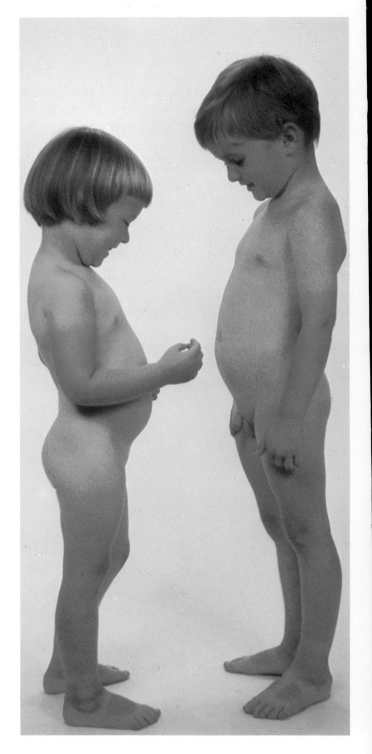

At a very early age children will become curious about the obvious physical difference between the sexes. If you have young children of both sexes, these questions will be inevitable. This will be the time when you will probably want to introduce some elementary sex education into their upbringing.

important, too, to persuade your daughter to discuss with you openly any feelings she may have about changes in her body and her growing interests in boys, and to give honest answers to her questions about how the opposite sex functions.

Puberty usually starts later for boys – at any time from 10 to 16 – but it is on average two years behind the girls, at about 13. The voice breaks and then

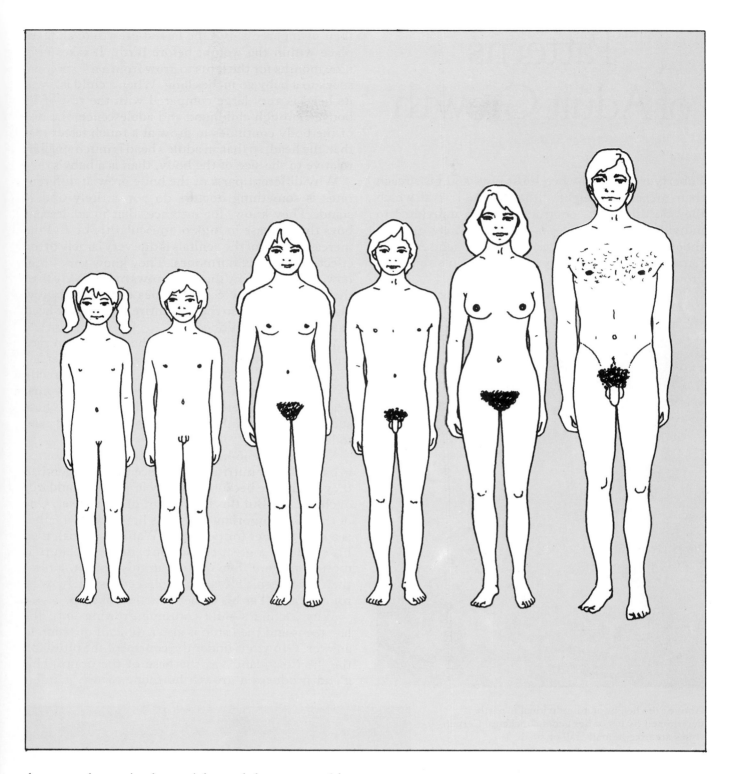

deepens; the penis, the testicles and the scrotum (the sac containing the testicle) enlarge; and he will develop body hair. After about two years, the boy's body will have almost completed its transition to that of a man. Unlike girls, however, who have finished most of their growing before their first period, a boy will usually get taller after he has matured sexually.

About midway in this period of bodily development – usually around age 14, but sometimes earlier – a boy will experience his first ejaculation. It is important to explain to him in advance that he will have seminal emissions at night ("wet dreams"), and that these are a perfectly natural result of the accumulation of seminal fluid in his body. As with your daugh-

There is a normal range of variation in adolescent growth. These drawings were made of girls aged 12 years, 9 months, and boys aged 14 years, 9 months. Those on the left of their group had not yet reached puberty, the ones in the middle were part of the way through, and those on the right had completed their development.

ter, your son should be told the facts about his own growth and developing interest in sex, and about the growth and feelings of girls. Both boys and girls should also be told at this time that masturbation is a perfectly normal activity that most teenagers – and many adults – engage in, that it can do no harm whatsoever, and that it is nothing to be ashamed of or feel guilty about.

Patterns of Adult Growth

Puberty is the time when most boys and girls reach their maximum height, although the rate at which they do this varies enormously from individual to individual. Thirteen-year-old Jerry may quickly shoot up to 5 feet, 9 inches, while his friend Andrew remains for a couple of years at preteen size before growing to 6 feet.

The speed at which children grow often surprises their own parents, but the fastest growth of all takes place within the womb, before birth. It takes only nine months for the fetus to grow from a microscopic speck to a baby 20 inches long. When a child is born, its head is very large compared with the rest of its body. Through childhood and adolescence, the rest of the body continues to grow at a much faster rate than the head, so that an adult's head is much smaller, relative to the size of the body, than is a baby's.

Why different parts of the body grow at different rates is something doctors do not entirely understand. They know, for instance, that in adolescent boys the increase in bulk of muscular tissue and the increase in size of the genitals is due very largely to the effect of male sex hormones. They know very little, however, about why the head grows more slowly than the body, and why certain bones of the skull grow faster than others, so that the entire shape of the head changes during childhood.

It is now an undisputed fact that the human race has slowly grown taller over the years. This belief has been borne out by many surveys, and more directly by examinations of old suits of armor worn by men who were considered large in their times. These suits would certainly not fit an average-sized man today.

This increase in height can certainly be attributed in part to better nutrition. Adolescents are bigger than they used to be because of vastly improved standards of child care. But this is only part of the answer. One of the most important factors is heredity. If a father is a high jumper (or perhaps a Watusi warrior), then his child has a great chance of being tall. Nature is more important than nurture in this respect. Unless there has been illness, an adolescent is likely to be roughly as tall as his or her genetic make-up.

Why a child should continue growing until the late teens and then stop is also a difficult question to answer. Growth is under the control of the pituitary, the "master gland" at the base of the brain. This gland produces a growth hormone, which is inter-

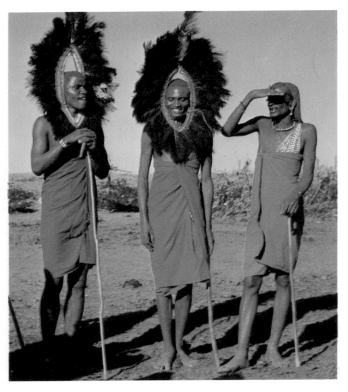

Above: the height of an individual is partly determined by his or her genetic makeup. Certain tribes are exceptionally tall or small.

Right: a son can expect to be as tall as his father, a daughter the same height as her mother, unless there are marked differences in nutrition.

Far right: the pituitary gland secretes growth hormone. This is in turn controlled by growth hormone releasing factor from the hypothalamus.

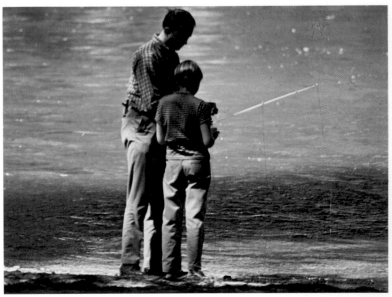

178

cepted by some "biological clock" within the body a few years after puberty. The growth plates of the long bones then cease to function. The sex glands and the adrenals also contribute to growth. The effects of these glands is most readily observed when they become either overactive or underactive. For instance, overactivity of the pituitary gland may be the result of a particular type of tumor. In children this causes a condition called *gigantism*, and in adults it produces *acromegaly*. Sufferers may have enlarge-

ment of the nose, mouth, hands, and feet, or may simply be excessively tall.

The majority of cases of *dwarfism* are due either to a disease, or to inherited disorders of the bones. *Achondroplasia*, a typical example commonly seen in dwarfs, occurs in families. An achondroplastic dwarf has a short body and even shorter limbs, but a normal sized head and brain. The cause is unknown but dwarfs have no other disabilities and are of normal intelligence.

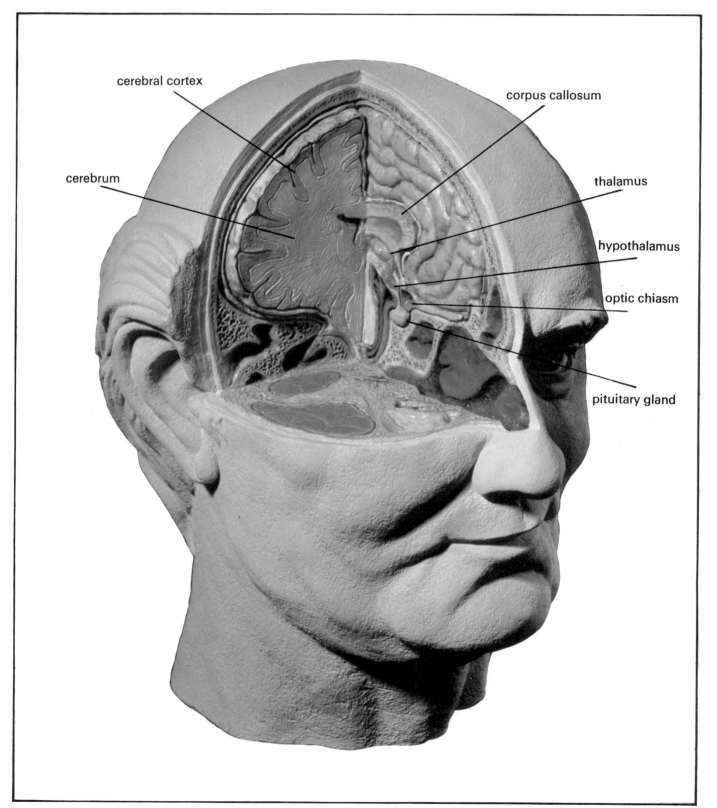

Increased Bodily Needs

Doctors are greatly interested in why some children eat more than others. A person's weight is initially controlled by the hypothalamus, a tiny nerve center in the brain that regulates appetite. Eating habits, nevertheless, are of primary importance. A contributing factor to excessive early weight gain in children is the old-fashioned if understandable idea that big babies are healthier. Some mothers feel that overfeeding their child is a safeguard against disease. Others, talking about their fat, overfed, child, defend themselves by saying: "He is so big, it is difficult to fill him!" However, obesity does cause excessive bone growth, so that most fat children become tall for their age. Yet puberty tends to occur early for them, and growth stops sooner than usual. So the eventual height of most fat children is less than the average.

Since they are often embarrassed about their weight, fat children generally tend to be hypersensitive. They may indulge in self-pity and be overly dependent on their parents. At the start of puberty their sensitivity about their appearance can increase and be quite painful. They may then genuinely try to diet on their own, but are hampered by inflexible family meals and pressure to eat because of a still prevalent belief among some parents that the child "needs to grow." However, once a child has become fat, it is difficult for him or her to reduce their weight by dieting. Considerable emotional disturbance may result from determined efforts to cause a child, particularly an older one, to reduce weight. It is therefore far better to prevent obesity than attempt to treat it once it has fully developed. But if you do decide that your teenage son or daughter should go on a diet, you should seek your doctor's advice. A crash diet could deprive your child of the nutrition needed for health.

In an affluent society the problems of children who are too chubby deserve as much attention as those who are "skin and bones." For the child who starts life as a fat baby there can be serious consequences. Robert Hughes, from Illinois, who weighed 400 pounds when he was ten years old, died in 1958 at the age of 32, weighing over 1000 pounds. His waistline was over 120 inches. Although this was an extreme case, mothers who take pride in and cater for their children's big appetites may be doing great damage. One such mother, replying to a doctor's questions about her child, anounced: "Oh, she's got a marvelous appetite. She never stops eating." The girl was 60 pounds overweight – which is nothing to be proud of.

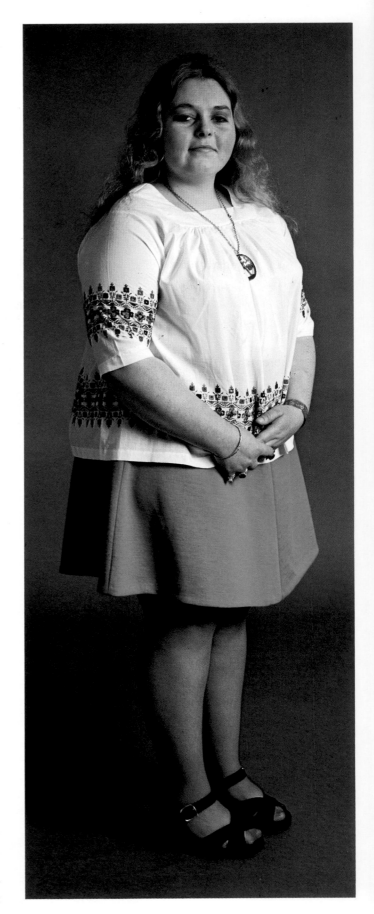

The majority of teenagers are overweight because they eat far too much – not because they are hungry but because their excess weight makes them feel depressed and insecure. The difficulty in buying fashionable clothes, and uncooperative parents, aggravate the problem.

An extreme form of poor appetite, or self-starvation, is the condition called *anorexia nervosa*, most often seen in adolescent girls. It is accompanied by a severe weight loss and, in girls, by delayed periods. Anorexia nervosa frequently starts as an attempt to lose weight by dieting and develops into an inability to eat, often made worse by self-induced vomiting. A normal life may seem to be maintained despite the weight loss, but teenagers with this disorder often appear to have broken down in their ability to cope with life both at home and at school. They may become extremely unemotional and uncommunicative. If the condition is allowed to develop too far, then these children have to be treated in hospital. There

they receive intensive treatment and in most cases, usually after some psychiatric therapy, are brought back to a normal weight and are able to resume their ordinary lives.

One theory about anorexia nervosa is that teenagers develop this condition because subconsciously they cannot cope with the problems of life and their developing sexuality. It is looked on as an attempt to retreat from these problems and a return to childhood dependence on others.

This girl is recovering from anorexia nervosa, a disease in which the victim refuses to eat enough food. If untreated, she may starve herself to death. A refusal to accept adult sexuality is often cited as the reason.

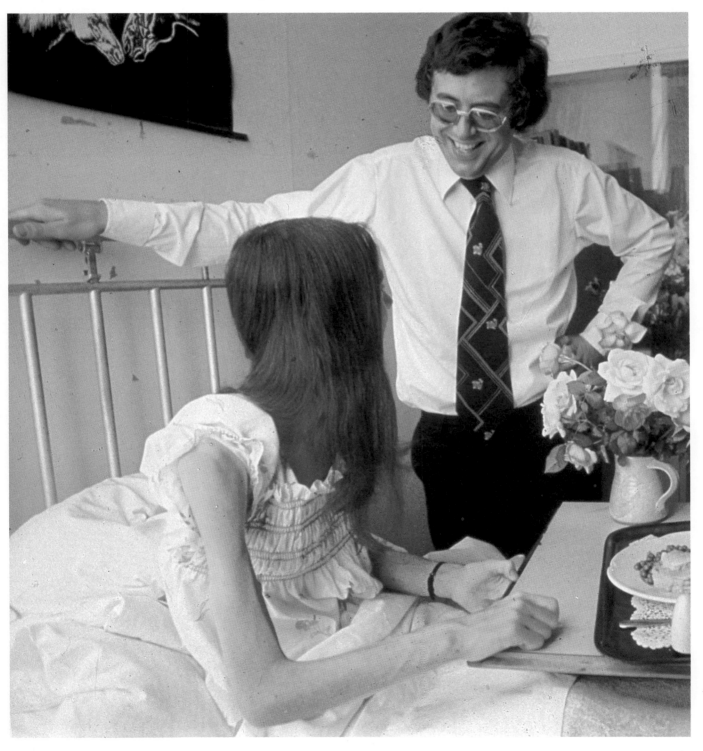

Drugs
and Alcohol

What do you do if you find that your teenager is taking drugs? The average parent's reaction to this discovery varies. They are shocked and unbelieving, numb and hopeless, resentful, quick to blame others for the problem; or else they reject their child altogether. All of these very human reactions provoke equally emotional counter-responses in the adolescent, and parents and child find themselves caught in a blind alley of hostility and aggression.

It is far wiser not to confront your child at the moment of discovery, but to allow a cooling-off period before discussing the problem with them as calmly as you can, and letting your son or daughter give their own justification. Keep a sense of perspective, and try to find out how seriously your child has been experimenting with drugs – and why. Finally, make sure you know where to turn for help if you feel that you cannot handle the situation alone. Check out the resources available in your community, such as schools, churches, mental health clinics, hospitals, or self-help groups that organize drug-counseling for the young. This is particularly important if it turns out that the child is physically addicted. Addiction is a physical dependence of the body on a particular substance. When this substance is no longer available the body experiences intense withdrawal symptoms which in some cases can be fatal in themselves. An addict should always be weaned off the drug under medical supervision.

It is important, however, for parents not to lose their heads over the question of teenagers and drugs. Adolescents are persons in their own right, and must eventually decide for themselves whether or not to use drugs. If parents respect the individuality of their children and are ready to support and advise without bullying, the teenagers will probably dismiss drugs as not for them, even if they have tried them once or twice out of sheer curiosity. But the teenager who persists in drugtaking probably has deep emotional problems that would have manifested themselves in other ways had drugs not been available. So parents should not focus their attention on the drugs alone, but should try to discover the underlying reasons for the anxiety that may be causing the young person to seek escape through drugs.

Drugs of abuse are generally classified as narcotics, hallucinogens and dangerous drugs, though this is a legal rather than a medical classification, and what it covers varies from country to country and from state to state.

Narcotics include cocaine, opium and its highly

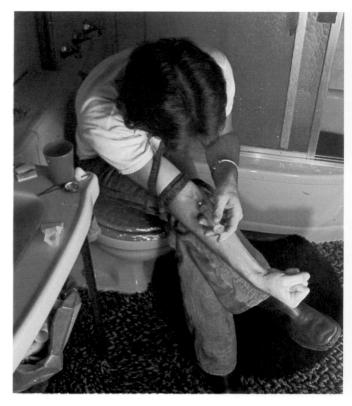

Above: heroin addition is increasing rapidly. If you suspect that your child is using this drug you should talk to him or her and try to arrange skilled medical treatment.

Below: pills such as depressants and stimulants are relatively easy to obtain, either on the black market or via the doctor. Their dangers, however, should not be underestimated.

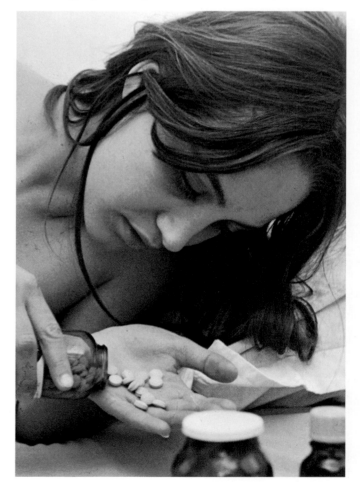

182

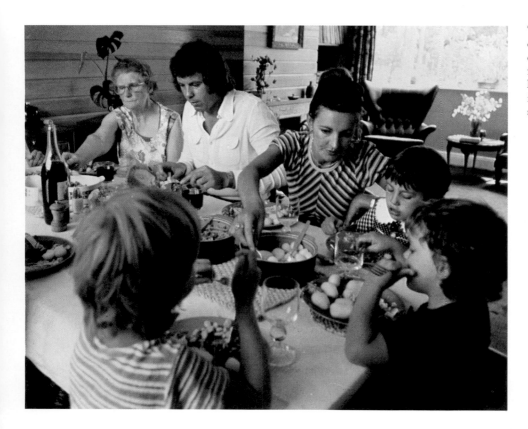

The young are more liable to develop drinking problems if they endow alcohol with an adult forbidden status. They are more likely to drink wisely if they are introduced to alcohol in the social setting of family meals.

addictive derivatives – morphine and heroin. The last is particularly dangerous; in many Western countries the number of addicts is growing at an alarming rate. Addiction is as much a social problem as a medical one. As the addict's tolerance to the drug increases, so his or her tolerance rises. Obtaining the drug becomes an obsession, and many addicts have to turn to crime to finance their habit.

Hallucinogens include lysergic acid diethylamide (LSD), mescaline and psilocybin. These induce a "trip" – vivid colored hallucinations, but can also push a user into a psycotic state.

Marijuana is the most controversial of the abused drugs, and this controversy is illustrated by the fact that in some of the United States its possession is regarded as a misdeamenor and in others as a felony. Smoking the drug produces a number of symptoms, including drowsiness, hallucinations, and increased awareness of sound. It can distort perception, which makes it unsafe when smoked before driving, but generally it is not considered dangerous. It is not addictive.

The most commonly abused drugs are the depressants, especially barbiturates, and stimulants, in particular amphetamines. They are usually taken orally, as pills, sometimes combined together to produce a state of euphoria. The "Purple Hearts" of the 1960s were such a combination. Some users inject the drugs, a practice which can lead to hepatitis and gangrene. Both amphetamines and barbiturates are addictive.

The dangers of barbiturates are neither appreciated nor stressed sufficiently. Overdosing with barbiturates depresses the respiratory center of the brain and can lead to death. They are a popular means of committing suicide. There is no home treatment for barbiturate poisoning and recovery is only possible in an intensive care unit. Other abused tranquilizers and sedatives include Mandrax, Valium and Librium.

Amphetamines were originally developed to overcome fatigue and were once widely prescribed as appetite depressants. Colloquially they are known as "speed," which is a good description of their effect. Mainly used by young people to stay awake, they can induce violent aggressive behavior and paranoid psychosis.

Many teenagers smoke cigarettes and despite warnings about the dangers it is unlikely that their parents can persuade them to stop, especially if they themselves are heavy smokers. Appealing to a teenager's vanity and informing them of the bad breath, stained teeth and reduced stamina will be more successful than an outright prohibition.

The dangers of alcohol will almost certainly have come up during talks with your teenager about drugs. Again, you have to know the facts and be consistent in your attitudes. Surveys have shown that the teenagers who misuse alcohol are usually those whose parents have mixed feelings about drinking or who are excessive drinkers themselves but forbid their children to drink until they reach a certain age, usually 21. Some authorities believe that problems might be prevented if children learned to drink wisely in a social setting at home. If you do have alcohol in your home, it seems advisable to allow your children a little beer or wine on special occasions when you consider them old enough, rather than issuing a strict veto that provokes them to clandestine drinking with their friends.

183

Teenage Health Problems

For many parents the adolescent and teenage years of their children present the biggest problems. Medically, their children will have fewer complaints than their previous years, but they are more likely to be involved in road accidents than any other age group – this is, after all, the age when many young people take to the road as motorcyclists or motorcar drivers.

Adolescents and teenagers need a healthy, balanced diet to help them grow. Unfortunately, because of typical teenage habits, such as skipping breakfast and surviving for the rest of the day on cake, candy and hamburgers, they very rarely eat wisely or well.

Nevertheless, to avoid the dangers of overnutrition or undernutrition, mothers should insure that their teenage children are receiving the minimum of what is good for them, including high-protein foods, fresh vegetables and fruit.

Eye troubles generally have their onset during adolescence, and therefore it is especially important at this stage that your child's eyesight should be checked regularly by a qualified ophthalmist. A constant squint, for example, should be investigated immediately. Adolescence may also see the beginning of some spinal conditions, leading to abnormal curvature of the spine. These conditions can be arrested with due medical attention.

Much to the disgust of at least 80 per cent of

Teenagers are very conscious of their appearance, particularly their complexion, and cosmetic manufacturers take advantage of this. Many of these products will merely aggravate existing problems, which could be the result of a lack of fresh air and exercise, regular cleansing, adequate sleep, or a sensible diet.

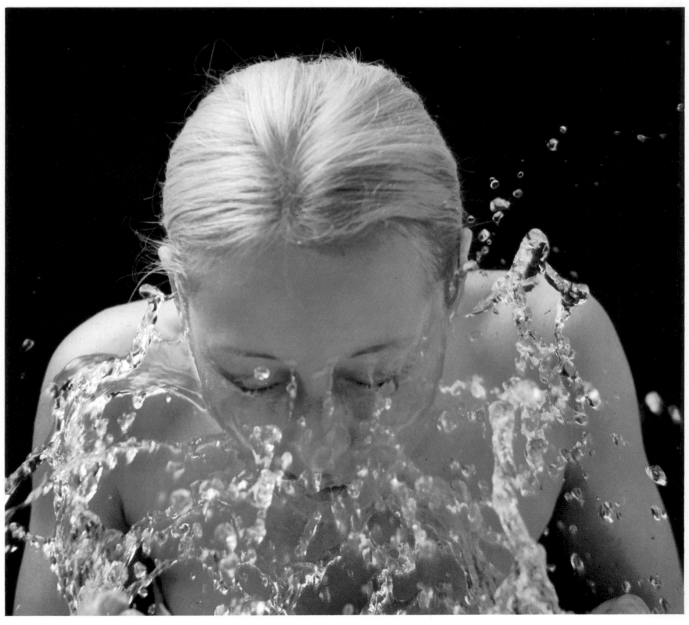

adolescents, this period is also marked by that scourge of the teenage skin known as acne. This is directly caused by the hormones that bring about sexual changes, but it will be of little comfort to your teenager that acne is a sign of maturity, and that it will eventually disappear. Time will probably take care of acne, but it may not take care of the damage acne can do to a teenager's self-esteem.

A severe or persistent case of acne should be handled by the family doctor or a skin specialist. Proprietary acne cures are unlikely to bring more then temporary respite, and may have no effect at all. Each teenager is different, and a remedy that works for one may be totally unsuitable for another. It is far more advisable, therefore, to obtain a prescribed medication to meet the specific needs of your child.

With or without medication to back it up, the best treatment for acne is careful cleansing and attention to diet. The skin should be kept free of excess grease by washing with hot water and soap and drying with a rough towel, three or four times a day. Blackheads or pimples should not be squeezed as this will only help to spread infection and may result in deep-pitted scars. Some foods may obviously aggravate the acne – chocolate is a common offender – and these should be eliminated from the diet. In certain cases antibiotic therapy may prove successful.

Adolescent acne should never be dismissed as "part of growing up." The teenager must be assured that something can and will be done, but that improvement is slow and the therapy may need careful and continuous attention over a long period. Vigorous daily exercise, sufficient sleep, fresh air and direct sunshine seem to do wonders for many complexions.

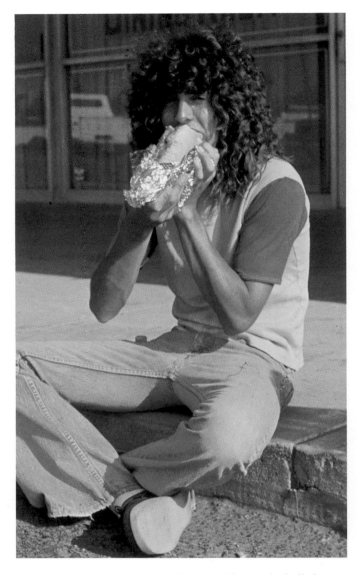

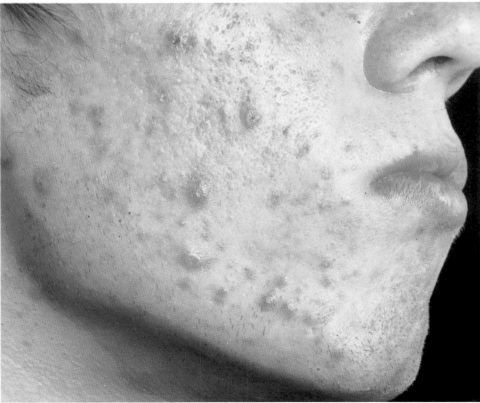

Above: with seemingly little time for proper meals many teenagers settle for fast food of dubious nutritional value.

Left: acne is a common skin disorder in teenagers and there is little at present that can be done about it. At that stage it is of little comfort to the individual to know that most acne disappears in adulthood.

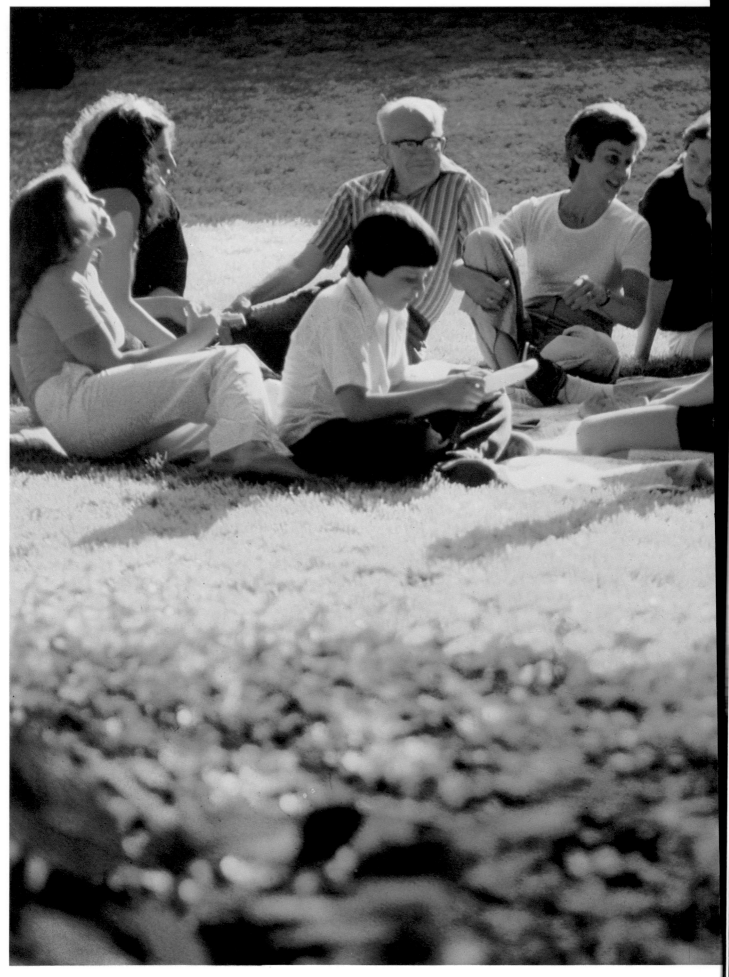

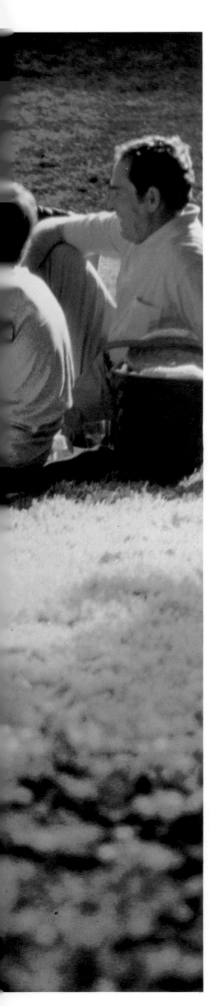

Chapter 10

Trouble in the Family

Throughout the ages, in every society, the family has been a major factor, not only in insuring human survival, but in shaping the life of each of its members. Part of the family's function has always been to give help and support to any of its members whose health has broken down. But when the illness is longterm, or involves problems such as alcoholism, mental instability, or violent behavior, then the giving of this help invariably puts a strain on the healthy members of the family – a strain which can often reach breaking point. The way in which a family responds to such a problem will test and prove its strength.

Opposite: every member of family desires unity and harmony. This ideal is often threatened, usually by minor problems. But sometimes there occurs a major catastrophe, and this is the time when the rest of the family must give support.

Family Relationships

Every family is different. Its success or failure will depend on the personality of each of its members, on its capacity for growth and handling periods of crisis, and a variety of other interacting factors.

The first two or three years of marriage are important. The new couple is immediately faced with a number of difficult decisions. At its simplest level the new husband may be used to his mother running the house in a certain way and he may not realize that his wife may have quite different ideas – based on her mother's system. Often such differences are the basis of the first quarrel. The husband may be quite willing to help with certain jobs about the house, like fixing shelves or gardening – jobs which his father traditionally did, and it comes as a shock when the wife suggests that he does his fair share of the cooking and washing up. Newlyweds can feel overintense about how a home should be run as these ideas are bound up with their background and past way of life, but if their background is a straitjacket, then it must be cast off. The past must be seen in perspective, the new family unit creating its own life, independent from – and yet achieving a happy relationship with – parents and in-laws. This is difficult to accomplish, but is well worth the effort.

This harmonious relationship becomes even more important when the first baby arrives and in fact this is one of the times when special understanding and tolerance is needed. The new baby is going to complete a picture of ideal family life the parents have had in their minds. But later when the young mother finds herself left alone in the house with only the baby for company, sometimes sleeping contentedly, sometimes screaming, she may feel depressed, lonely and even frightened. This is a time when the husband should give his wife as much support as possible and accept that she may not have had the time or the stamina to do the house chores.

It is unavoidable, but parents nearly always have

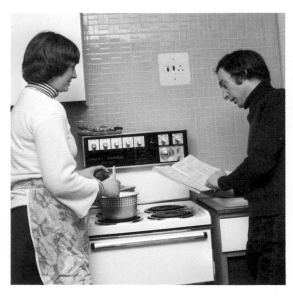

Above: no household skill should be regarded as the preserve of one sex. Although many men were not given the chance as boys to learn how to cook, they can easily remedy this by helping their partners in the kitchen.

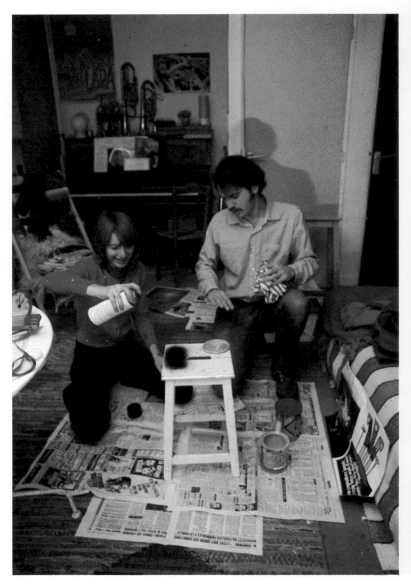

Right: daughters, as well as sons, should be encouraged to help their fathers in what are considered the husband's household duties. This will enable them later to lead independent lives.

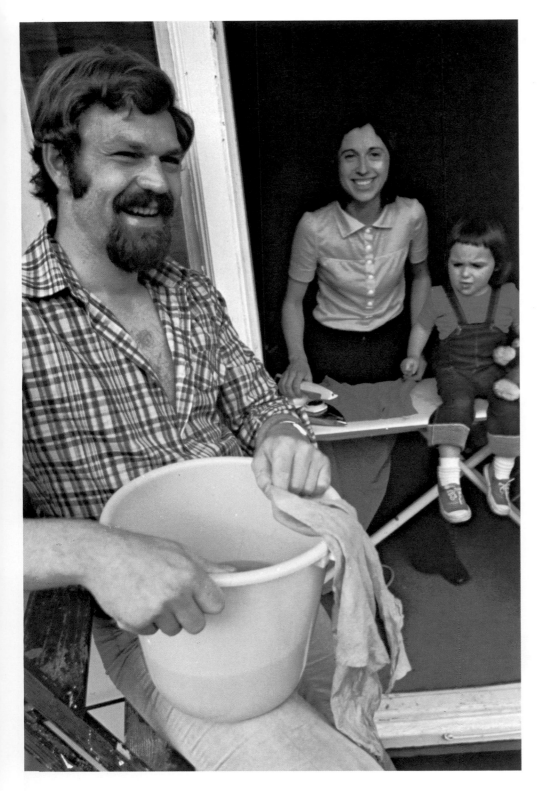

A large number of household tasks are mundane, boring and unpleasant. They can also take a long time to perform. It is unfair to expect one partner to shoulder the burden. But when they are shared by everyone, they take on a new meaning as a communal family activity.

to make some sacrifices in their leisuretime activities when the baby arrives. There may also be a considerable cut in income if the wife was working before the baby arrived. Misunderstandings between husband and wife at this stage – so easily leading to long-lasting resentment – should be strenuously avoided and budgeting should be a combined effort with each partner willing to make compromises.

When a woman has her family is also important. Studies have shown that there is an age band in the fertility span of a woman during which the reproductive risks are at a minimum; on either side of this relatively safe age band, the risks increase progressively. Because there is some controversy among experts as to the exact limits of this age band, women who are in doubt should consult their doctor.

The family is the most basic social unit, the one closest to us. The famous anthropologist Geoffrey Gorer has written that a relationship that includes "give and take, understanding, love, mutual trust, equanimity, sexual compatibility, comradeship, a decent income, mutual interests, happy home life and no money difficulties" would seem to be most people's ideal – but it has to be worked for.

Humans as Social Animals

It is only necessary to watch someone walking into a crowded room to realize that human beings are social animals. Their movements, their dress, their first words of greetings on entering a crowded room all have been shaped to varying degrees by myriads of past interactions with each other.

In studying relationships, social psychologists have used as a central concept the notion of the social group, which they define as: "two or more people who interact more with each other than with other

other and have developed a social instinct. But this theory cannot be tested and the facts may be accounted for more simply by saying that humans join social groups in order to survive. Thus every social group is formed because a number of people have the same objective and none of them can achieve it alone. This is the *group goal* which members share in common. In addition different members stand to gain a wide range of subsidiary advantages. To achieve the group goal, different members must restrict their behavior to roles which complement each other, and they are also expected to conform to certain standards of behavior, beliefs, opinions and attitudes, which are called *norms*.

In the majority of societies, the family is the most powerful social group. When born into a family, we are without any choice exposed to and conditioned by a particular set of cultural norms and role expectations. The leaders of the family control desir-

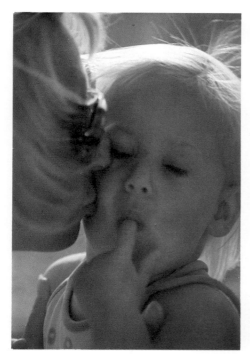

Above: kissing is a gesture of intimacy, and can range from the loving or paternalistic kiss of a parent for a child, and the passionate kiss of a lover, to the formal social greeting.

Right: role expectations are developed very early in life, and many parents foster them unwittingly. Toy household gadgets have no educational or practical value, and they limit a girl's ambitions.

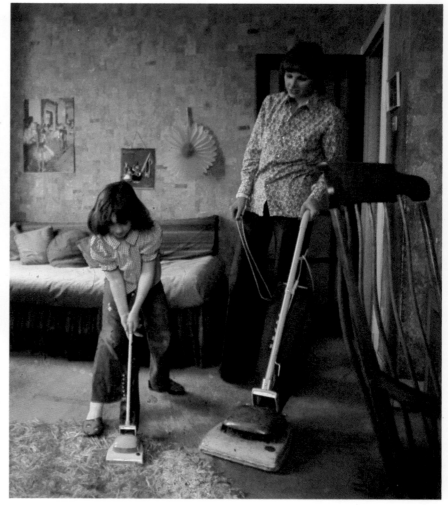

people." Such interactions must occur in order to achieve any objective beyond the reach of an individual. Early examples of prehistoric social grouping must have been moving rocks or lifting logs, hunting for food and building.

It is tempting to say that evolution of humans has been influenced by living in herds for such a long time that people now naturally enjoy living with each

able rewards, such as love and affection. It is hardly surprising, therefore, that in spite of the rebelliousness of the young, attitude surveys show a fairly high similarity between children and their parents on public issues. Also, because it is obvious, it is easy to overlook the fact that the language we first learn is the one spoken in our family and this is probably the richest heritage of a transmitted culture. Although this language is a vehicle of exploration, it also, to a certain extent, selects and limits our attitudes and experience.

The way we are brought up exerts a vital influence on our personality. An important American study of the effects of different types of child rearing was carried out in a New England suburb. The family life of nearly 400 five-year-old children was studied in

them, and were abnormally aggressive. The study also found overwhelming evidence that punishment, in contrast to reward, was quite ineffectual in the training of children.

So we can say that to a certain extent we are all indoctrinated by our own families into behaving in a certain way and believing in a certain set of values. And of course families are bound together by the

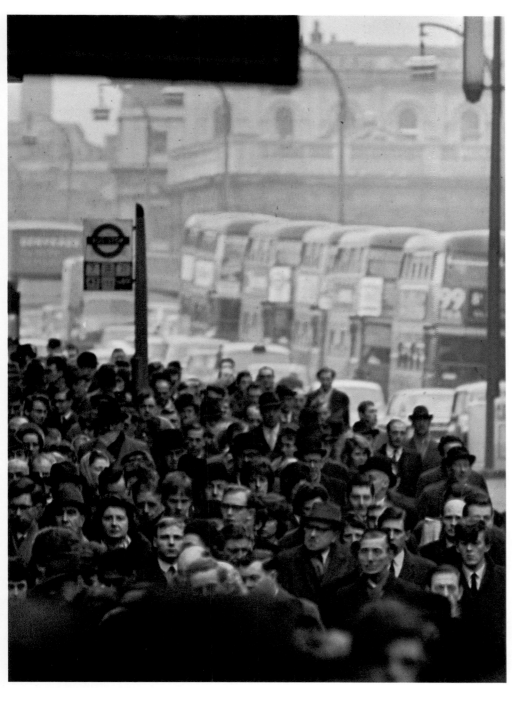

To a greater or lesser extent humans are expected to conform to the social group to which they belong. Societies tend to punish those who deviate.

the home by trained interviewers. They used a schedule covering 72 items of behavior and everything that occurred was tape recorded, transcribed, and subsequently converted into scale form for statistical analysis. The findings showed that in homes where the mother was cold and unresponsive, children often had eating difficulties, bed-wetting problems, did not fit in easily with the people around

group goal. But some people find it distasteful and a reflection on the essential dignity of the human beings to accept that they are products of the processes of social conformity. However, there are no grounds for a prevalent cause of anxiety, which is the idea that conformity reduces us all to dull uniformity. On the contrary, convergence to one group sharpens the divergence from another.

Kinship and Bonding

Why does society take so much care to sanction the union of a man and a woman by transforming it into a legalized marriage? The most obvious reason is that society in this way recognizes a unit through which it can perpetuate itself. Children receive names, status, and material goods from their parents, as well as the culture which they, too, inherited.

The ties of man and woman in marriage, between parents and their children, and between brothers and sisters, make up a network of relationships by kinship and affinity. If we examine our own patterns of kinship and affinity, descent, inheritance, and family behavior, we find many similarities of situations which prevail in other parts of the world, regardless of color, race, or religious convictions. Kin relations are those traced through parent-child or brother-

sister links and are recognized for social purposes. This element of recognition is particularly important in tribal societies.

The family unit has shrunk since Victorian times. Today, a couple and their children make up the usual family unit: it is relatively rare to find more than two generations under one roof, and this unit may have too many loads to bear. There may be too few relatives to turn to for the satisfaction of different kinds of needs. It may be for such reasons that the family unit today is under such stress, why there is so much divorce, so much conflict between parents and children. The shrinkage of the family unit can bring with it other social problems. The old are often relegated to loneliness because their children have no time for them. New forms of social planning often involve the breakup of family units which physically separate old from young, making their former closeness impossible.

On the other hand, small families do have positive benefits. One advantage of a small-scale family may be privacy. Several studies have shown that the physical development of children from large families compares unfavorably with that of children from

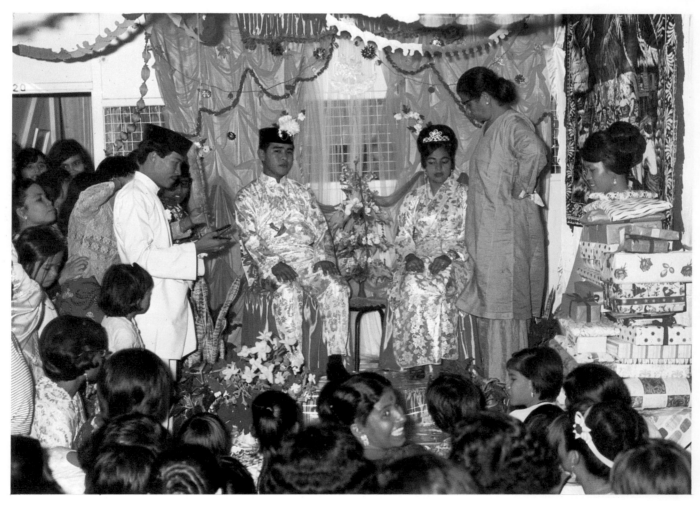

In most societies marriage legalizes the beginnings of a new family unit, and formally unites the families of both partners. For this reason, the marriage may be arranged, as is the case in Islam, which in addition permits polygamy.

small families. And intellectual development tends to be quicker in children from small families.

The children of large families may be prone to disorders not usually experienced by the small-scale

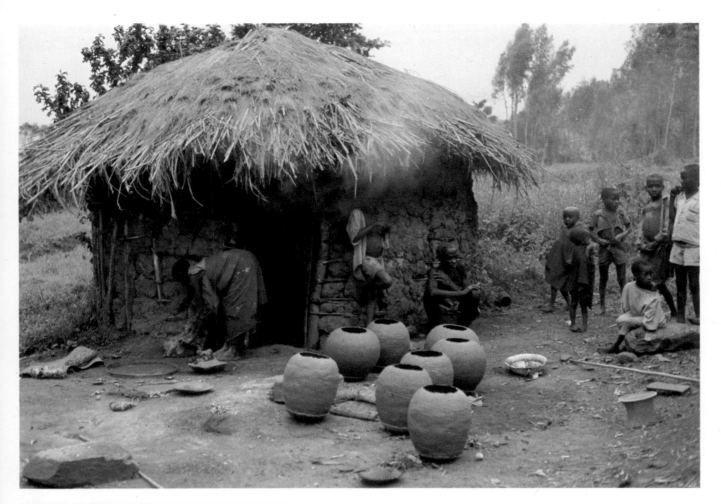

Above: the Tutsi tribe of Rwanda are one of the many tribes for whom the clan is the fundamental social unit. They are a cattle-owning people and have established social and political dominance over the other tribes in the area.

Left: in the West, the nuclear family is the basic social unit. It consists only of the parents and their children. The exceptions are eastern and southern Europe, where the extended family prevails.

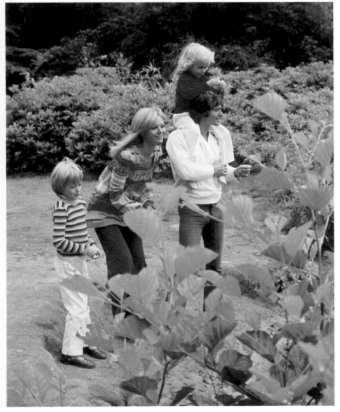

family unit. These include congenital malformations, physical handicaps, malnutrition, dental problems, infectious diseases, emotional problems, and mental illness. Some conditions – such as malnutrition – can

be related directly to the increased strain on family financial and maternal resources that accumulate with each additional child. In the case of common infections, larger families may simply lead to more frequent exposure to infective agents through other members of the family.

The place where one lives has a great importance in many aspects of family life. In some societies a young man goes to live with his wife's family; in others the young wife goes to live with her husband, or the young couple may immediately, or after a period of time, acquire a home of their own. In some primitive societies "home" is where the whole community lives under one roof – complete with all its livestock.

Robert Frost, the American poet, described "home" as "The place where, when you have to go there, they have to 'take you in.'" In Western society parents, spouses, or children are regarded as the people to consult over really serious matters that have to be "kept within the family."

Genetic Legacies

If a person, or one of his close relatives, suffers from a congenital defect, he may be anxious to know whether any children he may have could be in danger of inheriting this defect. Of course the final decision whether or not to take the risk may be influenced by reasons other than medical, such as the parents' desire to have children, the size of the family, economic circumstances, and religious convictions.

Not all congenital defects are hereditary, and not all hereditary defects are congenital. The defects produced in the fetus by the mother having had German measles or other infections are congenital, but not determined genetically, and therefore not hereditary.

The widespread belief that defects that occur repeatedly in a family are hereditary, whereas those that appear sporadically are not, is not necessarily correct. The person with the defect may be the first to show a genic mutation. Or several members of a family may be exposed to the same environment that

Similarly cleft palate and other congenital defects may be due to genetic mutation, to environmental modification, or to a combination of the two.

If a disease-producing trait known to be usually dominant appears in a family, and if the medical history of that family suggests a dominant inheritance, it is possible for a doctor to give a member of that family a good indication of what to expect if he or she has children. An affected man who marries a normal woman would probably be advised by a geneticist that his children have a 50 percent chance of being normal. But if the man comes from a family affected by a dominant disease-producing trait, but does not himself have it, he can be assured that he will not transmit the trait to his offspring. With such cases it is important to have a special and thorough examination to reveal any abnormal trait.

Laboratory tests can often help in detecting carriers of an abnormal trait that hardly manifests itself. A member of a family affected with a disease called hemolytic jaundice may appear free from illness, but have an increased fragility of the red cells, which is revealed only by special tests. "Carriers" of gout can be discovered by tests that show an excess of uric acid in the blood. In addition, before any members of an affected family are declared safe, they must be sure that they have reached an age after which the onset of a hereditary disease is unlikely. Since cerebellar ataxia (an inability to coordinate voluntary

Mendelian inheritance. 1. The gene for brown eyes is dominant over blue and all the offspring of a match between a blue-eyed and a brown-eyed parent are likely to have brown eyes. 2. However, in the next generation blue eyes have a one in four chance of reappearing.

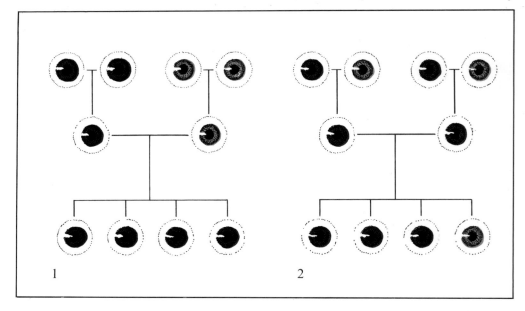

produces the disease. Thus endemic goiter, ricketts, pellagra, and the like, often occur within families, but they are not hereditary and may be prevented by a change in diet and living conditions.

Differentiating between hereditary and non-hereditary defects is further complicated by the fact that a nonhereditary condition may closely resemble a hereditary mutation. Thus congenital cataract is hereditary in some families, but cataract in an infant whose mother had German measles during the early months of pregnancy is of environmental origin.

muscles) may not begin before the age of 40, no member of an affected family should be considered safe before reaching that age.

The behavior of a recessive trait is often difficult to determine. A recessive gene can be carried through many generations without causing visible effects and then the abnormal trait can appear in about the fourth of the children of normal parents who are both carriers. Such traits are sometimes so sporadic that distinguishing them from similar nonhereditary conditions may be very difficult. A man who mani-

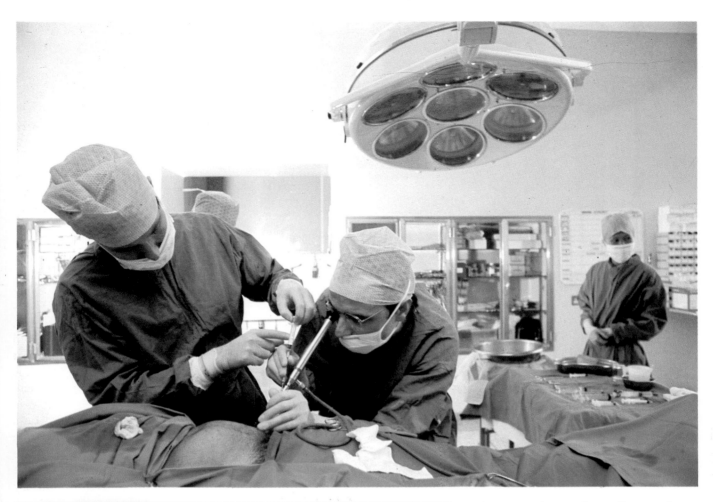

Above: amniocentesis can diagnose the development of the fetus. A sample of amniotic fluid, which will also contain fetal cells, is drawn off from the womb.

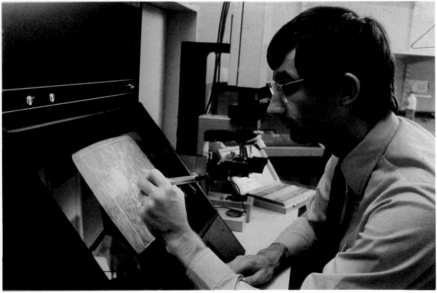

Left: computers are now being used for much faster chromosome karyotyping. This is a systematic arrangement of a cell's chromosomes to show up any abnormalities.

fests an X chromosome-linked recessive trait will – with a normal wife – have sons who neither show nor transmit the trait, but all his daughters will be carriers. The sons of such female carriers will have a 50 percent chance of showing the abnormal trait; those sons who do not manifest the disorder do not transmit it. All the daughters will appear normal, but have a 50 percent chance of being carriers, like their mother. There is usually no way of distinguishing the carrier daughters from their normal sisters unless their offspring reveal their state.

Possible inheritable defects present in an unborn child can be discovered with the aid of modern techniques such as amniocentesis (surgical puncture of the amniotic cavity), tissue culture, biochemical analysis, and chromosomal analysis. Many chromosomal disorders are potentially diagnosable with these techniques, as are many enzyme deficiencies and disorders. If parents are in any way concerned about hereditary defects, then they should see their doctor who will put them in contact with a genetic counseling center.

Mental Subnormality

Mentally subnormal or backward children will show marked signs early in life, as they lag behind normally developing children of the same age. The child whose intelligence is lower than average cannot keep up with normal school work, and therefore needs special educational provision. Extensive studies of the nature of intelligence have shown that mental ability can be classified by regular, graded, stages from the genius to the person with almost no intellectual capacity. Standardized intelligence tests make it possible to group children according to their educational capacities. But intelligence testing is a highly complicated procedure and to have any real validity these tests must be carried out by an expert who knows their limitations, as well as their value.

Among the mentally subnormal whose defect is inborn, the best known are the children with the condition known as Down's syndrome. Children with this disorder have one more than the normal set of chromosomes – 47 instead of 46. Described as "mongols," they make up about five percent of mentally subnormal children. They are usually easy tempered and friendly, and fit happily into normal home life. There is no cure for their mental subnormality, but their abilities can be increased by special training and encouragement. Even if the causes of Down's syndrome remain uncertain, it can be hoped that increasing medical knowledge will eventually help to prevent mongoloid births.

Phenylketonuria is a rare disease caused by the absence in the person's tissues of the enzymes that digest the amino acid phenylalanine. The excess of phenylalanine reduces the amount of oxygen available to vital brain cells. They are poisoned and the growth of the brain is permanently retarded. But if the disease is diagnosed early enough through a blood test, the child can be given a diet low in phenylalanine. In this way the chemical balance of the body is maintained and the brain will develop normally.

Most people are of "average" intelligence. Children with a level of intelligence far below average, may well be happier and better catered for in a special school. The best of these special schools try to provide a friendly atmosphere in which the mentally handicapped can progress up to the highest level of their ability without experiencing the constant pressure of competition with their brighter fellows. Students can learn skills or trades and will probably grow up to be self-supporting members of their community. Advances in research on the learn-

Although the great majority of mentally subnormal children cannot be cured, skilled therapy and specialized education can make the greatest use of their limited abilities.

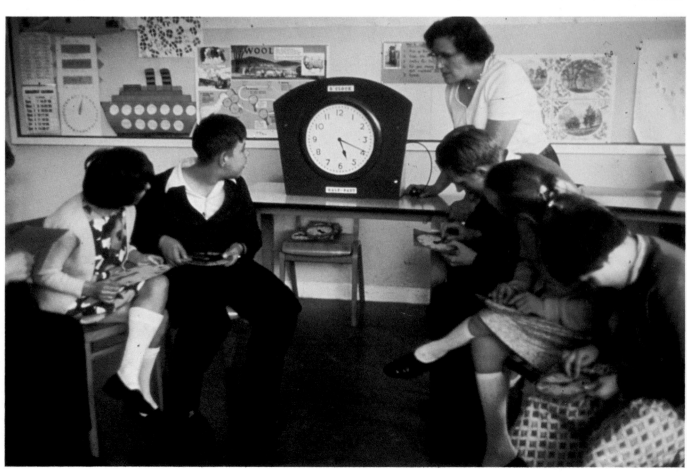

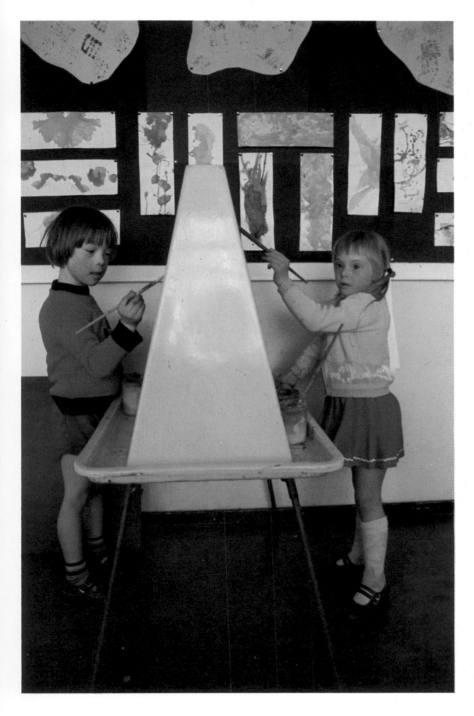

Children with Down's syndrome. In addition to being mentally subnormal, they may have heart or kidney defects, and about half do not survive the first year. Although their mental subnormality is incurable, and they cannot lead independent lives, they are generally happy and contented.

ing processes of backward children have shown that even the severely subnormal can respond to specially planned learning programs. Today emphasis is placed on what children can learn rather than what they cannot. Exciting new teaching techniques are also contributing to the rapid progress in schooling for the backward child.

Care and training for mentally handicapped children must be suited to the capacities and temperament of each individual. Whenever possible, it is best for the child to live at home and attend special day schools or training centers. The effect the retarded child has on the other members of the family must also be considered when making this decision. The child is likely to become a source of emotionally destructive tension in the home and parents may tend to forget that their "problem child" is a human being,

sensitive and full of his or her own needs. Sometimes the family as a whole cannot adjust to the abnormality of the child and cannot establish a satisfactory relationship, in which case everyone will benefit if he or she is placed in a special home. Often a severely subnormal child, very much loved, demands more attention than the mother can give without adverse effects on the rest of the family. It is sometimes possible to place such a child in a simulated family-type unit near enough to home for the family to visit frequently, preserving an important emotional link.

The large amount of medical and education research that is being devoted to mental subnormality and its problems is providing facts and solutions which will gradually dispel many of the superstitions and innacurate popular beliefs concerning mental backwardness.

Coping with Alcoholism

Stephen was a very capable hotel manager. He succeded in increasing the profits in his hotel immensely but since he was obliged to remain in the hotel after his official hours he found it pleasant to have an occasional drink, first in his office offering it to businessmen, later in the bar being offered it by guests. Within a very short time Stephen was drinking a beer with a brandy in the mornings and was hardly ever sober again. In the meantime he and his wife were planning to go into the motel business. His wife invested all her money and the local bank gave them a large loan. Everything was going well at first, but the alcohol took over. Gradually Stephen lost all interest in the new motel, then his wife left him and took the children with her, as she could no longer live with this completely changed person. Then the bank took over the motel and sold it. He was now drinking heavily, mostly strong and cheap liquors. He died a year later, totally emaciated, from a bleeding vein in the lower part of the esophagus; an obvious sequel to the damage done to his liver by alcohol.

This true story is a vivid illustration of how alcohol is the most dangerous drink that man has invented. It is a drug. Used in moderate amounts, its effects are pleasant and harmless. Taken in excess it can lead to both physical and mental breakdown – it can even kill.

Alcoholic content varies widely from drink to drink. Beer is relatively weak in alcohol; wine may be a bit stronger; and hard liquor, such as gin, whisky, rum, brandy or vodka, may contain more than 40 percent of alcohol. Different people react differently to the same amount of alcohol, and this is why it is impossible to lay down precisely what is a "safe" amount to drink. But one thing is certain: even the smallest glass of any alcoholic drink affects the delicately balanced functioning of your body.

Most of us know that a glass or two of wine, a cocktail, a whisky, or a couple of glasses of beer produce a temporary sense of warmth and wellbeing. The alcohol in these drinks dilates the blood vessels of the skin and brings an increased flow of warm blood to the skin surfaces. The pleasant relaxation

Alcohol is a socially accepted drug and consequently the dangers it presents are not taken very seriously. Yet in large quantities, taken regularly, it has a number of deleterious effects, including irritation of the stomach lining, inflammation of the liver, cardiovascular disease, and mental and emotional disorders.

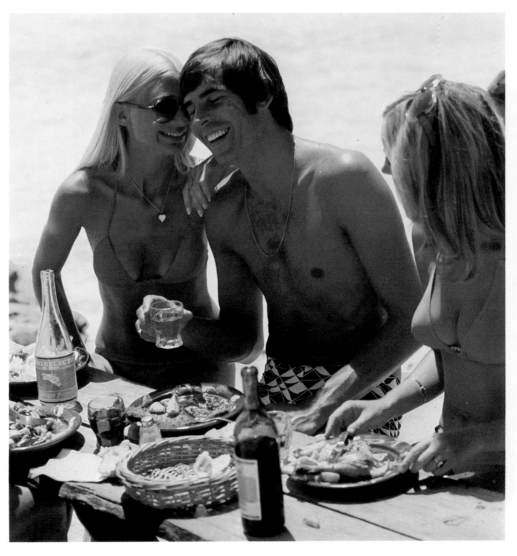

USE AND ABUSE OF ALCOHOL		
stage	blood alcohol level (per cent)	observations of alcoholic intoxication
No apparent change	0.0-0.11	Normal by ordinary observations; slight changes detectable by special tests
Emotional instability	0.09-0.21	Decreased inhibitions; emotional instability; slight muscular incoordination; slowing of muscular responses to stimuli
Confusion	0.18-0.33	Disturbance of sensations; decreased pain sense; staggering gait; slurred speech
Stupor	0.27-0.43	Marked decrease in response to stimuli; muscular incoordination approaching paralysis
Coma	0.36-0.56	Complete unconsciousness; depressed reflexes; subnormal temperature; anesthesia; impairment of circulation; death possible for some persons
Death	over 0.44	Death possible when blood alcohol concentration reaches this level

Source: Adapted from B.S. Bergersen et al., *Pharmacology in Nursing*, St. Louis, C.V. Mosby.

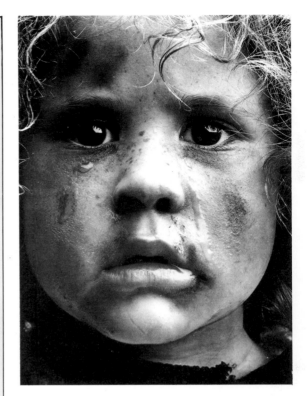

Above: this British Health Educational Council poster was designed to emphasize the neglect suffered by the children of alcoholics.

Left: the acute effects of alcohol. A number of other factors influence the state of intoxication. These include weight, duration and dilution of drink, and whether or not the subject had eaten beforehand.

and sense of feeling good is created because alcohol depresses the central nervous system. It acts as an anesthetic on the cerebral cortex which exercises conscious control over behavior. With the cortex lulled into happy lassitude, the primitive brain has a freer rein. So if you brighten up after a drink, or speak and act just a trifle more freely than usual, you do so because the restraining influences which usually monitor behavior have been diminished. The more you drink, the greater is the effect of alcohol on the nervous system. This eventually disturbs balance, so that the drinker begins to stagger and may pass out. The long-lasting effect of persistent excessive drinking is the creation of the alcoholic.

The effects of an alcoholic in the family are devastating. Apart from economic loss, the burden is oppressive to such an extent that without treatment and good counseling the outcome is grim. If the father drinks, he may soon become a menace to the rest of the family. If the wife takes to the bottle, the disorder at home will make life unbearable.

What can be done? Treating an alcoholic is difficult. One method that has proved successful is the type of group therapy practiced by the Alcoholics Anonymous organization. Under the guidance of a psychotherapist the group can help its members, all alcoholics, to overcome individual weaknesses and if they are able to talk freely about their addiction and visualize the outcome, then there is still hope for them.

The family itself can sometimes help its alcoholic, but this is difficult as it has the natural tendency to forgive mistakes too easily and thus encourage the alcoholic to start drinking again. Indeed, the drinker's immediate family often needs help as well, to cope with the emotional problems of which the alcoholic may be both creator and victim. There are specialized agencies that as well as helping to rehabilitate alcoholics also help the stricken families. To any family coping with an alcoholic in its midst the following words of encouragement from one US agency will be of help: "Through successfully resisting alcoholism as a threat to the survival of family life, each member may find new ways to improve his or her own daily life. When the ill member has embarked on a course of treatment which may bring about total recovery, and the other members of the family are aware of their proper roles in stabilizing family relationships, the rest becomes only a matter of time, and effort. The family is on the right track again."

199

An Invalid in the Family

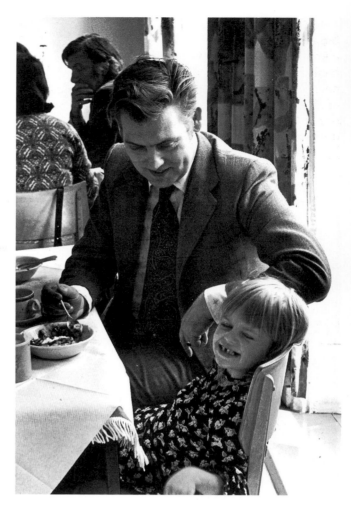

Probably you know from your own or your neighbor's experiences that the family problems raised by long-lasting disability are numerous. They are well illustrated by a study made in New York City of the families of children with rheumatoid arthritis. Almost all these families were heavily burdened financially and more than a quarter of them went into debt. Others had to reduce their standard of living drastically, cutting out every possible expenditure on such things as clothing, furniture, recreation, or vacations. Some fathers took extra jobs, and the mothers also had to find employment. Some were given assistance by the state agency for aid to dependent children, the Red Cross, fraternal organizations, employees' benevolent organizations, or the Arthritis and Rheumatism Foundation.

Above right: a disabled child should be included in as many outside activities as is possible.

Below: you may have to make certain adjustments in your home, particularly in the kitchen and bathroom.

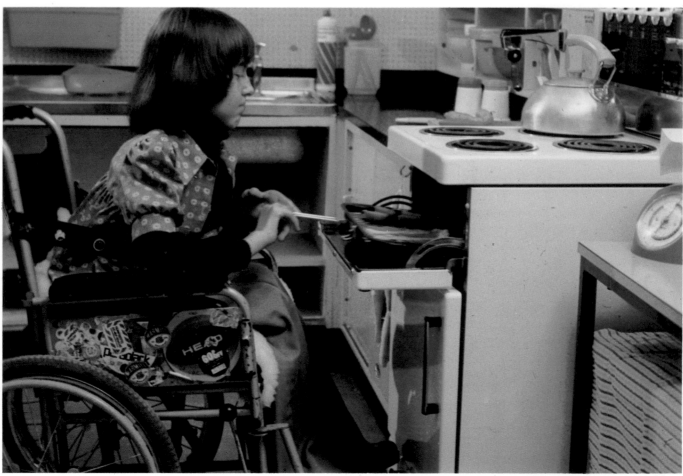

In the hope of aiding their invalid's recovery, some families moved to larger homes, some to a warmer climate, and others to a location nearer to medical facilities. In several instances, grandparents moved nearer in order to be of assistance. About one-third of the mothers suffered serious physical and emotional strain as a result of their anxiety and extra duties. Some of them became sick enough to require

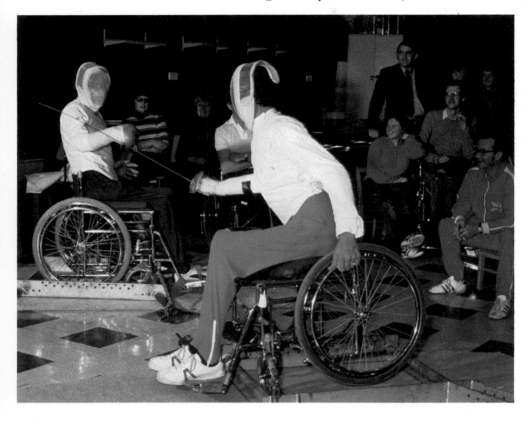

Partially disabled people can compensate for the immobility of some of their muscles by overdeveloping others. Many have been able to participate in their favorite sports, with only a few modifications. There are even Olympic Games devised for paraplegics.

medical care. Transportation to the doctor or clinic was a serious problem. If the child was wearing a cast, a taxi was necessary, and there was rarely any outside assistance with this expense. The amount of time consumed in medical visits added to the mothers' problems.

Many of the children were depressed, anxious, irritable, socially withdrawn or overdependent at some time during the illness. Some of the families had difficulties with the brothers and sisters either because of actual neglect of the healthy children or because of jealousy. However, many other parents observed that brothers and sisters were sympathetic and understanding toward the sick child.

Families that have problems with an invalid are often unaware of the potential help that is available. And some families are slow to take advantage of community resources because of timidity or pride. But families should make an effort to find out exactly what and where the community services are before they decide whether or not to use them. Families themselves have taken the initiative in different parts of the country and formed groups to secure community help where it did not previously exist. A number of the large organizations for helping handicapped children grew from just such beginnings.

As far as is possible, the handicapped child or adult invalid should be included in family activities. But what is taken for granted with other members may require special thought. For instance the schedule should be planned so that the invalid is not resting or having therapy at the time when the others want to be active. Being with the rest of the family at meals or as they watch television, sharing the morning goodbyes as others go to work, receiving guests – these are only a few of the normal home-life situations in which a disabled member of a family can participate. Naturally there are family activities in which handicapped people cannot participate, but the important point is to be conscious of the needs of the disabled members of the family so that they do not feel excluded.

When the family of Peter, an adolescent who was mentally handicapped, moved into a new neighborhood, his parents soon noticed that neighbors called their young children inside when he tried to join them. Peter's parents asked the president of the local association for handicapped children to come to their home for afternoon tea with the neighbors. He explained the meaning of mental retardation to the group, told them about the training Peter has received, and assured them that they need not worry about their small children. The neighbors had a chance to ask questions and to get acquainted with Peter. Soon afterwards some of them invited him to their homes and, when they saw that he cut the grass at his own home, offered him a chance to earn money by mowing their lawns. Before long, both the parents and the children of the neighborhood were Peter's friends.

Violence and Aggression

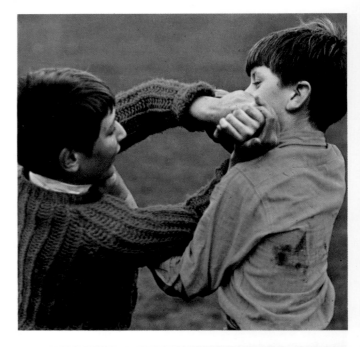

The problem of human aggressiveness has always been with us. But violence within the family, especially violent acts committed by parents against their children – often leading to permanent injury or death – and by parents against one another, is causing growing concern. Our newspapers and television screens are crowded with images of bloodshed, violence and brutality, both on a global level with reports of wars and communal strife, and on a domestic level with the increasing incidences of muggings, vandalism and baby battering.

Above right: physical aggressive behavior is frequently encouraged between boys, in sport and in play, as a training for the competitive adult world.

Right: there is a strong correlation between social deprivation and crime.

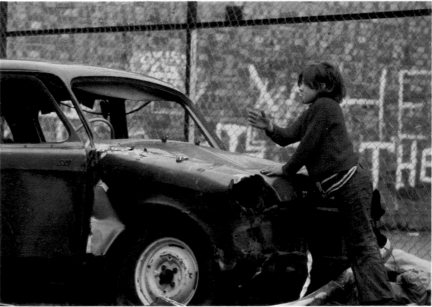

There are of course biological factors, such as brain malfunction and genetic errors, that contribute to violent behavior, but nevertheless today it is widely accepted that social factors, such as upbringing and the example set to children by parents and by the mass media, and the quality and frustrations of life, all contribute to a person's aggressive patterns of behavior.

Restraints are placed upon children in the process of socialization, and severe deprivations and frustrations occur throughout our adult lives. It may be that aggressive impulses could thus accumulate and merge. Sometimes chronic irritation builds up a vast amount of vague "unattached" protest; whereas when life is smoother, there may be relatively little of such free-floating aggression. In an attempt to understand the roots of aggression, the vital role that parents play in the development of a child's personality, and in the transmission of cultural attitudes and values, has led researchers to look closely at how children are brought up. A proneness to violence has been found to depend to a great extent on a child's identification with, and imitation of, the parents' behavior, in particular the father's. Persistent rejection by one or both parents often triggers off aggressive behavior. Children who have received harsh physical punishment over a long period of time tend to react to this kind of discipline with aggressiveness in their everyday behavior, and when they grow up often inflict the same kind of punishment on their own children.

In humans and higher species of animals, the males are habitually more aggressive than the females. Most crimes of assault are committed by young men in their late teens, twenties or early thirties. Some authorities believe that the biological difference in aggression between men and women makes for the stability of the family and for sexual

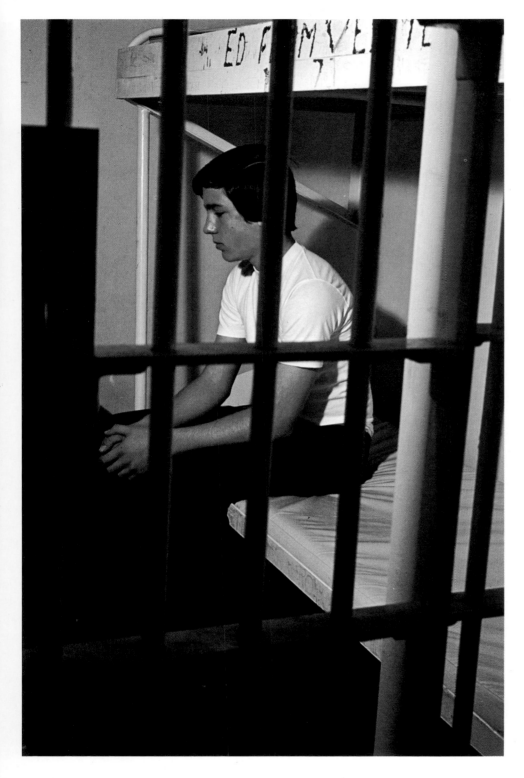

Prison is society's solution to crime. But imprisonment in a rigorous, strictly disciplined institution has been shown not to be the answer for young offenders. They invariably return to crime, often with tips picked up from professional inmates.

happiness between couples. Aggression is said to provide the impetus for the child to throw off the long period of helplessness and dependence on parents, for the striving toward a sense of identity and autonomy. Aggression would therefore be necessary to achieve one's ambitions in a competitive world.

Can anything be done to reduce the hostility which exists between and within people? Moral vetoes on violent behavior, or the application of harsh punishment, do not seem to work. In fact they can have just the opposite effect as has been found by parents, schools, and – in a wider context – societies which

have tried to suppress the aggressiveness of their members in this way. Comparisons of various institutions – such as one using harsh discipline and others using the philosophy of understanding – have proved very illuminating. Violent boys were unchanged by the "hard work and harsh discipline" regime, but those who were treated with understanding showed important and desirable changes. One of the directors of such an institution has pointed out: "Punishment teaches the child only how to punish; scolding teaches him how to scold. By showing him that we understand, we teach him to help; by cooperating, we teach him to cooperate."

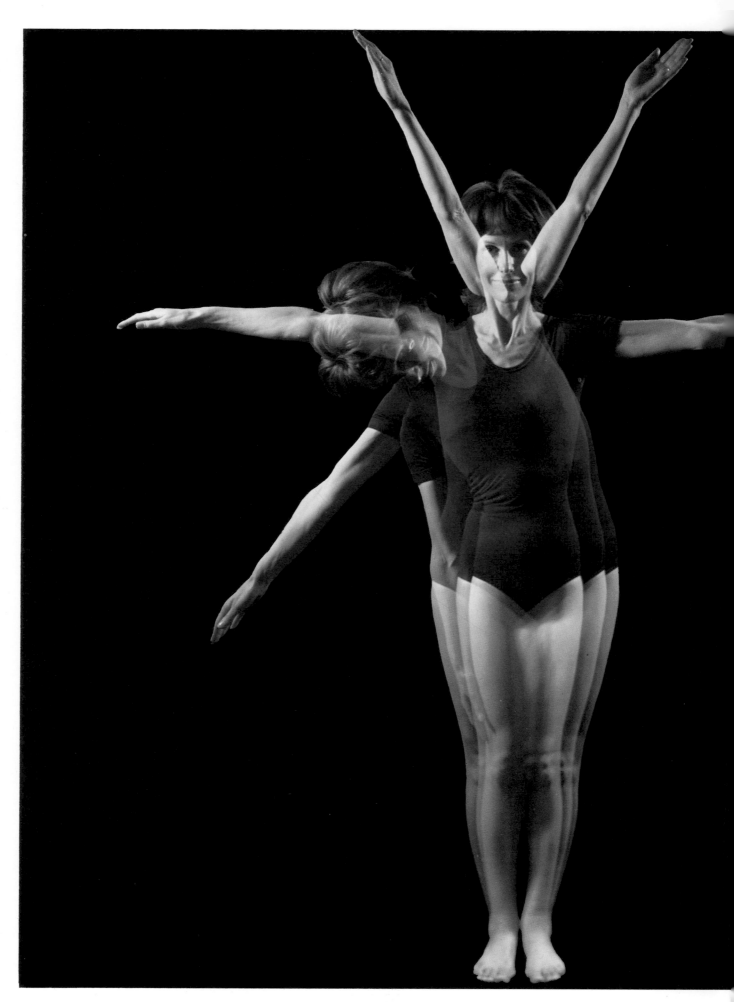

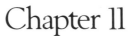

Chapter 11

Keeping Fit
Every Day

One dictionary definition of exercise is: "Regular or repeated appropriate use of a faculty, power, or bodily organ." Thus even if we never run, jog, swim, or play sports, we are nevertheless indulging in some sort of exercise: the mere act of living insures this. But the key words are "regular" and "appropriate." Whatever exercise program you choose – either to achieve real fitness or to remain fit – you must make sure that the exercises appeal to you enough to make you feel that you can face doing them regularly, and that they are right for your age, weight, and present level of fitness.

Opposite: keeping fit is not unnatural; it is our life-styles which are not suited to our bodies. Yet it is easy and painless to incorporate a minimum of physical exercise into our daily lives.

Health
is Beautiful

The process of living has two dimensions. One is the sheer number of days of our lives. The other is the quality of the life experience itself – what we get out of it and what we put into it in return. If we maintain our bodies in top physical condition through proper eating, sensible exercise and adequate rest, then both dimensions should be enlarged. We will stand a good chance of living longer, and be able to make a greater contribution to the overall happiness of our families

Right: a demanding occupation brings job satisfaction, but too much pressure can build up stress.

Below: a healthy life is one which is enjoyed to the full, and this enjoyment should be shared with others.

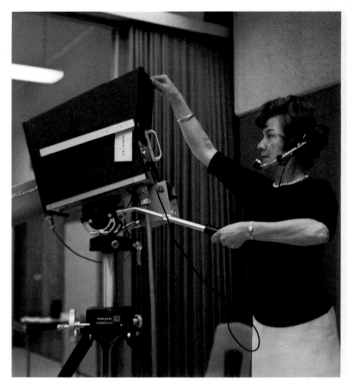

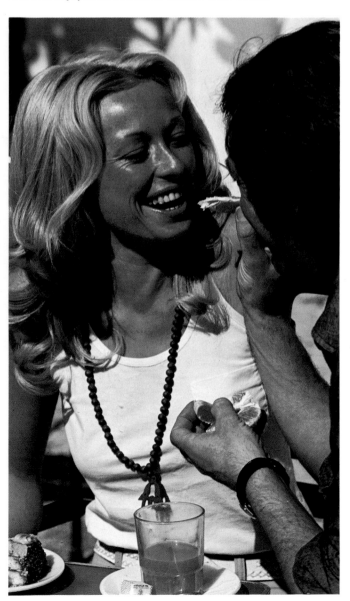

and ourselves. We will feel good and – equally important – our inner health will manifest itself through our outward appearance.

One essential part of any program for healthy living is daily exercise. Exercise can make you look, think, sleep and feel better. It can help release tension and stress, prevent aches and pains, improve circulation, and keep your heart and lungs in good order. Work alone is usually not enough, because it exercises only certain muscles – and often not in the proper way. Exercising for health, however, is like eating for health. Both work best when you follow a regular regimen, and least well when you try to beat past abuses with crash programs. If you lead a sedentary life, are overweight and feeling stale, do not embark on a vigorous fitness campaign first thing tomorrow. The most you will get from a sudden bout of strenuous exercise is sore muscles and you will probably give up there and then. Instead, make it a rule to do at least 10 minutes of mild exercise three times a week. The benefits of small amounts of exercise do mount up, and a minimal exercise program is enough to keep you fit, healthy and vital – provided you follow it regularly.

Many of us have one particular point of our body that we would like to change for the better. This can be done – but there are limits. Your basic skeleton cannot be altered. You have only fat and muscles to work with, and unfortunately you cannot take the fat off just in one spot. Fat is lost by burning more calories than are consumed and it comes off the different parts of the body that store it, all at the same time. Muscle, however, can be built up selectively to keep you in proportion and give you a better shape. For example, a woman may have pleasantly proportioned legs, but heavy buttocks and waist.

An isometric exercise for tightening the breast muscles. Place your right fist in your left palm and push with the left arm to the right, while resisting with the right. If you are performing it correctly, you will feel your breast lifting. Then try it with the right arm pushing the left.

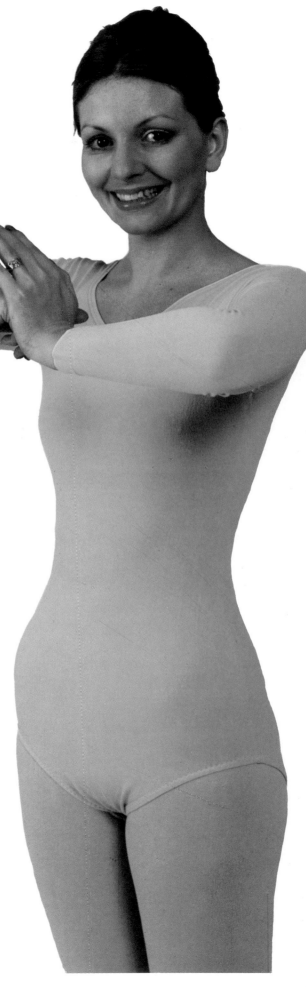

She can remedy this situation. First she should go on a diet to get rid of the extra fat. But then her legs above the calves will be too thin, because she will have lost weight there too. So, while exercising her whole body to keep it trim, she should concentrate on leg exercises that will build up the muscle tissue in order to bring her legs into proportion with her now slimmer buttocks and waist.

But there is one important exception to this sytem as far as women are concerned – the breasts. These are composed of fat tissue and contain no muscle. Breast size is almost entirely due to fat deposits and exercise can only tighten the muscles around the breasts to give a firmer breastline. One such exercise, which is particularly helpful for sagging breasts, is to stretch the arms out in front, bend the elbows, and grip your forearms as if you were pushing up both sleeves at once. Push several times in sharp jerks, then relax. This exercise should be repeated about six times a day.

Good posture is important. Apart from being vital to your appearance and comfort, the way you stand, sit and move is also important to your health. Good posture aids breathing, circulation, digestion, and puts far less strain on muscles and joints; it even helps the nervous system to function efficiently.

Exercise and diet are vital to good inner health, but they must be combined with adequate rest and relaxation. If your body and mind are tense, you will feel and look tired. For the way you look depends just as much on what is going on inside your body as on anything you do to the outside. No amount of exercise can right the havoc caused by fatigue and tension. But exercise can help to relieve tension and make you relax. And knowing that you are physically fit and attractive will give you added confidence.

Everyday
Fitness

Most experts today emphasize that health and physical fitness are interdependent. And even if your "health," in the traditional sense of the word, becomes impaired, keeping as physically fit as possible will often help you to fight your illness much more effectively than if you are totally unfit.

A person's position on his or her "health scale"

Below: the symptoms of profound fatigue are muscular and nervous exhaustion. There may be headaches, and a yearning for sleep. Mental fatigue is very similar to boredom, and is more common after a boring, repetitive task than an equally demanding but interesting one.

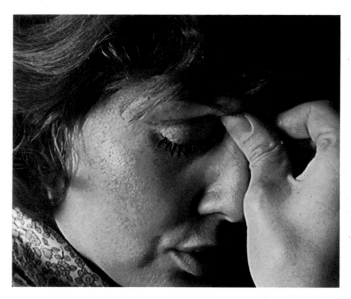

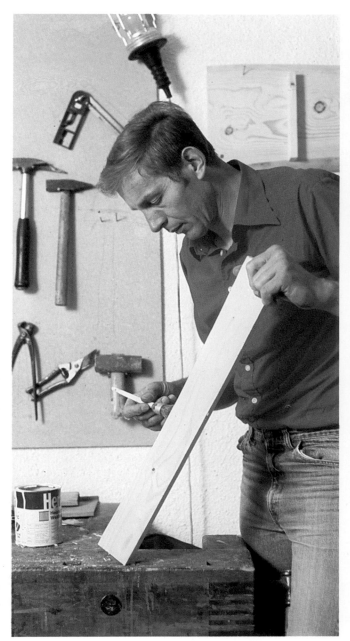

Above: physically demanding work exercises the muscles to full capacity but does little for the brain. People engaged in such work often need a creative pastime to compensate for this lack.

may fluctuate slowly as a result of subtle, unobservable changes. But this position can be controlled to some extent by the individual. If a person neglects the body's needs for physical activity, this may shift that person's position to the "unhealthy" side of the scale, whereas a suitable exercise program may result in a shift to "healthy." Although so many factors affect a person's position on the "health scale" that it may be impossible to know exactly what that position is, he or she can actively increase the probability of being as far to the "healthy" side as it is possible.

When a person reaches a level of what is called "minimal functional fitness," he or she has the ability to respond physically and emotionally to the typical daily activities and problems of life in such a way as to maintain the mind and body in good order and to function effectively in society. But it is not always possible to maintain this desired standard of fitness. Some changes in our bodies may not be

noticeable and thus beyond our control until some symptoms occur. However you can determine whether you are responding to the challenge of life in such a way that you are not constantly tired, and you should know if you are happy and generally relaxed and whether you have the capacity to enjoy life. On the other hand, if you are constantly fatigued, often gloomy, prone to temper, unable to relax, and can see little purpose in life, it takes only a bit of self-analysis to become conscious of the state you are in. And if this happens then it is quite likely that you have not attained the minimal functional fitness level and should be actively remedying the situation.

A functionally fit person has the capacity to respond to near maximum, short-term effort or sustained work without bodily or emotional distress.

Such a person will then have an increased capacity to enjoy life and is also capable of carrying out a number of common physical tasks without undue discomfort or injury.

It is obvious that minimal functional fitness varies from person to person. Because people are engaged in such differing kinds of work, and because any given situation may produce very different responses in different people, plans for achieving and maintaining fitness must be extremely flexible so as to suit the individual. Whereas someone engaged in a physically demanding occupation may need a creational pastime, a more sedentary person may well need a relatively energetic activity. Thus some people may find fulfillment and emotional release in hobbies, while others need sporting activities. The ultimate decision must be left to the individual and may or may not involve vigorous exercise, relaxation techniques, or even a change of job.

One of the immediate effects of physical fitness is what it can do for your sexual performance, both in terms of frequency and quality. The more responsive your body, the more heightened will be your sensual sensations. Sexual activity makes demands on the neuromuscular and cardiovascular systems, and it produces an elevated heart rate and blood pressure. If you are tired out and flabby, your responses will match your physical state.

How do you avoid, after a weekend's work in the garden or moving heavy furniture, being so sore and stiff that you can hardly move your aching and supersensitive body from the bed next morning? It is not a simple question, and exercise is only part of the answer. But in order to arrive at your minimal functional fitness level, you must expend more energy, and in different ways, if you are to avoid the more serious consequences of unaccustomed, occasional, near maximum work or play efforts. The best form of prevention appears to be a personally designed, never-ceasing plan for attaining this fitness – and you do not have to be a competitive athlete with a high level of sporting skills in order to achieve this.

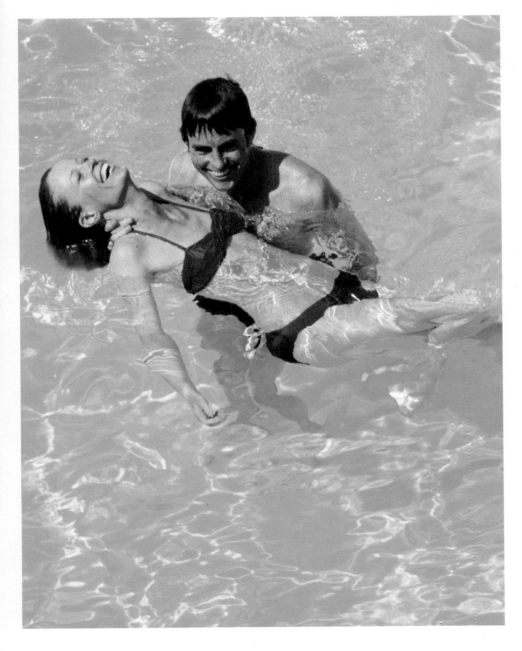

Many of us have sedentary occupations and do not get sufficient exercise. Muscles become flabby, posture suffers, and the heart and lungs deteriorate from underuse. We should therefore take advantage of any local facility for sport or other physical activities.

The Benefits of Exercise

Many people believe that exercise can damage the heart. A newspaper gives an account in its obituary column of the death of a 52-year-old man – cause of death: heart attack while shoveling snow. It would seem that for this man exercise at that particular time was not beneficial and was the direct cause of his death. According to up-to-date statistics, out of every 100 fatal heart attacks, nine occur during heavy physical activity, and in these cases it could be argued that exercise was the direct cause. However, by the same token neither is being fast asleep in bed beneficial for the 13 percent whose fatal attacks occur at this time. Standing and talking are even more dangerous: 37 percent have fatal attacks under these conditions. It is not necessary to labor this point. Properly conducted exercise will not cause heart attacks.

A similar misconception – that too much exercise causes a condition known as "athlete's heart" – has been discounted. An athlete may well develop a larger and stronger heart than will the average person for his size, but this is not the enlarged heart seen in certain kinds of heart disease. The larger heart of the athlete appears to be a perfectly normal and useful adaptation to the demands placed upon it.

There is little doubt that regular and at least moderate exercise will reduce the resting heart (pulse) rate. This means that the heart rests more often and there is evidence that its total work is decreased and its efficiency increased. Based on the law of use and disuse, the increased blood pressure during exercise might exert some beneficial influence on the elasticity of the blood vessel walls. Taking this line of thinking a stage further, it is possible that disuse hastens the hardening of the arteries. Although this is a controversial area, there is evidence also in support of the claim that regular exercise does increase red blood cell count, hemoglobin and total blood volume. One of the obvious benefits is that exercise increases the oxygen-carrying capacity of the blood.

We could make a long list of the obvious physical benefits of regular exercise. And it would be pleasing to add to the list that exercise helps us to live longer. But unfortunately, there is little direct evidence to support this claim. However, some serious studies have revealed startling and dramatic longevity differences between groups taking regular exercise and those taking none at all. In one study, even in the 45-49 age group, there were 4.6 times as many deaths in the group taking no exercise. Even if, to quote the study, "ill health may reduce the ability or the desire to exercise," it would appear to be an important piece of evidence for this theory.

The claim had been made that athletics and physical education activities can improve a person's self-image and thus help with personality problems. It seems more reasonable to say that exercise, athletic competitions and physical education can contribute in improving personality, but there is no assurance that this will happen. There are wonderful opportunities in competition and physical education for positive personality growth, but the benefits actually derived are more dependent upon the individual's

Physical exercise should not be viewed as a penance for an overindulgent life, but an enjoyable activity for all the family. For their children's sake as well as their own, parents should set a good example.

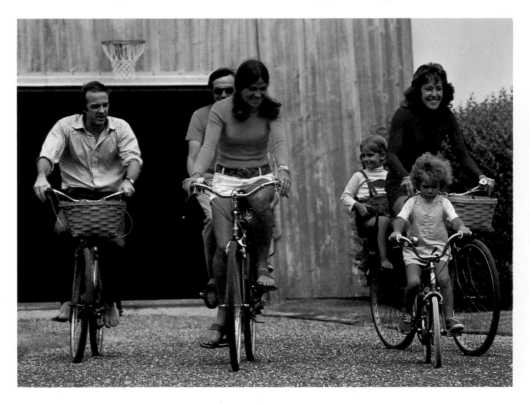

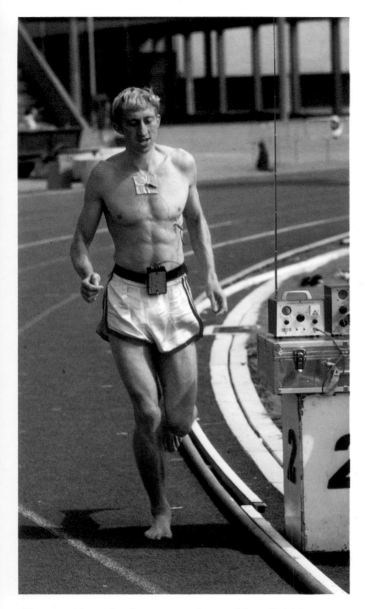

Above: athletes develop stronger hearts. Here, British athlete David Hemery is having his heart-beat monitored.

Right: a huge muscle mass has limited uses and for the average person puts extra demand on the heart.

response than upon the activities themselves.

There are conflicting reports as to whether regular exercise will help a person to integrate better into society or reduce aggressive tendencies. Nearly all the studies carried out on specific groups of athletes have concentrated on such factors as athletic ability, size and intelligence, and have not been concerned with the regular everyday activities of the athletes or whether they are happy, well-adjusted members of society. However, in school and college life the successful athletic performers are often accorded a higher social acceptance than they possibly deserve.

Although exercise can help to relieve tension and depression, it is not possible to say catagorically that regular exercise will prevent mental illness. There are too many factors involved to make any sweeping statements on the matter. But it is known that exercise can be of great help to those people recovering from a mental breakdown.

Strength is often equated with fitness, but this is not necessarily true. Firstly, strength does not depend solely on muscle size or how much they bulge – the so-called "definition" of the muscles, although there is little question that people with large and well developed muscles are usually physically strong. In attempting to achieve health and fitness the emphasis is not entirely on appearance, but functional capacity and individual needs. Secondly, strength is quite often confused with muscular endurance. But the measure of true strength is the maximal amount of force that a muscle or muscle group can exert. It is not properly measured by determining the maximum number of repetitions of a certain activity, such as push-ups or sit-ups. Maximum strength is evaluated by determining the maximum one-effort force. However, a minimum level of strength is obviously necessary for you to be fit.

You can get stronger without enlarging your muscles, and you can also enlarge your muscles without much increase in strength. Indeed big muscles might not be such a good idea in the first place, except for those who need massive bodies to put against heavy loads, such as weightlifters. Ironically the popular Tarzan-like symbol of fitness for men – a massive chest, shoulders, arms, and legs – can be a physical drawback. A large muscle mass means an extra weight to carry around. In a sense, it is like being obese. But beware of the other extreme. If you do not use your muscles they will waste away, but when you move them every muscle becomes an auxiliary heart, helping to pump blood. When a muscle contracts, it squeezes blood toward the heart; when it relaxes, it allows the muscle to be filled with blood – exactly like your heart.

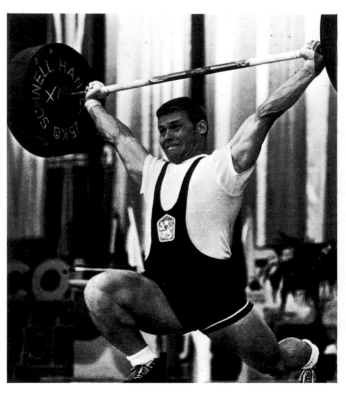

Smoking
or Health

"Smoking *or* Health" was the title given to the third report from the Royal College of Physicians of London, published in 1977. The choice is that blunt – a smoker may live a relatively long life, and appears to be quite well, but he or she is certainly not healthy, and not as fit as they are capable of feeling.

Any other drug which produced or was implicated in the number of diseases that smoking is would find itself banned. But many of the dangers of cigarettes were not realized until long after smoking had been established as a socially acceptable drug, a highly profitable industry, a psychological crutch and a symbol of adulthood and sophistication. But whatever the reason for starting, most smokers soon get addicted – to a habit which proves to be more and more dangerous on each investigation.

Many heavy smokers start when they are still children, and their parents are usually smokers themselves. To the young, cigarettes appear as a symbol of adulthood and sophistication, an image often fostered by advertising.

The dependence of smokers is due to the presence, in tobacco, of nicotine. Nicotine has widespread effects on the body, including nausea in a novice smoker, raising of the blood pressure, increase in heartbeat and constriction of the surface blood vessels. Like any addictive substance, its cessation brings on withdrawal symptoms, and the so-called pleasure from smoking is as much due to answering the body's craving for the substance – the "soothing" effect of tobacco. Nicotine is also a poison.

Tobacco smoke contains tar, which has been found to contain at least 20 carcinogens and more seem to be discovered on each investigation. Tobacco tar is also an irritant; it clogs the lungs and prevents the mucous membranes from doing their job of clearing out particles efficiently.

The third culprit in tobacco smoke is carbon monoxide, the poisonous gas present in exhaust fumes. Carbon monoxide combines with the hemoglobin in the blood and thus reduces its capacity for carrying oxygen. The effect is thus that of oxygen starvation – the smoker is less able to do any strenuos exercise and tires easily. It is estimated that in heavy smokers the oxygen-carrying capacity of the blood is reduced by 15 percent.

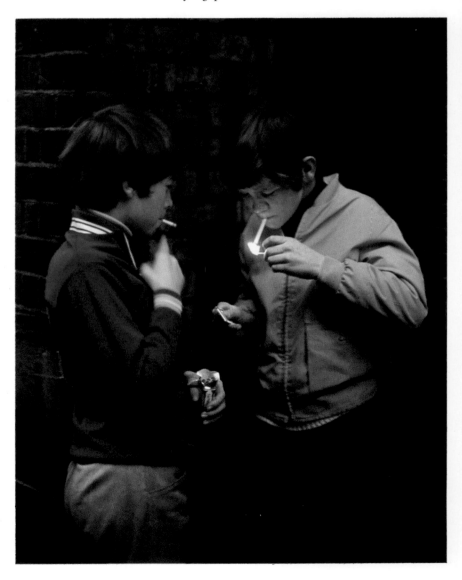

The link between lung cancer and cigarette smoking is so strong that it cannot be dismissed as a statistical coincidence nor can it be ignored. Lung cancer takes a relatively long time to develop but is commonly incurable. As a killer disease in the West, it comes second only to coronary heart disease. Smokers run a far heavier risk of contracting the disease, even more so if they inhale deeply, take many puffs of each cigarette and do not put it down after each puff. Tobacco smoke also increases a person's chances of developing cancer of the mouth, throat and windpipe, and has been implicated in cancer of the bladder and urinary tract.

The inhalation of cigarette smoke is a direct assault on the lung, and apart from cancer other lung diseases are far more common in smokers than nonsmokers. *Chronic bronchitis* (gradual inflammation of the passages in the lungs), often accompanied by *emphysema* (breakdown of the air sacs), are invariably the result of long-term heavy smoking and the familiar "smoker's cough," which is an attempt to clear the excessive amounts of phelgm produced by the lungs, is a prelude to chronic bronchitis. In general the lungs of smokers are more susceptible to infections of various kinds.

of non-smoking mothers. The frequency of still-birth and death in the first week of life is 30 percent more common in mothers who smoke heavily after the fourth month of pregnancy.

The risks of smoking are so great and also very well publicized and yet smoking is still a very common habit. There are some who either ignore the warnings or claim they enjoy the habit too much, but many do indeed find giving up extremely difficult. Part of the problem is that cigarette addiction is not purely physical but involves a number of psychological factors. Smokers smoke to indulge, to be stimulated, sedated, or for oral gratification. Many heavy smokers are so habituated that they light up automatically even when they already have a cigarette on the burn. The obvious advice to a smoker is to give up, but how to is not so easy to answer. For some the easiest way is to stop altogether; others succeed by a more gradual method – cutting down or changing to safer alternatives such as filter cigarettes, ventilated filters, cigars and pipes. The smoke produced by cigars and pipes is alkaline and thus the nicotine can be absorbed through the mouth, unlike the acid smoke of cigarettes which has to be inhaled.

There are no "cures" for smoking, other than a

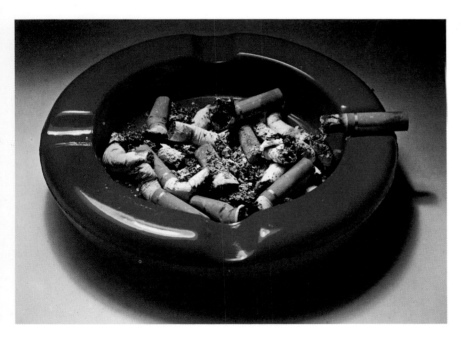

If this is your ashtray at the end of the day, then you are a heavy smoker. But think of what it is costing your health, as well as your pocket.

Not content with ruining their lungs, smokers run an increased risk of death from cardiovascular diseases such as stroke, coronary thrombosis, and heart failure. Diseased arteries in the legs which can lead to gangrene are also more common in smokers.

The children of smokers are exposed to several risks, not least being the likelihood that they themselves will grow up to be smokers. Most heavy smokers start young – before the age of 20, and some as young as five years old. In addition, children are not going to be impressed by warnings of health hazards from parents who are obviously ignoring the risks themselves. Mothers who smoke give birth to babies who are, on average, 0.5 pounds lighter than babies

genuine desire to stop. The various therapies available are not intended as a substitute for willpower, but are merely adjuncts. Giving up will be easier if you avoid smoking compartments, other smokers – who will invariably offer you cigarettes – situations of stress which will make you smoke more. Put aside the money you would normally spend on cigarettes and treat yourself as a reward. Develop a positive attitude to your health and a liking for fresh air in your home. Give yourself a clean start by having your teeth scaled at the time that you give up.

Remember that each cigarette you smoke shortens your life, and may be hastening you to a slow lingering death.

A Good Night's Sleep

In our modern world, full of noise and stresses, disturbed or inadequate sleep is experienced by all of us at some time in our lives. Insomnia is a growing problem as can be seen by the enormous consumption of sleeping pills.

Insomnia seems to attack the old more than any other age group. Several surveys show that the older the person investigated the more likely he or she is to suffer from insomnia. In one survey only 7 percent of the 40-year-olds reported sleeping generally less than five hours a night, as opposed to 22 percent of the 70-year-olds. As age increases so does the incidence of early wakening (before five in the morning) and interruption of sleep by waking during the night. Women complain of inadequate sleep more often than men and also of difficulty in getting off to sleep. Other surveys show that unmarried people suffer less from bad sleep than married couples – perhaps because of their different degrees of responsibilities. And those people with mental problems fare worse than those with only physical disabilities.

Sleeplessness or insomnia is caused by the brain's overactivity, due to disturbances that are either mental, chemical, or physical. Also, you cannot store sleep. If you try to catch up by sleeping 12 hours or more, this will be of no benefit at all. Many people claim that they benefit from 12 hours of sleep after several days with too little sleep, but the slight gain they might get in terms of repair and renewal is more than canceled out by the fact that the longer you stay in bed the more unfit you become. Bed rest has a severe deconditioning effect. All the physiological processes slow down, circulation becomes sluggish, the muscles become flaccid, and the whole body begins to lose its tone. Remaining in bed for half a day diminishes the time you can be active; thus the longer you remain in bed beyond a maximum of nine hours, the weaker you become.

Although the exact purposes of sleep are not clear,

During sleep the chemical processes of the body slow down. The activity of the brain also changes but it does not actually stop. In fact, during sleep there are periods of electrical activity in the cerebral cortex, the area of the brain concerned with conscious and intelligent activity. These dream periods constitute REM (rapid eye movement) sleep.

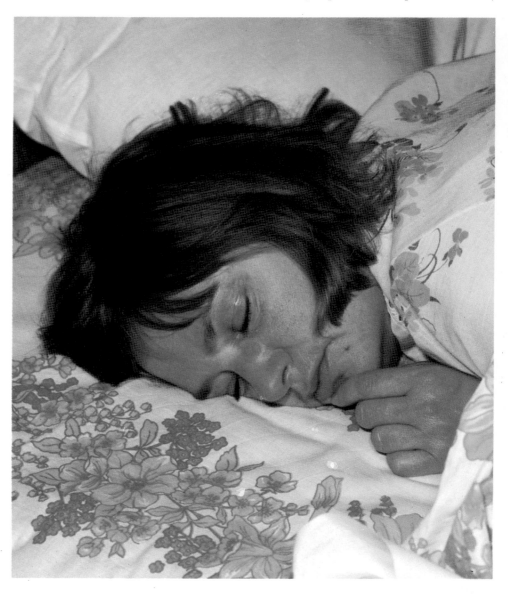

it is obvious that adequate sleep is essential to health. Insufficient sleep results in a diminished work performance and a loss of concentration, while sleep deprivation causes vivid and unpleasant hallucinations. The brain as well as the muscles have to rest.

Insomnia is not a recent phenomenon; for centuries hypnotics such as opium have been used to induce sleep. A vast range of sleeping pills have since been developed. In the past barbiturates were commonly prescribed for insomnia, before their dangers were fully appreciated. By that time many were totally dependent on them and could not go to sleep without their dose. Also, barbiturate-induced sleep is not very satisfactory because barbiturates suppress the dream periods of sleep (REM sleep) which serve an important psychological function. One serious problem is the potential danger of overdosing; some people forget that they have taken their dose and repeat it.

Below: insomnia is a very common problem, and for many a sleeping pill appears to be the obvious solution. But regular use of such drugs can lead to dependence. Often insomnia may be cured by tackling the actual cause. This may be depression, anxiety, physical discomfort, illness, or simply a lack of need for sleep.

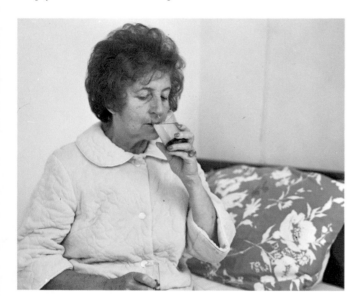

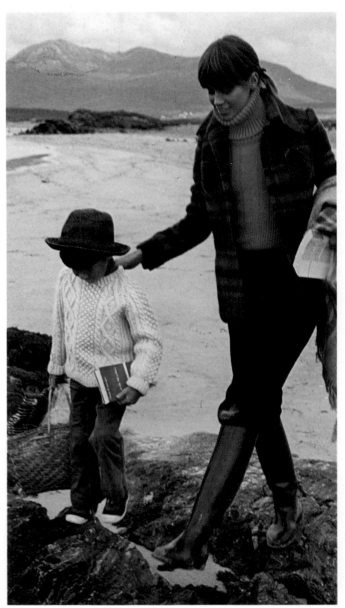

Above: fresh air, plenty of exercise and relaxation seem to be time-honored cures for insomnia. On vacation we all seem to sleep longer and more soundly. At home a walk directly before going to bed, or brief period of yoga or similar will have the same effect.

And barbiturate overdosing can be fatal.

Other types of sleeping pills are available which are invariably preferable to barbiturates. These include tranquilizers which calm the nerves and thus, hopefully, induce sleep. Antihistamines and sea-sickness tablets also induce sleep as a side-effect. However, all pills, if not actually addictive, carry with them the danger of dependence.

There are nonchemical methods of combating insomnia. Hypnosis, carried out by a qualified person, can be as successful as a sleeping pill; but it works well for some and for others not at all. Some people can be bored into sleep (counting sheep) while for many physical exercise such as a walk before bed, a spell of yoga or sex do the trick. A new development is the electronic sleep machine, which sends small electric charges to the brain to induce

sleep. These can only be used under medical supervision, although there is now a do-it-yourself version on the market. These are, however, a very expensive form of self medication. Instead, teach yourself to relax.

The most sensible way to treat insomnia is to analyze its cause and remove it. It may be that the bed is uncomfortable or the room too hot. The cause may be hunger, in which case an apple or warm drink will help; or overeating, which is not so easy to overcome. If depression or anxiety are the causes of your insomnia then seek medical treatment – overcoming the sleeplessness is merely treating the symptom.

Finally, do not worry. People have differing sleep requirements, and some need far more than others. You may even be one who would benefit from intermittent catnaps rather than a full period of rest.

Sensible Eating

Compulsive eaters who turn to food when they are worried; hard-pressed executives who will not stop for a proper meal, and made do with a high calorie snack; housewives alone at home who cannot be bothered to prepare lunch, and have a candy bar and a cup of coffee instead – these are only a small proportion of people who slip into bad eating habits. The long-term result can be that the individual is overfed – but undernourished. The body may be calling out for essential nutrients, but is forced to accept excess calories in their place.

If you have been eating the wrong foods for any length of time, it is inevitable that your health and looks will have suffered. Most bad diets are based on eating too many sweet foods, and too little protein, milk, fruit and vegetables. The poor often cannot afford the kind of diet they should have. But, even among the affluent there are cases of malnutrition, not because of lack of food, but because of too much of the wrong kinds of food.

It is all too easy to fall into bad eating habits, and the habit of eating too much is, perhaps, the easiest bad habit of all. People overeat from a number of different reasons. It may be simply that they enjoy their food enormously, or it may be that they have a deep-seated psychological problem they are not fully aware of. Whatever the cause, overweight is the most common sign of poor eating habits. The giveaway signs are bulges around the waistline, zippers that strain, and buttons that pop. If you are surprised to find that you have put on a few extra pounds you do

This patient is being examined with calipers designed to measure the amount of adipose tissue (fat) underneath the skin. It is the amount of fat rather than the body weight which is a true measure of obesity.

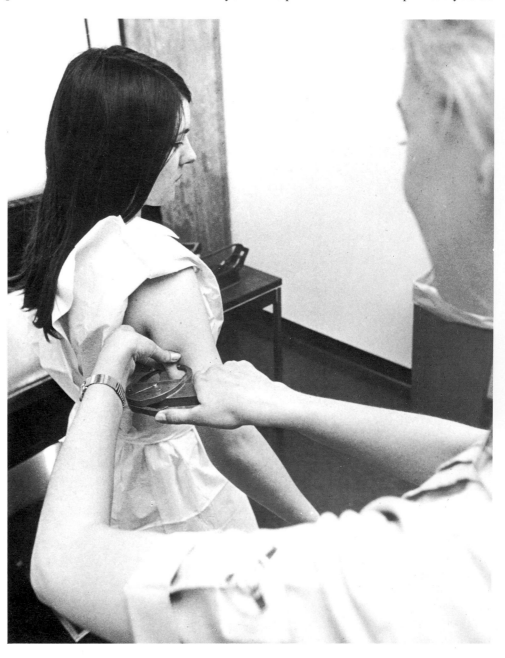

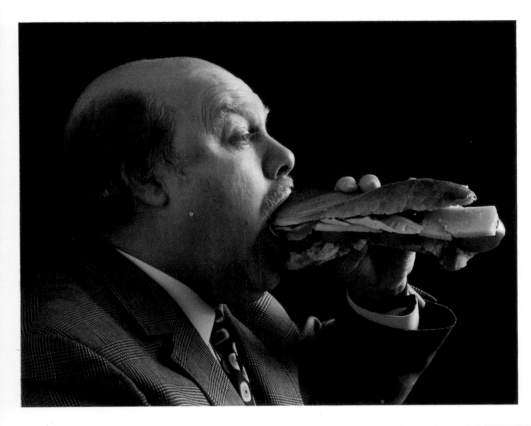

Left: obesity is the result of bad eating habits: excessive portions of food which is usually high in refined carbohydrates and calories, and low in nutritional value.

Below: during the week lunch need not be a high-calorie snack. A salad, yoghurt, fruit and cheese are healthier, less fattening alternatives.

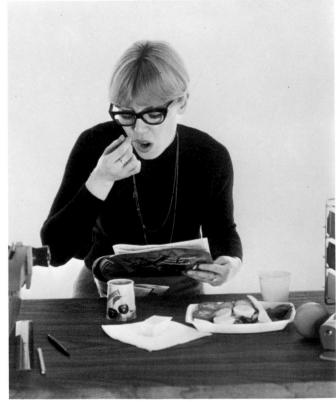

not notice, you should take an immediate grip of the situation. Remember that one pound of surplus weight can lead all too easily to another. So, if your weight begins to creep up, take stock of what you are eating.

Obesity is a problem of fat, not weight. It is the fat in your waistline, hips and thighs you should look at, not the poundage on your scale. The true index is your belt size and your skirt size or pants size. When your skirt of pants get tight, you are getting fat. You should forget your scales and attend to your waistline.

An excellent measure of fat is the "inch of pinch" test. Find a book that is one inch thick. Get acquainted with the feel of the book between your thumb and your index finger. Then grab the flesh at the side of your belly, waist, thighs, buttocks and the back of the arm. At no point of the body should the skin fold thickness exceed one inch. If it is more than that, then you need to diet.

Doctors have calculated that with every 10 percent of weight he gains over the desirable weight for his height, a man risks cutting his life expectancy by 13 percent. Even 10 or 15 pounds of extra weight make a person more vulnerable to serious diseases. Heart disease, high blood pressure and strokes, for example, are twice as common in people who are over-weight.

You can maintain your body in good physical condition by keeping three things in mind: do a reasonable amount of exercise; eat only when you are hungry; and follow a sensible diet. Grill, braise, or boil your food instead of frying or roasting it in fat. Wherever possible eat fresh vegetables instead of canned or frozen ones, and do not overcook them. Cut out high carbohydrate deserts, which have little nutritional value, and substitute fresh fruit instead. Do not rely on artificial sweeteners and the like but try to reeducate your palate and eliminate your "sweet tooth." Fats have a high calorific value and should be watched. The much maligned potato is not fattening in itself but the butter or cream that usually accompanies it is. Finally, reduce your consumption of coffee, tea, cola and, of course, alcohol, and drink more fresh water.

217

Skin, Hair and Nails

If you have a spotty, or blemished skin, it may be the result of an inadequate or inappropriate diet. The high content of vitamins C and A in some fruit and fresh vegetables help to keep your skin healthy. Fresh air and exercise can also help to improve the blood circulation, and this will bring a sparkle to your complexion.

The most important factor governing the condition of our hair and skin is heredity. It also determines the color and texture. A healthy lifestyle, nutritious food and adequate sleep cannot improve upon nature, although their absence can have adverse effects.

Unfortunately you can eat a perfect diet, and have enough fresh air and exercise, but still not have the fine translucent skin that is considered ideal. Heredity is an important factor. If you have the right genes you will probably have a clear, smooth, troublefree skin. But although many women use face packs and a multitude of lotions and creams on their faces, none of these have any beneficial effect on the texture of the skin. Creams and lotions are only an efficient way of cleansing and lubricating the skin and prevent excessive dryness. The actual texture of the skin depends on the thickness of the different layers of skin. What your skin will look like is determined by two factors: the activity of the sebaceous glands that pour an oily secretion called sebum into the surface of the skin to lubricate it, and the level and balance of your sex hormones. These factors are outside our control—we are simply born with them and only time will alter their balance.

Another inherited trait is the thickness of the *collagen* in your skin. Collagen is a protein that is the

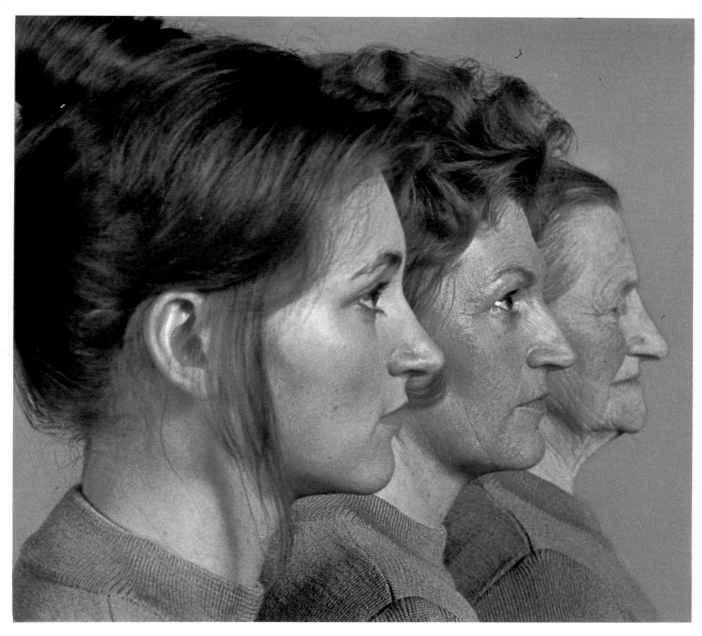

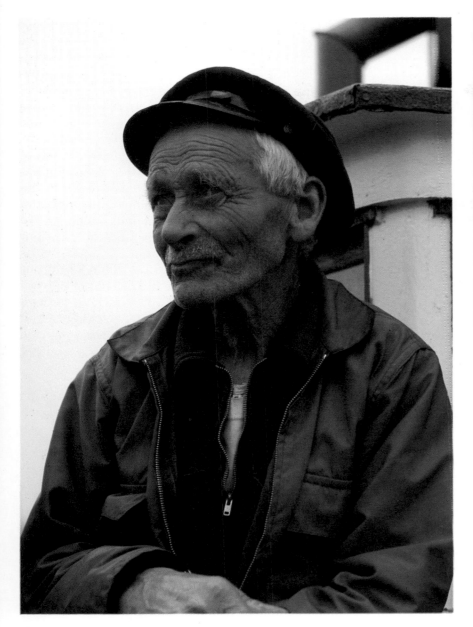

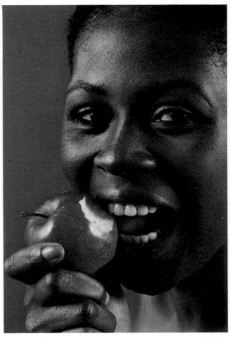

Above: fresh uncooked fruit is a rich source of vitamin C, a substance important for healthy skin. It is essential for the manufacture of connective tissue, which is necessary for the skin's elasticity.

Left: excessive exposure of a fair skin to the sun leads to premature aging, and possibly skin cancer. Dark skinned races contain the pigment melanin, which protects against the harmful effects of the sun's ultraviolet light.

chief constituent of bones and connective tissue. Whether you develop wrinkles early or late in life depends on the type of collagen you are born with and also on how you treat your skin. Generally speaking, the fine, thin skin that looks so wonderful early in life tends to wrinkle sooner than the thicker type of skin. Perhaps this is nature's way of giving us a chance of some beauty at certain times of life. But you can age even a good complexion prematurely by too much exposure to ultraviolet light. Older people especially should limit the amount of sunbathing they indulge in.

Hair and nails are both made up of modified skin cells, filled with a hard substance called *keratin*. When a person is in good health, the natural secretions of the sebaceous glands in the scalp coat the hair with a thin layer of oil, giving it a glossy and shiny appearance. But your hair can become what is often aptly described as "lifeless." It loses its gloss, bounce and depth of color if you are not in good health. If your hair does become "lifeless," rather than trying proprietary remedies you should consult your doctor.

Color fading due to ill health should not be confused with graying. Actually "grayness" is just a mixture of white and normal colored hair, but un- unfortunately it cannot be held at bay by good nutrition or exercise. Nevertheless, gray hair can look healthy and attractive. How soon you go gray, and if you go gray at all, depends once again on your genes. Baldness in men is also partly hereditary.

In some instances, malnutrition – or simply the lack of good eating and living habits – can cause the fingernails to become thick or brittle, or to split easily and break. But it is difficult to relate any single condition of the nails to a shortage of any single nutrient. Conditions of the nails are often affected by psychological stress. Unhappiness and worry seem to make the nails weak or easily broken. The same psychological factors tend to upset people's dietary habits, so diet may be implicated in an indirect way. It is impossible to pinpoint any method by which a particular change in diet can improve the nails; however, if you do not eat properly your nails could become worse.

Minimum Maintenance

In the late 1940s US Air Force medical experts were intrigued when they discovered that air transport pilots, as a group, did not live as long as other air force personnel, and had the shortest active careers of any occupation in the United States. The speculation was that their early breakdown in health had to do with vibration, poisonous gases in the cockpits, prolonged low levels of oxygen, or just plain fear of flying. When the problem was investigated seriously, all these early speculations were discarded. The answer was found to lie in what the pilots did when they finished flying. Their flights would put them down at lonely bases near isolated towns. There they would often have to wait long hours, even days, for their next flight. Invariably they would spend their time in bars getting drunk and eating fatty steaks, and generally indulging in an excessive lifestyle.

The lifestyle of these pilots is an extreme case of what confronts all of us to a degree: tension, boredom and fatigue drive us to seek release. We reward ourselves by seeking a lazy, overindulgent existence in as much luxury as we can afford. The consequences are devastating. Much of the human deterioration that we attribute to aging is simply the result of deconditioning caused by inactivity. The feeble, slouching, uncoordinated person who stumbles past us may be only in early middle age.

To avoid this perilous condition you have to have a fitness program. And before this can be devised you must first determine how fit you want to be. There are many levels of satisfactory fitness. A basic level is the very minimum below which you are going to experience physical and mental deterioration. But

This is one way to relieve boredom, tension and fatigue – pour yourself a drink and light up a cigarette. Unfortunately, although you may benefit psychologically, physically you will feel no better.

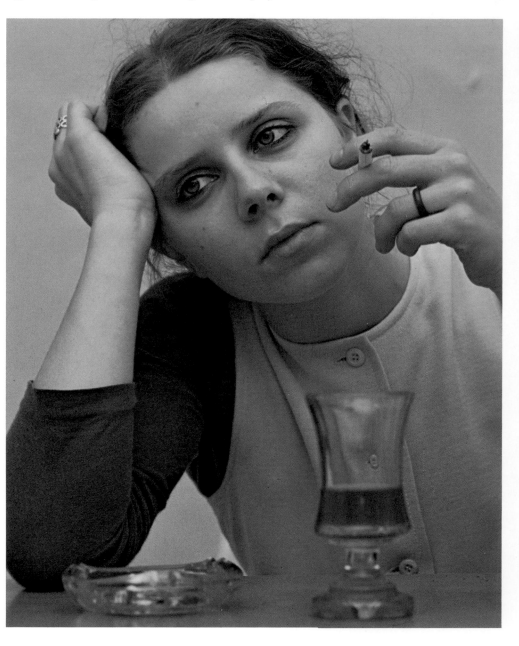

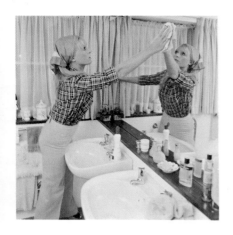

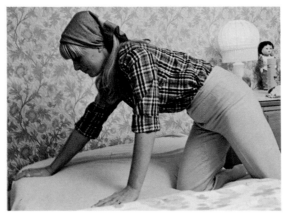

Left: simple household routines incorporating bending and stretching provide most of the requirements for minimum maintenance.

Below: if you have never taken walking seriously, get yourself a dog; then you will have no excuse.

only a higher general level of fitness will provide you with a safe margin of adaptation for change, including emergencies, and enable you to get through the day without an undue amount of fatigue.

The basic level of fitness, which we can call minimum maintenance (MM), requires nothing more than the incorporation of a few simple habits into everyday life. Minimum maintenance can be achieved by meeting simple requirements, such as turning and twisting your body joints to their near maximum range of motion, standing for a total of two hours a day, and lifting something heavy for a few seconds, perhaps a child, to maintain your muscle tone.

Shopping for groceries takes care of nearly all the requirements for MM, with just a touch of emphasis on your part: instead of turning around when you are looking for something, twist around. Bend for groceries on the bottom shelf. Stretch for them on the top shelf. That could be your mobility exercise for the day. When you go to work, take stairs instead of the elevator; walk up the escalator. During the day, whether you are in an office or at home, follow these maxims: do not lie when you can sit; do not sit when you can stand; and do not stand still when you can move.

For lunch, pick a restaurant some distance from your office or work place, and walk there. If you are running errands, park your car a distance from where you are going, or get off the bus one stop early. The more briskly you move, the more your heart and lungs will be working. Never hold yourself back – move with vigor.

At the end of the day, walk briskly from work to your car, train or bus. When you get home, play for a few minutes with your children or your dog. Help with the dinner. During the evening fix something that has awaited your attention. Put your desk or a section of your den in order. Walk the dog.

You do not need to create difficulties for yourself to achieve a MM level of fitness. Exercises for MM can be incorporated into daily life, performing the most mundane activities. The game is to be active as frequently and regularly as possible with elements such as twisting, standing, lifting, a brief burst of motion, and sufficient activity to burn some excess calories every day. If you have a predisposition to be physically active, then you never need worry about doing formal exercises. But if you want to move beyond the MM level of fitness, if you want a reserve of fitness so that you can meet challenges such as changing a tire in the rain or even snow, if you want to enjoy recreational activities such as a long hike, then you will need a more demanding program.

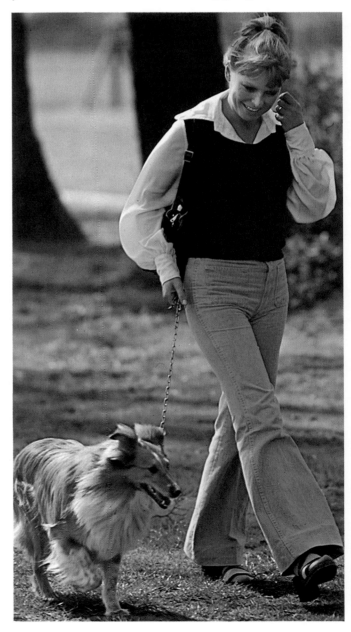

30-Minute Fitness

(Based on Laurence E Morehouse and Leonard Gross, *Total Fitness in 30 Minutes a Week*, 1977).
In our modern society an increasing number of people have so little time to spare that they can no longer keep fit through recreational sports. They are simply too busy. Moreover they are almost always on the move. For these people in particular Dr Morehouse has developed a realistic fitness program.

This program is divided into three stages, each lasting eight weeks. Stage one will help you to develop tissue, stage two will increase your endurance, and stage three will build up your strength. The chart gives you your training pulse rate in each eight-week period, which should be used as rough guides only. But do not become a compulsive pulse counter. Use your pulse as a checkpoint to gauge the accuracy of your perception of exertion, so that you can find the intensity which is just right for you.

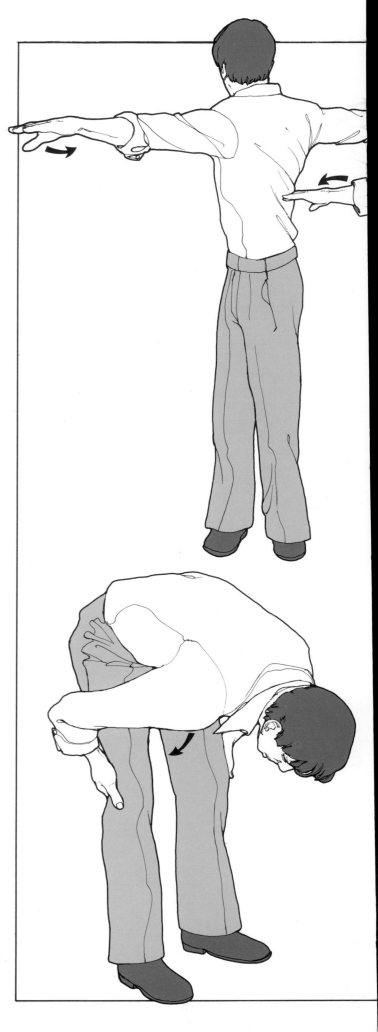

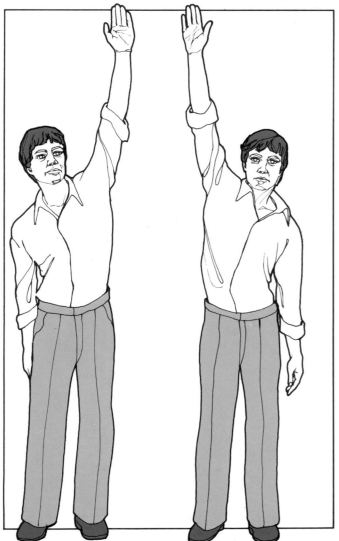

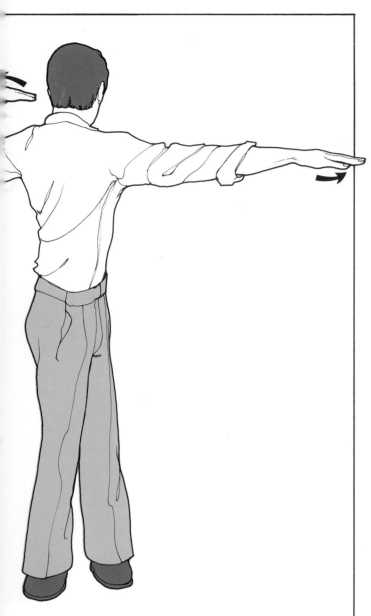

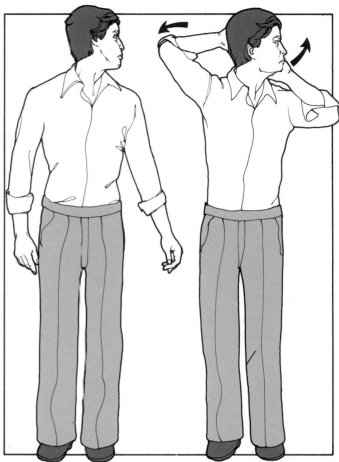

Step One

1-minute limbering warm-up: reach up as high as you can toward the ceiling with one arm. Feel the stretch all the way to your ankle. Repeat the exercise with your other arm.

Extend your arms sideways. Twist your trunk in either direction as far as you can turn.

Then lean over, grasp yourself behind the knees with your hands, and pull your shoulders gently toward your knees. Do not use force.

Turn your head to the side, with your chin over the top of your left shoulder. Now turn your head with your hands just a little further than it can turn on its own. Reverse sides.

1.5-2-minutes strength push-aways: stand a little beyond arm's reach from a wall. Put your hands against the wall at the height of your shoulders. Lean forward until your chest touches the wall. Then push back until you are in the starting position.

1.5-2-minutes strength sit-backs: sit on the floor with your feet hooked under a piece of furniture. Bend your knees. Work your chest up against your knees, or as closely as it will come. Once you are in position, move back away from your knees until you feel your stomach muscles being worked to some degree. Then go up to your knees again. As you get fitter your point of moderate effort will drop further and further backward. Eventually, your shoulder-blades will lightly brush the floor before you raise your trunk again.

2-10-minutes endurance lope: the most steady, easy endurance exercise is running in place. Or try the fitness hop. The only requirement is that your movements be energetic enough to get your pulse rate up to your moderate level by the end of the second minute.

Step Two

1-minute limbering warm-up: as in step one.

1-2-minutes 15-20 push-aways: now you do twice as many – and do them fast.

2-3-minutes 15-20 expansion sit-backs: while you are leaning backward, probe the abdominal muscles in all areas, low and high, with your hands. This helps to keep the muscles hardened.

3-10-minutes endurance intervals: the conventional method is to run for a number of seconds, say 30, then slow to walk for about 30 seconds, then run and walk alternately. During your endurance lope, in

the first eight weeks you should work to 60 percent of maximum. Now you should speed up so that your training pulse rate goes to 70 percent of maximum during the fast portion of the six-minute period.

Step Three

Now the element of relaxation should be perfected and you will be moving up to 80 percent of all-out effort. These are energetic, fast workouts. "Energetic" and "fast" imply relaxation.

1-minute limbering warm-up: as in step one.

1-3-minutes endurance push-aways: now we want to make things so difficult that we can do no more than five. So we not only go to the floor but the best way is to have someone put his hand on your back while you do your up to five push-aways.

3-5-minutes 40-50 endurance sit-backs: now

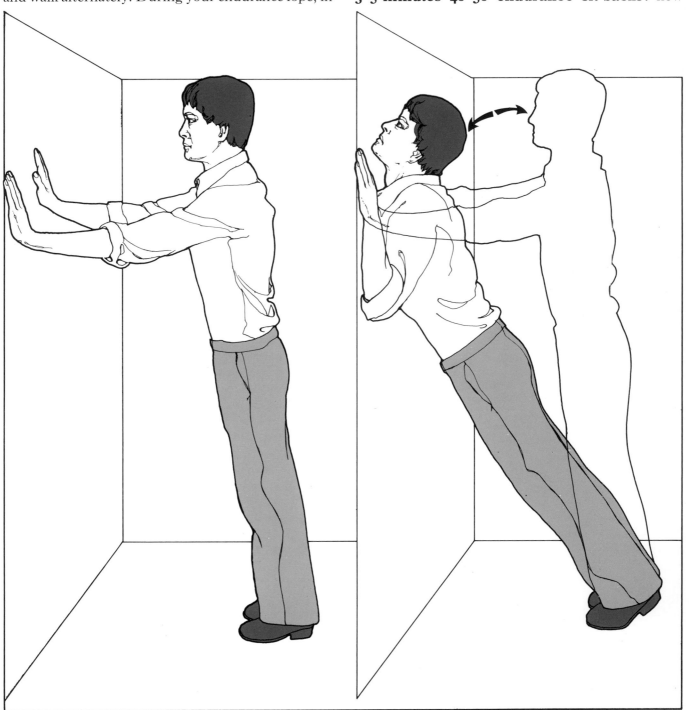

assume a position you can hold without trembling for only five seconds. There are two basic ways to create that much difficulty for yourself. The first is to extend your arms over your head. The second is to hold a weight either in your hands or in your arms, folded across your chest. Do not exceed your training pulse rate. It is now 80 percent of 220 minus your age.

5-10-minutes sprint intervals: alternate slow and fast periods of sprinting level each 15 seconds for eight minutes. At 80 percent of maximum a 50–60-year-old person can exercise now at a training pulse rate of about 130 beats a minute. A 40-year-old person can go to around 140 beats a minute. The key to activity at this level is relaxation. Begin with a normal amount of tension. Then deliberately in-crease the tension, the objective being to get below the level of tension with which you began.

Your training pulse rate

Age	TPR 1	TPR 2	TPR 3	TPR 4
Under 30	120	140	150	150-160
30-44	110	130	140	140-150
45-60	100	120	130	130-140
over 60	100	110	120	120-130

TPR 1 = TPR for the first 8 weeks about 60 percent maximum rate (220 minus your age × 0.60).

TPR 2 = TPR for the second eight weeks about 70 percent maximum PR.

TPR 3 = TPR for the third eight weeks about 80 percent maximum PR.

TPR 4 = "maintenance level" for the fourth eight weeks and beyond.

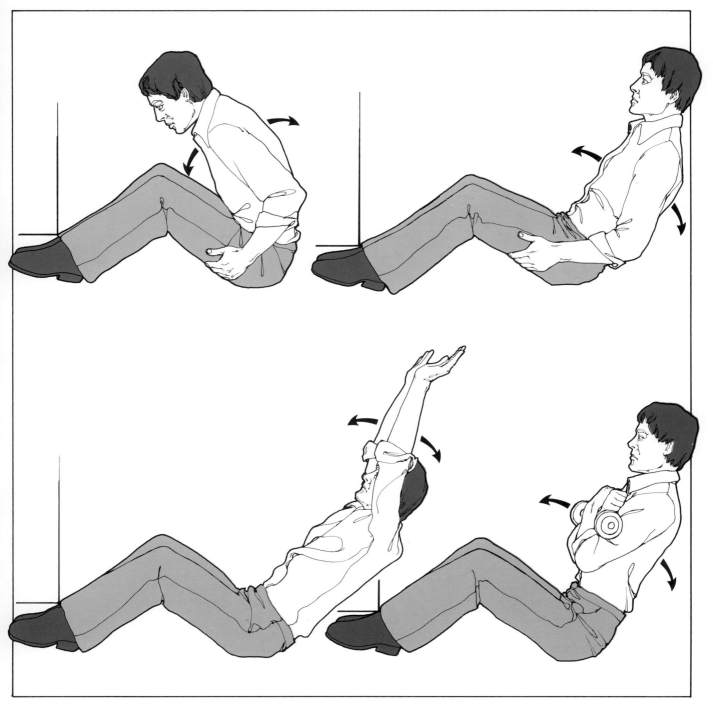

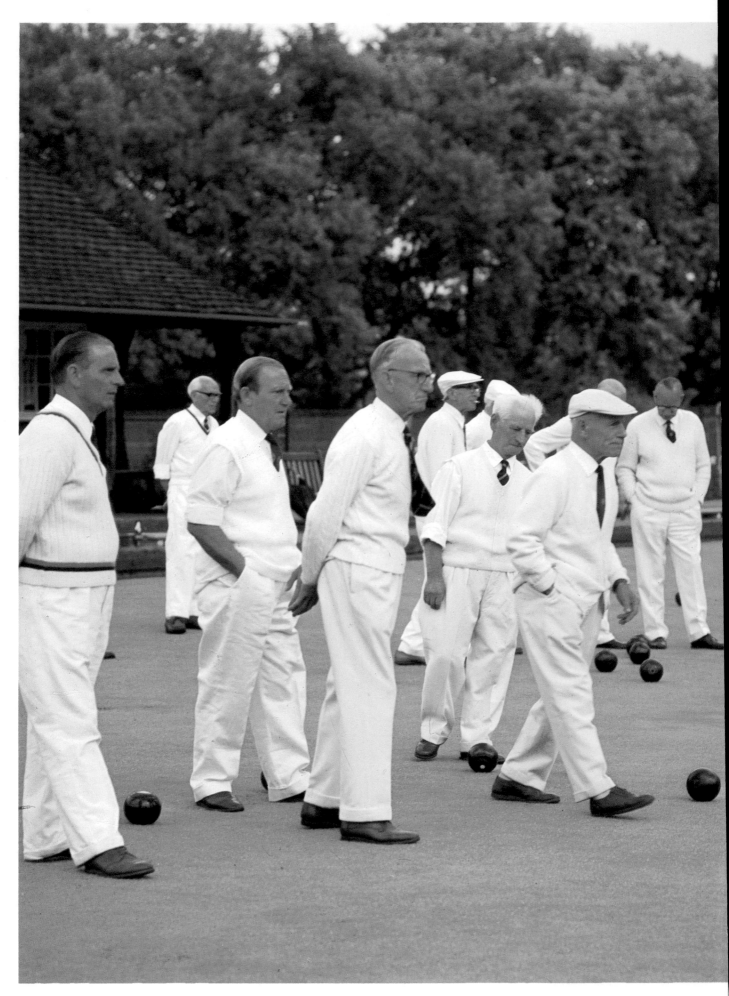

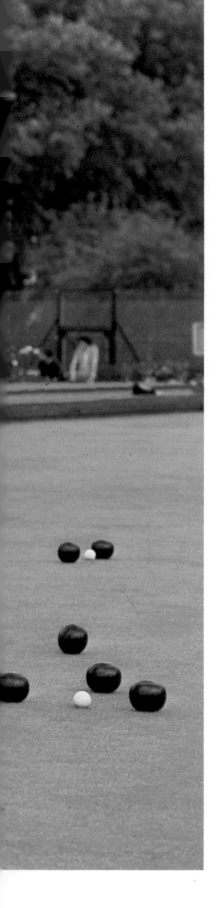

Chapter 12

Health in Retirement

Sooner or later most of us will face the realization that someone close to us is getting old and may soon become dependent on our care and support. The wheel turns full circle until it is our turn to care for those who once looked after us. But it is not easy to be old in our society. In a culture that is youth oriented and that places a high value on productivity, the old may feel underprivileged and unwanted. Doctors who work with the elderly know that the mutual support of family members is a major factor in prolonging physical and mental health in older people. Here, then, is how we can care for the elderly best – by showing them the loving concern that will bring happiness and comfort to their lives.

Opposite: although the body does deteriorate with time, all the evidence indicates that by maintaining an active and interesting life, the elderly can enjoy their retirement rather than endure it.

The Process of Aging

Why does a mayfly live for only one day, a human being for over 70 years, and a tortoise for up to 150 years? Aging is still not fully understood, and there are many factors that contribute to this inevitable process. What is known is that the rate at which we age has not changed since prehistoric times – but because of the benefits of civilization, and especially

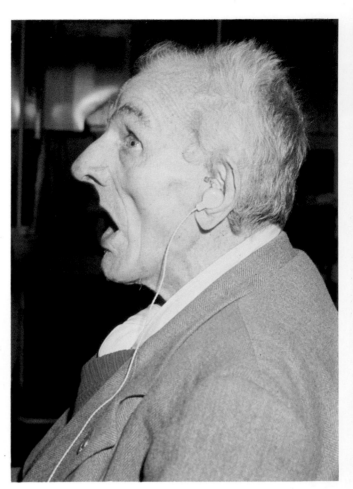

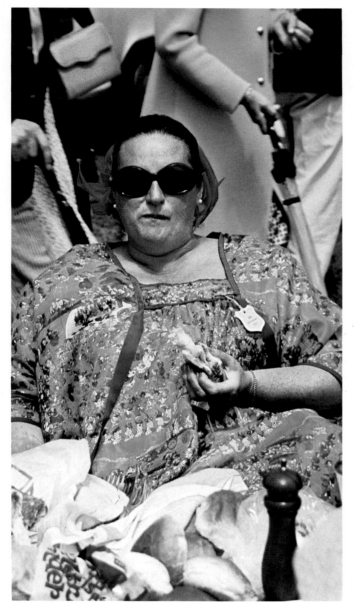

Above: eating her way to an early grave. Obese people are more prone to diabetes, cardiovascular disease, kidney problems, damaged bones and hernias.

Above right: aging involves the deterioration of the physical faculties. Many elderly people will need to pay attention to their diminishing sight and hearing.

modern medicine, we stand a much greater chance of dying naturally. In other words our life expectancy is greater.

We know that certain anatomical changes indicate that the aging process begins at birth. Thus our life-span depends to a great extent on the speed of this process. Each tissue, or tissues, in the body may age independently at its own rate and according to its own built-in program. Someone in their seventies may have certain organs which show practically no evidence of aging, while other organs or structures show extreme deterioration. In a woman, for example, the ovaries age at the menopause long before there may be obvious evidence of aging in other parts of the body. On the other hand, all the body tissues may age together – but by different processes.

There are so many factors that determine our life-span that it is impossible to list them all. The type of organs and body structures that a person inherits are important factors but so are the many illnesses, stresses, and the degree of wear and tear to which the body is subject throughout a lifetime. A person with a frail body who has not been afflicted by ravaging illness, organ damage, or other stresses, may outlive someone with a stronger body who has experienced serious and repeated assaults of disease and injury. But even if your anatomical structures are to a great extent inherited, longevity will depend on what happens to these organs in the course of a lifetime. For instance, strong blood vessels will afford no protection against the development of a fatal infection or malignant tumor.

But some factors that can aid or hinder longevity are known. Intelligent exercise will aid it insofar as it helps to keep your body fit; on the other hand if

regulated diet and may lead to diseases of vital organs. Smoking can have a similar effect, and certainly can contribute to premature death. Diet in general plays an important role in longevity. An inadequate diet often leads to defective body metabolism. On the

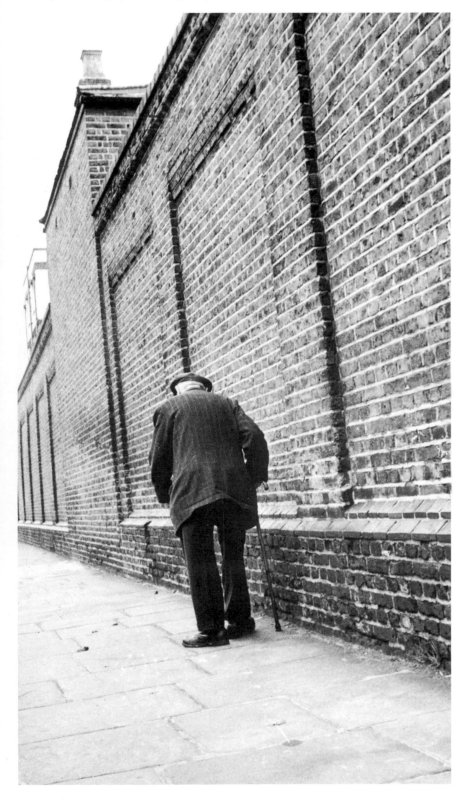

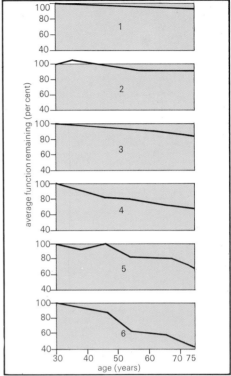

Above: the function of body organs decreases with increasing age. (1) brain weight; (2) nerve-conduction velocity; (3) basal metabolic rate; (4) cardiac output; (5) kidney filtration rate; (6) maximum breathing rate.

Left: bones weaken with age. The elderly are prone to osteoporosis – thinning and weakening of the bone tissue, and osteoarthritis, degeneration of the joints, in particular, in the legs and spine.

there has been serious chronic or recurrent disease in earlier life, exercise can damage important organs and lead to a premature aging. Excessive eating or drinking can shorten a person's lifespan. Large quantities of alcohol may interfere with a well-

other hand, overeating is a factor in premature aging in that it leads to obesity and places an inordinate strain upon the heart, blood vessels, and other organs. And it is well known that thin people tend to live longer than fat people.

Facing up to Retirement

Retirement is one of the best examples of role change for the elderly and at the same time one which illustrates the social implications of aging. The physical changes of aging make it more difficult for a person to work, but there is such a diversity of response among different people to these changes that it

For some elderly people retirement is the ideal opportunity to consolidate their savings and move out of the city to an area with a healthier, more temperate climate.

would appear unlikely that a single retirement age could be agreed upon. Besides, the range of types of work in our society, with different mental and physical demands, would again seem to make it unlikely that we should have a fixed retirement age. Yet most advanced societies do have such a retirement age at which people who stop work are entitled to a pension. Not everyone stops work at that age – but the great majority do.

What has contributed to the development of the concept of "retirement" other than physical abilities? One factor may be a lack of understanding between people trained and qualified at a past level of technology and their younger colleagues. Another factor is the attitude of employers to older workers: emphasis may be placed upon the importance of retiring older workers in order to provide opportunities for the promotion of younger men and women. Also a

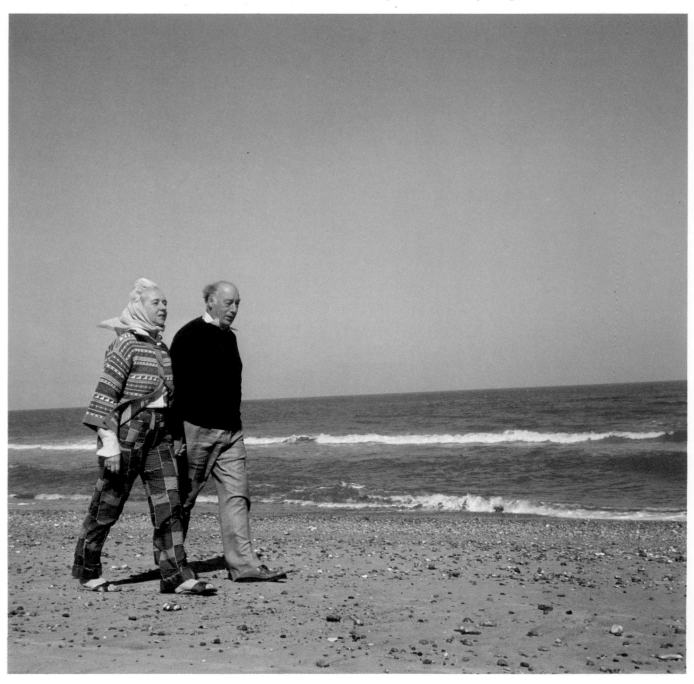

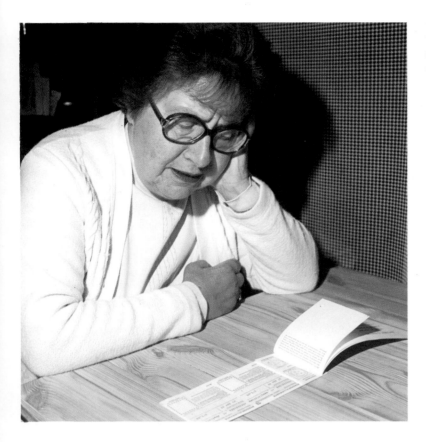

For others retirement brings the inexplicable bureaucracy of pension systems and welfare payments, where life from now on will be dependent on the charity of institutions.

further factor may be the attitudes of the elderly themselves toward work, for they may welcome a point in time when, given a choice, they can stop working. Another important factor is that it is administratively convenient, both for the state and for private organizations, to have a fixed retirement age.

Retirement has a direct effect on lifestyle. Only for infants up to five years old and for the retired is life largely unstructured by institutional requirements. With retirement suddenly most of the constraints and responsibilities of a busy working life are removed. How a person responds to this situation varies from individual to individual according to the type of work he or she did in the past, and depends also on their personality and other interests. Some people clearly miss work, others are only too pleased to stop working. There are undoubtedly people who once retired find their previously desired freedom from work a burden in itself.

At one time it was widely believed that there was a direct connection between health and an unhappy retirement, and even that the trauma of retirement could result in death. But recent research has called this theory into question. The most important single reason given for retirement is poor health, although it is run a close second by compulsory factors such as retirement age. But the physical condition which is incapacitating as far as work is concerned may not be incapacitating as far as general mobility and self-care are concerned. In fact a number of surveys have provided evidence that retirement often leads to an improvement in health.

A person's choice between work and retirement is obviously affected by financial considerations. As pension benefits increase, the proportion of older people who choose to retire will no doubt gradually increase over the long run, but there will be a residue of people with a strong desire to continue at work, particularly in those occupations in which interest in work is high. Making it possible for such people to continue work is an important social goal.

Some experts are prophesying that we are perhaps moving towards a period when retirement will be much more a question of an option on the part of the individual workers, coupled with an assessment of their employability based on factors other than age. Such a development would place a great responsibility upon the medical profession, for doctors would have to make a distinction between an illness which is a reason for a person not to work, and an illness which may be caused by the inability of a person to find a job.

A growing awareness of the problems of retirement has led to "preparation for retirement" programs being set up in several countries. Most programs include a discussion of income and health problems and activity for later years, and in addition include discussion of other considerations such as personal and social adjustment. Doctors often play an important role in such programs, for they can provide useful advice about nutrition and health changes in old age, together with practical advice about the different facilities and services available for the retired. Unfortunately in the United States and Great Britain experience has shown that an extremely small percentage of people have been willing to participate in such preretirement education programs.

How to Carry On

Every old person is, of course, unique, but elderly people do share certain problems and anxieties. Apart from any physical discomfort they may be suffering, they worry about becoming a burden, about losing their ability to care for themselves, about being useless or unwanted. They may be concerned about growing absent-mindedness, about being unable to cope with official papers, about lacking the money to meet their needs. They may find it difficult

Many old people are particularly good at caring for small children. They are often willing to tell the same story over and over again, to play repetitive games, or take time to help a toddler dress or eat. And, for their part, children are the best confidence-boosters an elderly person can have. They will listen to their grandparents' stories without being patronizing, happily pour out their own thoughts, and admire an older person's smallest talent.

The decision to bring a grandparent to live with the family should not be taken lightly. An elderly person may not be as physically active as their son or daughter, but that does not necessarily mean that they cannot take care of themselves. Like people of any generation, some will prefer their independence, while others would feel lonely by themselves. But no elderly person is going to feel comfortable in a situation where they are barely tolerated, let alone

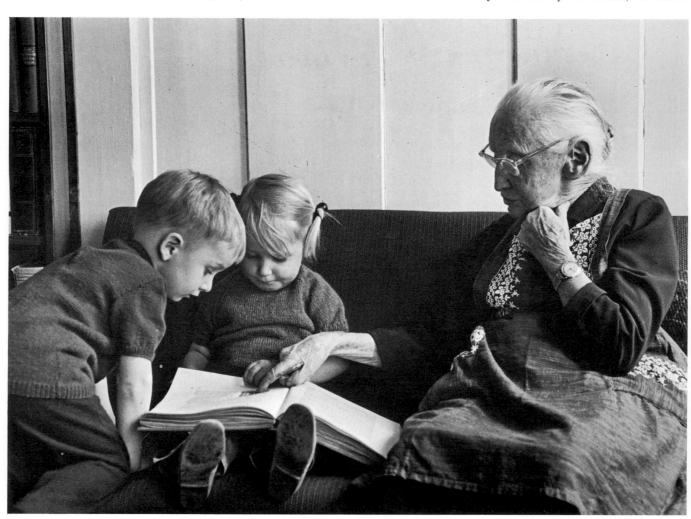

Grandparents can have a valuable role to play in the family, as is seen in the extended family systems of eastern and southern Europe. They often help in raising the children.

to make decisions, and be distressed by change.

Whenever possible, the elderly should be encouraged and welcomed into their childrens' families and made to feel useful. This is a highly beneficial feature of the extended family which has been lost to a great extent in Western countries.

made unwelcome. The strain will also be felt on the rest of the family.

An elderly relative should be encouraged to participate as much as possible in family life. Occasional mistakes and mishaps are bound to occur, but it does not help to criticize. Old people have their pride and dignity as much as anyone else, and criticism may make them lose more self-respect, even leading them to withdraw from all activity. In fact, old people may themselves look for scapegoats – their failing health, say, or even another member of the family – to take the blame when things go wrong, because they do not want to admit a loss of confidence in themselves.

is out, and exercise should never be continued after any signs of tiredness. Walking is still probably the best exercise for the elderly, but old people who have been used to swimming, dancing, gardening, bicycling, playing golf, or bowls, can safely continue this,

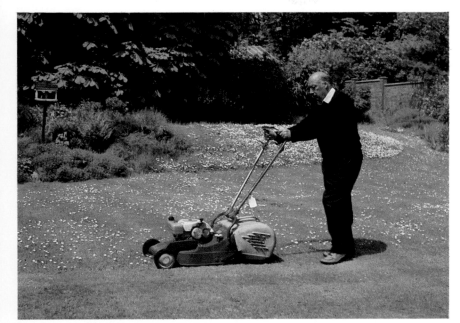

Left: elderly people should not be told to "take it easy" but should be encouraged to get as much exercise as possible, especially around the house.

Below: for many elderly men and women social clubs provide suitable sports facilities, as well as company.

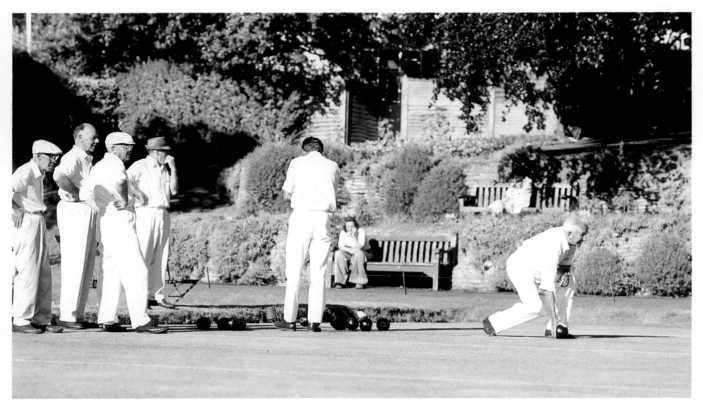

Older people are rarely either senile nor invalids, and should not be treated as such. They will tire more easily, but even so physical activities are important to insure that they get the exercise they need. For, although aging reduces reserves of strength and energy, exercise is still necessary to keep muscles active and maintain good health – and it will help an old person to get a good night's sleep. Moderation is, as usual, the keynote. Sudden or prolonged exercise

in moderate doses.

Even if an elderly relative does not move in with the family, contact should always be maintained. This is a time when widowhood may have struck and an elderly person's family may be all they have to offset loneliness and isolation. Increasing age does reduce mobility, and the elderly, more than anyone else, will greatly appreciate visits, letters and telephone calls.

Loneliness and Isolation

Isolation and loneliness are commonly thought to be among the main problems of old age. By comparison with the young and middle aged, the old are liable to a loss of attachments and activities. But their vulnerability may often be exaggerated.

There is an important distinction between isolation and loneliness in old people. Isolation refers to the nature and extent of contact with other people,

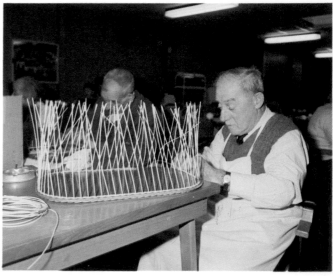

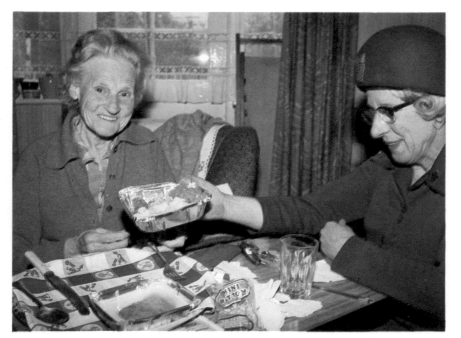

Above: many elderly people regard the extra time is an opportunity to learn new skills, and for the elderly who live alone, a group activity is especially important. Without an interest in life, the will to live disappears.

Left: certain countries operate a meals-on-wheels system for the elderly. This enables them to get nutritious food which they would otherwise not have been able to afford, or be able to cook. For many it is also their only outside company.

Opposite: for many elderly who live alone, a pet provides companionship, security and a sense of responsibility. Dogs need daily walking and therefore make regular exercise a pleasurable necessity.

loneliness to a psychological state. The percentage of the elderly who are found to be isolated depends very much upon how we define isolation. In a study in Great Britain it was found that between 2 and 3 percent of all elderly were isolated: they lived alone, had no visitors in the previous week and had no human contact on the day previous to being interviewed. However, when the criteria for isolation were changed, taking into account all the contacts with children and other relations and friends, eating of meals in company, etc., it was found that 21 percent of old people were classified as isolated and 4 percent as extremely isolated.

So we can see that isolation is a major problem for the elderly. Its full social significance has not yet been evaluated, but there are many practical measures that society as a whole – and individuals – can take to prevent old people from being socially isolated. Simply visiting an old person regularly is an obvious answer. But unfortunately social isolation and loneliness are not the same thing. Loneliness has

been defined as an "unwelcome feeling of bad luck or loss of companionship." Loneliness is an individual response to an external situation and each old person will react quite differently to it: many isolated old people do not feel lonely and some old folk living with their relatives or in homes for the old feel very lonely.

Bereavement is a major contribution to loneliness. A husband or wife may die, leaving an elderly person with no one to care for – and no one to care for them. Or old friends may die or move away, leaving them lonely and isolated and leading a sad and aimless existence. Without some meaningful involvement in day-to-day activities and regular contact with others, they may lose all interest in life. In fact the loss of a spouse often precipitates an elderly person's own death. That is why it is wise to encourage an elderly relative or friend to belong to a club – not necessarily designed for old people, but perhaps a special-interest club, where he or she can play chess or poker, discuss gardening, or local history, with members of various

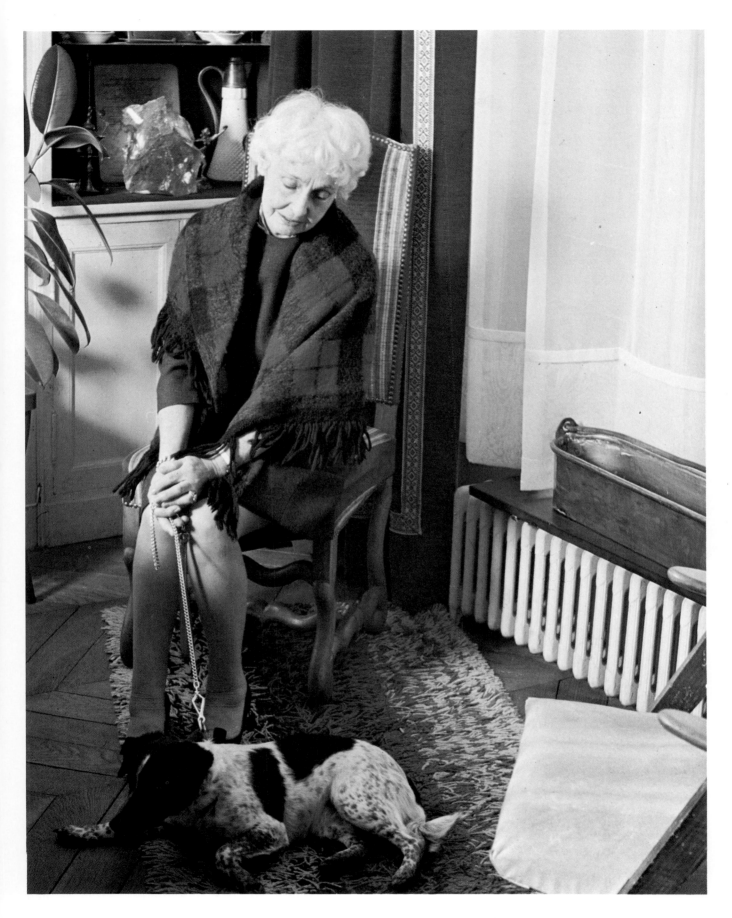

ages. Day centers for the elderly are also excellent for providing the companionship of contemporaries, as well as shared activities. Some senior workshops may even provide paid work for the elderly that can be a great incentive for an old person.

For an elderly person living alone, having a pet can be a great comfort. As well as being a source of companionship and affection, a pet can give that person the satisfaction of having something that depends entirely on their love and care.

Health and the Elderly

Geriatrics deals with the diseases and other medical problems of old people, and is a specialized branch of medicine and nursing. An elderly person may be slow to report signs of ill health, and others must keep an eye out for his or her welfare.

The elderly need less food than more active younger people, but they must eat the right things. A poor

eggs and milk) and an adequate supply of vitamins from fruit and vegetables.

Older people should cut down on fats, which may slow their less efficient digestion, and on carbohydrates (an old person needs less of the energy that these provide). Their diet should be rich in calcium (mainly from milk and cheese) and contain vitamin D sources like fish-liver oils and margarine to counteract softened or brittle bones. They also need plenty of fluids – around two quarts a day. Fluids aid digestion and help clear waste products from the kidneys. As appetite may lessen with age and the senses of taste and smell become less sharp, food should be as varied as possible, look attractive, and be well seasoned. And a glass of wine or jigger of alcohol before dinner can help stimulate a flagging

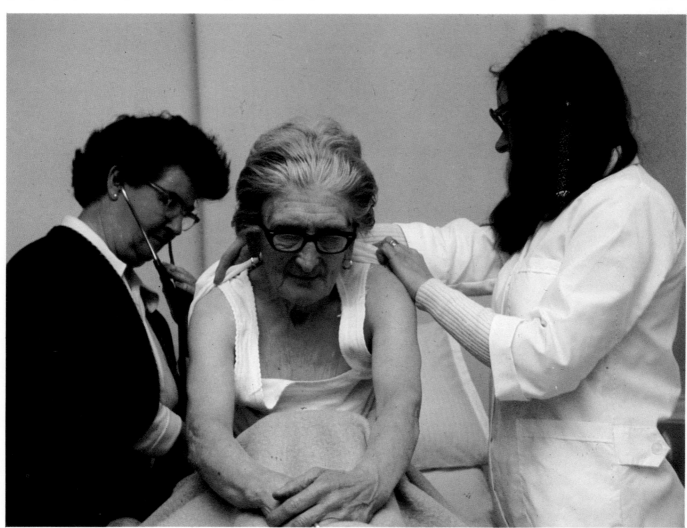

For the aged in particular, regular medical checkups are essential. Even a minor complaint, which in a young healthy body would cause little concern, can produce serious complications in a frail, aged person.

diet, especially one lacking in vitamins, can create many health problems, from difficulty in swallowing and digestive upsets to loss of appetite and fatigue. Finance will be a problem for many old people live on low incomes. Elderly people need plenty of protein (principally from meat, fish, cheese, pulses,

appetite and aid digestion.

Even a vigorous and healthy old person should have a regular medical checkup. Regular dental care is also important, and so are checks on vision and hearing. Dentures will have to be adjusted or replaced as the shape of the mouth alters. A home dental service is available in many communities. If a hearing aid appears necessary, the doctor should be consulted first before any commercially available aid is purchased.

Taking drugs can be a problem with the old. An elderly person can forget how many tablets he or she has taken, or get up during the night in a muddled state, because of sleeping tablets, and suffer a fall. Sleeping drugs – or any other type of drugs for that matter – should therefore never be taken except when prescribed by a doctor, and should not be left on a bedside table.

Incontinence, the lack of voluntary power to control the passing of urine and feces, can be distressing for old people and should be handled with a great deal of compassion and understanding by those that look after them. Drugs have been developed to help control incontinence, but if the condition is chronic then devices for catching the excrement and preventing the soiling of bed linen and clothes are probably the most practical.

Old people are often reluctant to report symptoms of illness, either from shyness, hopelessness, fear of going to a hospital, of upsetting relatives or being a nuisance, or perhaps because their doctor has seemed unsympathetic in the past. It is therefore important for you to be on the alert for any signs of illness in your elderly relative or friend. Do not put symptoms such as dizziness, breathlessness, aches and pains, indigestion, or tiredness, down to "old age" – they may indicate some illness that can be diagnosed and cured.

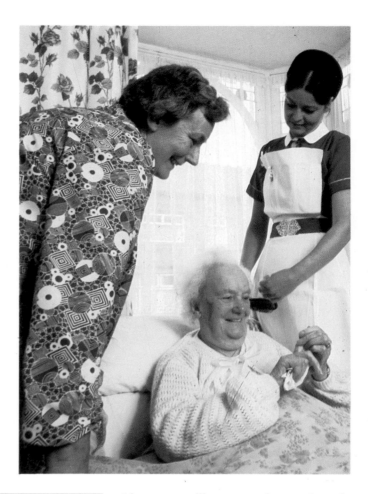

Above: some illnesses require a prolonged rest, and many elderly people would prefer to be bed-ridden at home than in the geriatric ward of a hospital. Their family should insure that the patient receives visitors, and regular nursing and medical attention.

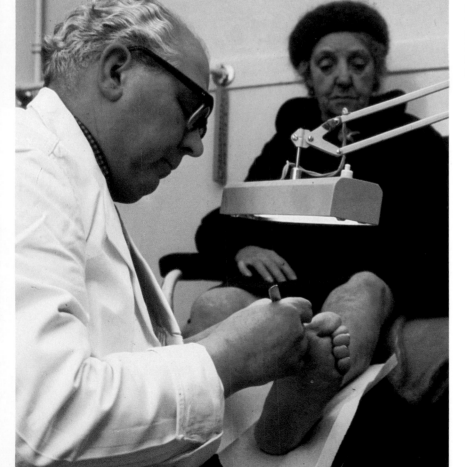

Left: in the old, the feet may develop painful problems, which will be aggravated by osteoporotic bones and arthritic joints. A regular visit to the chiropodist is advisable, and many welfare systems provide this as a free service for the elderly.

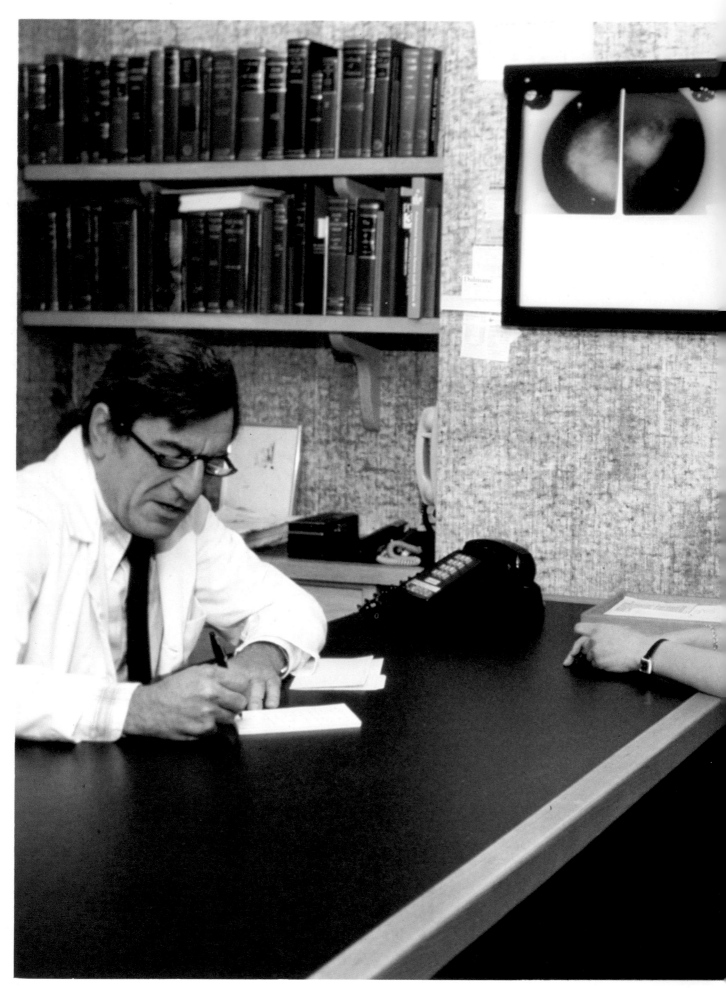

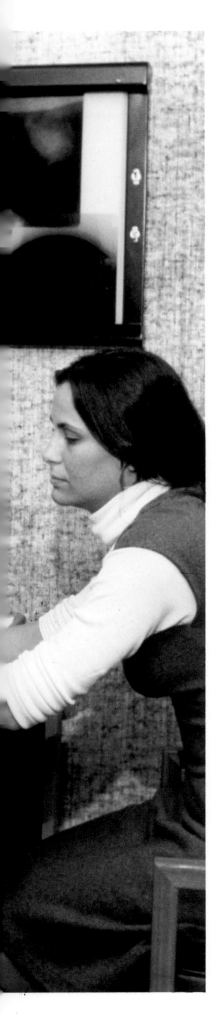

Chapter 13

Regular Checkups

Specialists in preventive medicine recommend that every adult woman – from the age of 18 – should have a medical checkup at least once a year. A man should have his first checkup at around 25 and provided everything is well, a further check every two or three years until he is 45 should be sufficient. Those men over 45 are advised to have an examination at least once a year. But the truth is that it is not always easy to get a checkup. Most doctors are so busy treating diseases that they may be reluctant to examine the bodies of perfectly sound people. But this attitude is changing, and it is really up to you, for the sake of your health, to see that you get a regular and thorough checkup.

Opposite: a routine checkup is the surest way to spot any incipient disease at a time when it can be treated easily. It will also allay any fears you may have about seemingly ominous symptoms.

A Visit to the Surgery

Most illnesses are caused by common, easily diagnosed diseases, and a visit to your doctor is usually a simple matter. You report your symptoms and he or she may possibly examine the affected area. The doctor will then prescribe a medicine or suggest a course of action that will clear up the trouble in a short time. But sometimes the matter is not so simple and requires a thorough investigation – and like many other forms of investigation, finding out what is

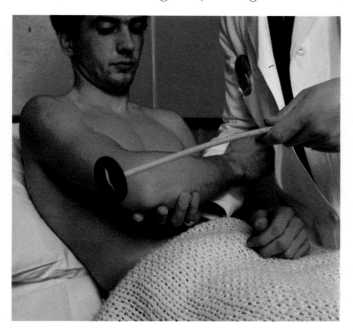

Above: a number of reflexes are examined to determine lesions in the nervous system.

Above right: an abdominal examination.

wrong with a person demands a methodical approach. The doctor has to discover all the patient's symptoms, and evaluate their significance. To accomplish this the doctor employs a comprehensive diagnostic routine, a physical inspection which follows a methodical pattern designed to eliminate error, for every good doctor knows that "more wrong diagnoses arise from not looking than from not finding."

First the patient's medical history has to be established. Has the patient had any operations or been in hospital. The doctor will inquire about the state of health or causes of death of immediate relatives. Some questions about the patient's home and family environment may follow as these could reveal the patient's mental attitude to his or her life and work. Once the doctor is satisfied that the background has been filled the patient can tell the story of the illness

concerned. The doctor then asks questions, using the symptoms as the starting point.

The examination proper can now begin. The patient's general appearance is noted; the weight and height are recorded. Then the doctor takes the patient's temperature and examines each physiological system in turn.

The neck, armpits and groin are examined to see if any glands near the surface are enlarged. Then the digestive system is investigated: in the mouth the state of the teeth and gums are noted, the abdomen is palpated (examined by touch) to see if there is any enlargement of the liver, gall bladder, spleen or kidneys, or any abnormal swelling of the bowel.

The doctor's hands and ears are delicately combined in the next stage of the examination. Putting the left hand flat on the patient's skin, the doctor strikes the back of the left middle finger with the tip

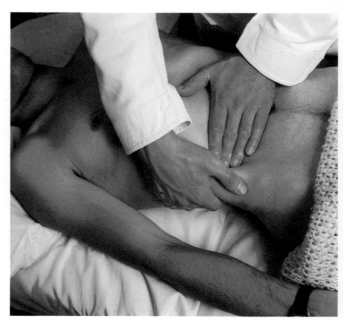

of the right middle finger. This form of "percussion" is used to sound out quantities of air or fluid inside the chest and abdomen and detect any abnormality.

Examination of blood circulation is a very important part of diagnosis. With visible inspection, palpation, percussion, and auscultation (listening with the ear or by means of a stethoscope) the doctor looks for any abnormal pulsations in the arteries and veins. The patient's pulse is checked for irregularities in the rate or rhythm of heartbeat. Blood pressure is then measured with a sphygmomanometer. Finally with the use of a stethoscope the doctor listens to the heart. Abnormalities of the heart sounds may indicate disease of valves or muscle.

Usually the respiratory system is examined next. The chest is investigated to see if the lungs move evenly, equally and at a normal rate – 15 to 20 breaths per minute. The nervous system is studied by testing each part in turn. The doctor examines the patient's eyes with a ophthalmoscope: the state of nerve endings and blood vessels that run across the retinal

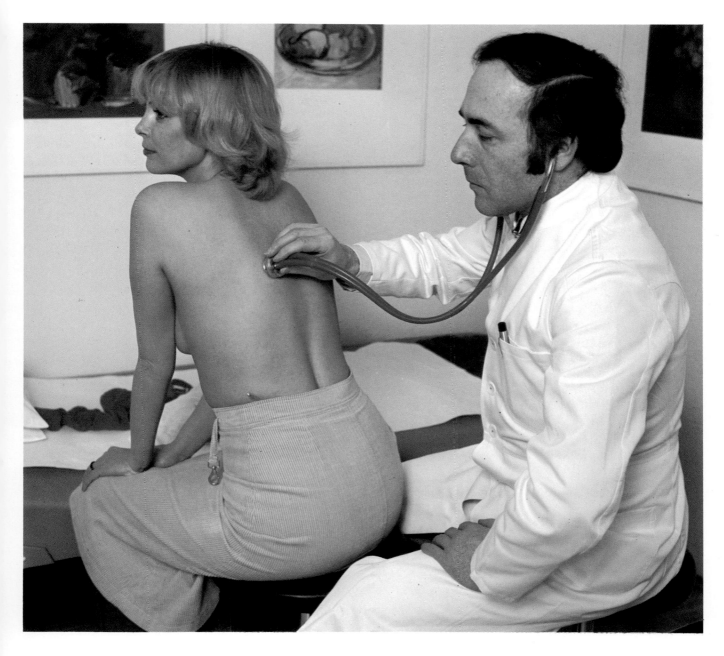

surface are very indicative of the general state of health.

Next the doctor insures that the patient can coordinate his or her movements and examines the arms for any nervous tremor. Skin sensations are tested by asking the patient, eyes closed, to say whenever he or she feels the skin being brushed by a wisp of cottonwool or pricked with a pin. Then the reflexes are examined by tapping muscle tendons at the elbows, wrists, knees, and ankles with a small hammer. The doctor completes the physical examination by looking in the patient's ears and investigating in greater detail any suspicious areas of the body. The patient is asked to provide a urine specimen which will be examined under the microscope and subjected to some simple chemical tests to determine its content of albumen, glucose, blood, and bile.

After the examination has been completed the doctor can nearly always make a "presumptive" or so-called clinical diagnosis. But if the doctor is not satisfied, a whole series of further investigations and

Examining the lungs with a stethoscope. The passage of air through healthy lungs produces a certain sound, and different diseases distort it in characteristic ways.

tests can help establish a firm diagnosis. X-rays may reveal disturbances of function and structure that remained undetected in clinical examination. A blood sample from the patient can be sent to a laboratory for a blood-cell count and chemical analysis. Some specimens, such as urine, feces, sputum, or throat swabs, can be sent to a microbiological laboratory for testing.

Even if the doctor suspects that the patient may be suffering from mental illness or neurosis, the diagnostic method follows the same pattern as that for physical illness. This is because mental symptoms, such as agitation or depression, may sometimes be symptoms of a physical disease, for example an overactive thyroid gland. And physical symptoms, such as diarrhea, indigestion, or even paralysis of a limb, may be symptoms of a mental illness such as an anxiety state or hysteria.

241

Regular Checkups

Even the most serious illnesses can be helped effectively if they are detected early enough. Illness usually does not happen overnight. It is more often the result of processes that have been developing for years. A thorough checkup can reveal conditions that might lead to illness long before any symptoms could be noticed – and at a point when there is still time to clear it up. By detecting health problems before they become serious, periodic checkups can save years of emotional, physical and financial strain. And then there is always the possibility that a health check may pronounce you 100 percent fit – a marvelous boost to anyone's wellbeing.

Right: chest X-rays, blood pressure measurements and pulse rate are three of the standard tests in hospital and general practitioner's checkups.

Below: this scanner builds up a color keyed picture of the internal organs as it passes over the patient. It also has facilities for storing pictorial and numerical data.

If you are reluctant to take up your doctor's time with a routine health check (and in any case the public health services of many countries do not provide this facility), it may be necessary to make an appointment at one of the special centers that exist in many major cities for this purpose. In these centers a whole battery of sophisticated tests are carried out that will plot a complete head-to-toe profile of

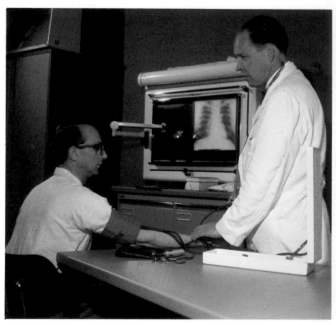

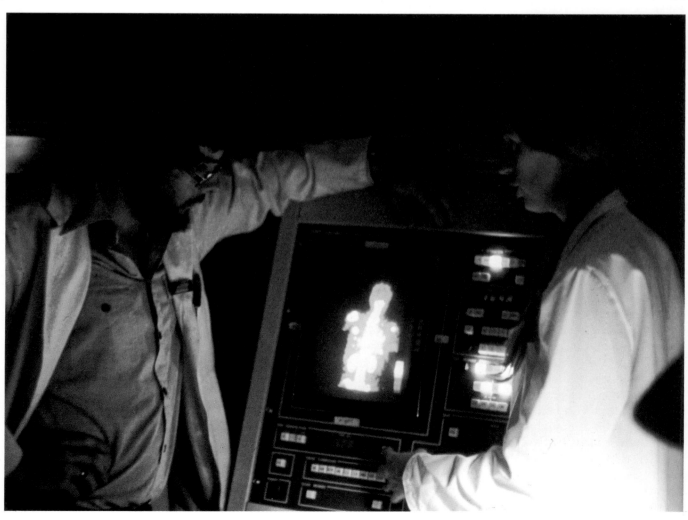

your health status. Apart from physiological measurements, physical examinations, and laboratory tests, some centers make use of computers to collect detailed information about every aspect of a person's life that may have a bearing on his health – facts about surroundings, work, home life, heredity and the entire medical history. Many people thoroughly enjoy telling the computer all about themselves, and find it much easier to give frank answers by pushing a button than by replying to a doctor or filling out a printed questionnaire.

The efforts of various public health services have started a whole new field – called *presymptomatic medicine* – to diagnose a patient's illness during the period before actual symptoms of disease manifest themselves. Sometimes this is tremendously important, because the disorder may well progress to quite an advanced stage before the patient realizes anything is wrong. In some illnesses, certain types of cancer for instance, it is already too late for a cure when the symptoms appear. Presymptomatic medicine today is the most developed in the United States, but in Europe generally the idea of a patient visiting the doctor for a regular checkup, regardless of whether there are any symptoms, has been regarded with some disdain until quite recently. Some doctors still feel that by the use of a multitude of tests many trivial abnormalities will be found that would make the patient neurotic. Problems of cost are also a great stumbling block to its widespread implementation.

Despite the problems, in most countries of the world some methods of presymptomatic diagnosis are being used – in the form of mass X-rays, routine checkups on children's teeth, routine blood testing for mothers during pregnancy, Pap tests, and many more. The advantages of mass miniature radiography is a typical example. X-ray unit housed at clinics, or in large mobile vans, enable vast numbers of people to have chest X-rays. The films are examined by a radiologist, and those people who have abnormalities are readily picked out. These will be asked to attend an X-ray department and any abnormalities in their lungs will be further investigated. This method has proved of great value in the fight against tuberculosis and also in the early detection of lung cancer.

Routine blood testing is often carried out, particularly in pregnancy. Thus anemia can be discovered and treated, and through the use of serological tests veneral disease may be discovered, often quite accidentally. Urine examination can reveal abnormal quantities of albumen, which may be a sign of kidney disease. A number of kidney diseases may be latent for many years before a person notices anything is wrong – and during this time irreparable damage may be done to this vital organ. Similarly the presence of glucose in the urine quite often indicates diabetes. Wherever routine testing of urine of all patients is started, a large number of cases of undiagnosed diabetics are discovered.

Routine testing for early detection of some forms of cancer has given astonishing results. In most countries a routine Pap test is saving the lives of many women with early cancer of the cervix (neck of the womb). Similarly routine medical examination of the breasts can detect early tumors or can give reassurance that cancer is not present.

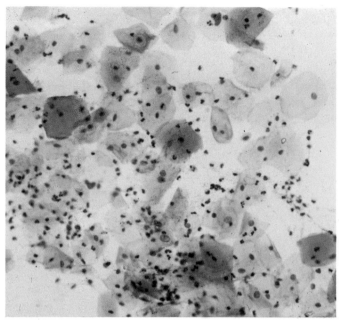

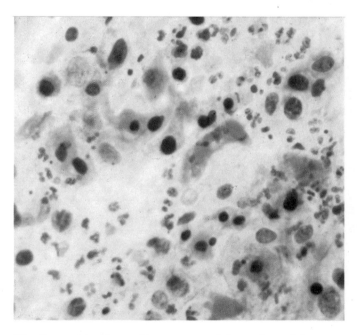

The Pap test involves taking a smear of the surface of the cervix and can reveal cells in a precancerous state. The top picture shows a healthy cervical smear, the lower one a precancerous sample. In this way, the cancer can be eradicated before it has had a chance to spread.

There can be no doubt that one day most countries of the world will realize the need to establish more and more presymptomatic clinics. Diabetes, glaucoma, cancer of the cervix, gastric ulcer – the number of diseases that can be detected at an early and curable stage is almost endless.

Examining
the Heart

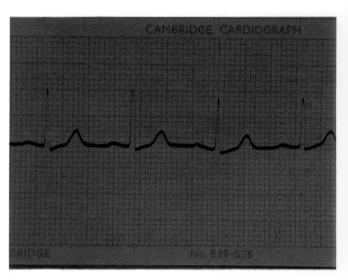

The most common failure of the heart function is when blood flow is insufficient. It happens when general circulatory pressure falls to 50 percent of normal (due to loss of blood or to abnormal dilation of the blood vessels); when the pulmonary artery is narrow (so allowing too little blood to leave the right ventricle) or leaks; when the pulmonary artery or

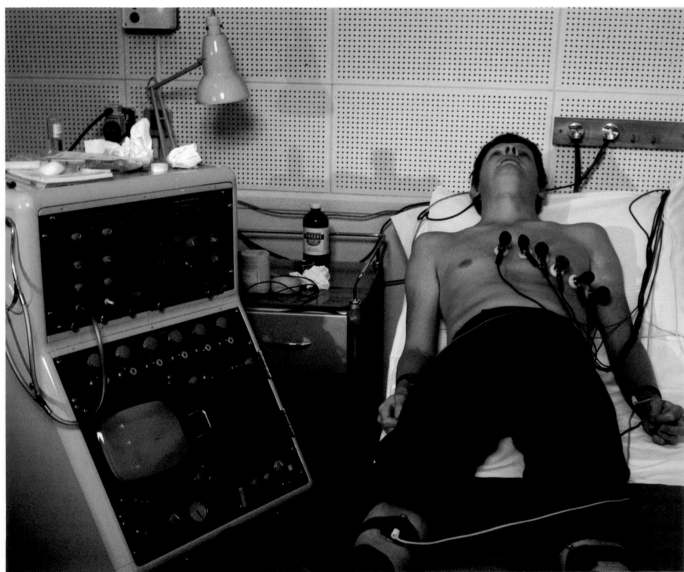

Above right: ECG of a normal heart. An ECG can reveal abnormal rhythm and damage to this vital organ.

Above: a patient wired up to an electrocardiogram.

veins are too narrow; when the capillary beds in the lungs are affected by lung disease; when the coronary arteries are diseased; or when the aortic valve is

either too narrow or leaks. Narrowness (called stenosis) and leaking often go together.

Except during major surgery the heart is so inaccessible and so well protected that doctors must conduct most of their tests at some distance from it. The *electrocardiogram* (ECG) can tell us a lot about the shape of the heart, the regularity of its rhythm, and the condition of its muscle and conducting system. An ECG is a tracing on a graph of the electric current generated by the heart muscle during a heartbeat, but it tells doctors little about the heart's output, or the state of its valves and internal walls.

The best external indicators of the valves and walls are the sounds the heart makes. The doctor can listen directly to the sounds by pressing his or her ear straight on the chest wall. The normal heart makes a double beat that can be transcribed phonetically as lub-dup – in other words, the first sound is softer and longer than the second. The "lub" coincides with the contraction of the ventricles and the "dup" comes immediately after the almost simultaneous closing of the aortic and pulmonary valves. A third sound, like a rapid echo of the "dup,"

catheterization plays a great part in the study of congenital heart abnormalities, in diagnosing heart disease accurately and objectively, as a prelude to surgery, and in correlating heart output with other bodily changes. The catheter itself is a radio-opaque, hollow nylon tube between approximately 0.04 to 0.2 inches in diameter. At frequent intervals the physician checks the course of the catheter on a *fluoroscope* – an apparatus used for examining internal organs and structures by means of X-rays. Catheterization, however, can be risky. In its early days and

Using Focussed Phased Array apparatus to monitor the action of the heart as it pumps blood around the body. The organ is scanned with ultra-high frequency sound waves, which are reflected back onto a screen. It is a useful method for studying valve defects and holes in the heart.

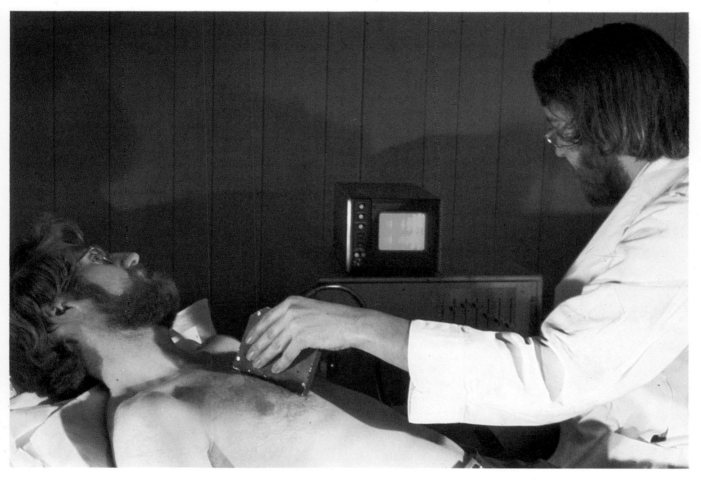

is normal in young adults. If any of the valves or walls leak, or if a valve is too narrow, then either the normal sounds will be modified or extra noises and murmurs will be heard. The timing of these extra sounds and their exact location on the chest wall give clues to the nature of the fault and to which parts of the heart are affected. The location is often easier to find with a stethoscope than with the naked ear. The *phonocardiograph* (PCG) can record several parts of the heart and the arterial and venous pulses in the neck simultaneously and display them all alongside an ECG. The PCG is particularly useful for diagnosing valve defects.

The highly specialized technique of *cardiac*

in some places still today, it was and is indulged in for its own sake, with meager returns in diagnosis.

Doctor Inge Edler, a heart specialist at the University of Lund, in Sweden, applied ultrasonics to diagnosing abnormalities of the heart. The technique uses the sonar echo principle: high frequency (and inaudible) sound waves reflected back from an object reveal its characteristics. Echo cardiography can for example, measure heart muscle thickness, detect valve abnormalities, and even show an image of the heart pumping on a television screen – without surgery or other invasive techniques. Ultrasonics has been used to explore other areas of the body, notably the developing fetus in the mother's womb.

Blood Pressure and Pulse

Checking the pulse is the medical test that we are most familiar with. You can feel it yourself on the inside of the wrist, on the thumb side. But what causes a pulse and what can it tell us about our state of health?

At each heartbeat a quantity of blood is pumped through the aorta and pulmonary arteries, and subsequently through the subsidiary arteries. The walls of the arteries are elastic and transmit the blood as a fluid wave, expanding as the blood flow increases and then regaining their normal size. Where the blood vessels lie deeply below the skin these waves cannot be detected externally, but at certain points, where the artery is near the skin and can be lightly com-

pressed against a bone, the pulse can be felt. These points are known as "pressure points", an example being the radial artery in the wrist. The actual pulse is not the heartbeat itself but the rebound in the artery.

When a doctor or nurse feels your pulse they are examining three factors – the pulse rate, its type, and its regularity. Pulse rate is not constant but in a resting adult it averages between 60 and 80 beats per minute, while in a child it is between 90 and 140 beats per minute. The pulse rate increases during and after exercise, and during eating, sexual intercourse and other states of excitement. It also rises during a fever, hemorrhage and anemia, and a rapid pulse rate called *tachycardia* (persistent rapid heartbeat) is often a sign of heart disease. *Bradycardia* (persistent slow heartbeat) produces a slower than average pulse rate and occurs during jaundice, typhoid fever and during convalescence following certain infections, for example pneumonia and influenza. Heart block also produces a slow pulse.

The type of pulse is also indicative of a person's state of health. In a person suffering from fever, a *dicrotic* pulse, where a wave immediately follows the

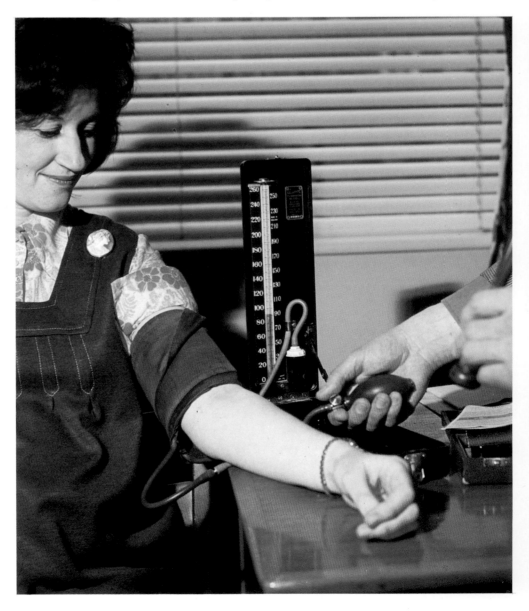

Testing blood pressure with a sphygmomanometer. The rubber cuff is inflated and a stethoscope is applied to the brachial artery pulse point. As the pressure is increased the pulse disappears. This is the pressure at which the heart contracts.

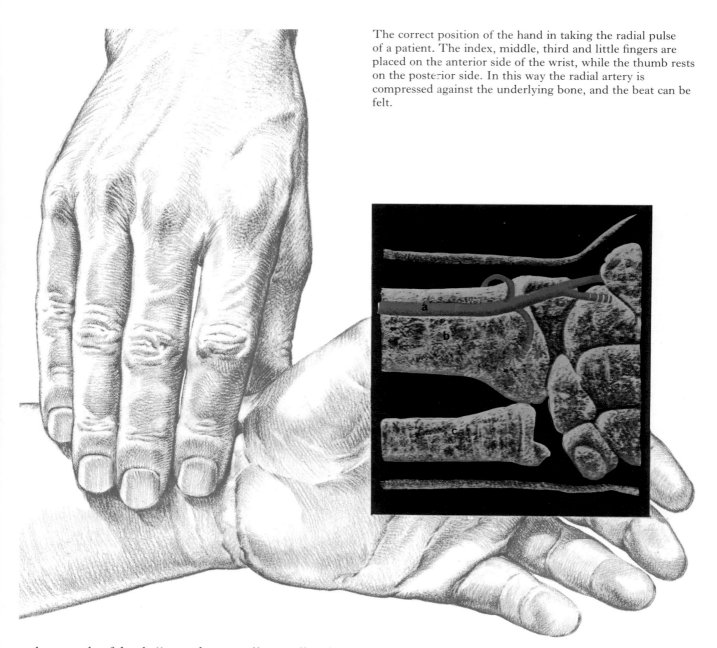

The correct position of the hand in taking the radial pulse of a patient. The index, middle, third and little fingers are placed on the anterior side of the wrist, while the thumb rests on the posterior side. In this way the radial artery is compressed against the underlying bone, and the beat can be felt.

pulse, can be felt. A "waterhammer" or collapsing pulse often indicates aortic disease. In children, because the wall of the arteries are thin, the pulse can barely be felt. As the arteries harden with age, and in most cases thicken, the pulse wave becomes more noticable. Thus the strength of a pulse can tell a doctor much about the state of the arterial walls. Meanwhile, an irregular pulse indicates possible fibrillation (rapid, uncontrolled twitching of muscle fibers) of the heart.

In addition to feeling your pulse, your doctor will also want to measure your blood pressure. Strictly speaking, the blood pressure is the pressure which has to be applied to an artery to stop a pulse beyond that point. It corresponds roughly to the pressure at which the heart pumps out blood and also to the elasticity of the blood-vessel walls. It can be gauged roughly by applying pressure with the finger to the point where the pulse is obliterated.

A more accurate measurement can be obtained using an instrument called a *sphygmomanometer*. This consists of a hollow rubber cuff, the inside of which is connected to a pressure gauge and an air pump. The cuff is strapped onto the patient's elbow, just above the crook, and pumped up. Meanwhile a stethoscope is applied to the brachial artery which is just below the elbow. As the cuff is inflated, that is, the pressure inside it is increased, the pulse disappears. This occurs at the point known as the *systolic* pressure, the pressure at which the heart contracts. In practice a more accurate reading is obtained if the cuff is inflated and then the pressure gradually released to the point where the pulse reappears.

As the cuff is allowed to deflate further the beat becomes louder. Then it starts to get weaker, eventually disappearing. This is the *diastolic* pressure or pressure between heartbeats. The pressure readings are gauged in millimeters of mercury, in the same way as barometric pressure.

Like the pulse the blood pressure can vary within an individual, but a significant deviation from the average is a distinct sign of disease or impending illness.

Lungs
and Respiration

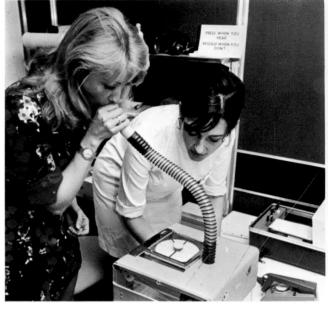

The lungs may cease to function efficiently either because air cannot circulate around the system efficiently or because there is a fault in the process of gas exchange. Inadequate air flow occurs when the air passages are physically blocked with solid particles, dust or smoke for example, or mucus; when the air passages contract in a spasm under the influence of certain reactions; when the passages and alveoli lose some of their elasticity so that they are unable to expand fully or contract naturally; or when the joints and muscles of the rib cage or diaphragm lose their mobility or strength. Inadequate gas exchange occurs when the alveoli begin to break down and join together to form enlarged sacs (a condition known as *emphysema*); when the alveolar walls become diseased and thicken; when the alveoli fill with fluid – as in pulmonary edema; with anemia; with a disturbance called respiratory acidosis; or when the blood flow is inadequate.

A peak-flow meter is an instrument used to measure the amount of air inhaled and exhaled by the lungs. If a healthy person is connected to the instrument and asked to breath normally, the machine's indicator will produce a reading on a dial. On breathing in as deeply as possible and out again to a normal level, the reading increases. When the person forces as much gas from the lungs as possible, the test is complete. The normal volume of lung available for pumping gas to and from the atmosphere is called the *tidal volume*. Extra inhalation is the *complemental volume*, and extra exhalation is the *ex-*

Above right: testing the volume of air inspired and expired with each breath. The tidal volume, complemental volume, breathing rate and vital capacity are altered to varying degrees by different lung diseases.

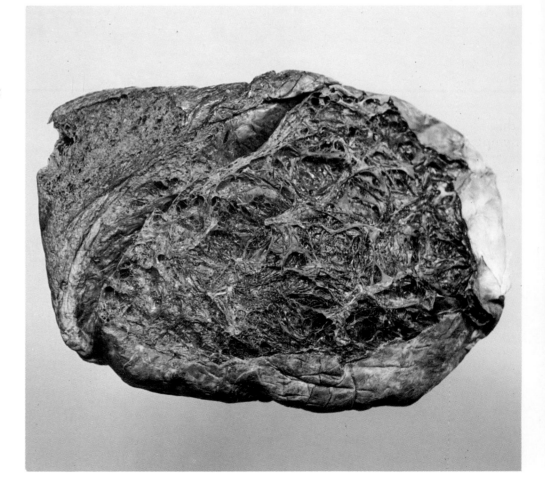

Right: a lung specimen from an emphysema victim. The lungs become abnormally distended with air and the partitions between the alveoli may be destroyed. The condition often accompanies chronic bronchitis.

piratory reserve volume. But even at maximum exhalation there is still plenty of air in the lungs. Most of it is in the alveoli, the rest in the air passages; collectively it forms the *residual volume*, which has to be calculated because it cannot be measured directly. The residual volume of the air passages is called the *anatomical dead space* – because there is no gas exchange there. The dead space becomes significant when a person's breathing grows shallow. If his breathing fell drastically, even this effect would not be sufficient to get fresh air into the alveoli each time.

The readings produced by the peak-flow meter allow doctors to determine the degree of lung incapacity. Most lung conditions increase the residual volume (the volume of air that cannot be cycled in and out) two- or threefold. In asthma and emphysema the lungs are working at the top end of their capacity; the patient's chest feels very tight and he or she has to fight for each breath. With emphysema the tidal volume is normal, but with the slightest exertion (the amount of air that can be forcibly expressed after a full inspiration) the patient breathes to the full range of his or her vital capacity which is much reduced. With asthma the bronchioles contract so much during breathing out that each cycle takes much longer. To compensate, the person is forced to breathe more deeply, so even without exertion breathing covers the full range of the vital capacity – which again is much less than normal. If the patient is given drugs to relax the bronchioles, the pattern returns to near normal.

With edema (an abnormal accumulation of fluid) the lung tissues often grow less elastic, so their total capacity is reduced. Much of the residual volume is filled with fluid. The effect is to squash the normal pattern; but the tidal volume is near normal and in its right place. In other words the person's chest is not always near its maximum expansion. The result is that – except during exertion – the patient has no symptoms. But even moderate effort can bring on breathlessness and rapid breathing over the full range of the again restricted vital capacity.

Another test, this time using a spirometer can help to clarify the nature of the condition. The operator asks the patient to inhale deeply and to breathe out as fast as he can. This reveals the rate of the breathing cycle. Asthma patients will breathe in normally, not much more slowly – so that a maximum 30 percent, say, of their vital capacity is exhaled in one second. People with emphysema or edema will have their so-called forced expiratory volume at 80 or even 85 percent of their (much reduced) vital capacity.

Such tests can tell us what is wrong with the lungs but not where the seat of the trouble lies, for only rarely is the condition uniformly spread throughout the lungs. Where obvious techniques (listening with a stethoscope, tapping the chest to locate dull, airless parts of the lung, looking down the trachea with a bronchoscope or listening down it with microphones, and so on) fails, chest doctors turn to special

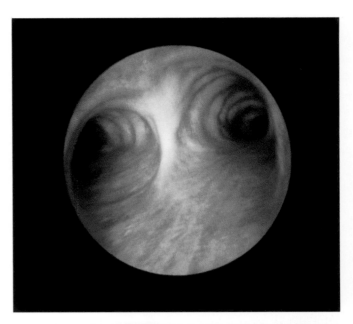

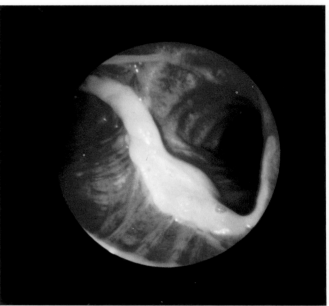

The bronchoscope is a fiber-optic tube which illuminates the interior of the lungs and enables the doctor to see inside. The top picture was viewed at the point at which the trachea divides into the two bronchi. The bottom one shows the bronchi of a patient with chronic bronchitis.

types of X-rays and radioactive gas tests to help locate the problem. In one type of X-ray study, a rubber catheter introduces iodized oil (which is radio-opaque) into one lung; the oil spreads to coat the trachea and bronchi and the whole bronchial tree is thus revealed to X-rays. If the trouble lies in the bronchioles or alveoli, an atmosphere is passed into the lungs in which some of the nitrogen is replaced by a radioisotope of the rare gas xenon. An instrument for estimating radioactivity, called a *scintillation counter*, is trained on the chest to reveal which parts of the lung this atmosphere does not penetrate or areas in which it is present in abnormal volumes. Readings can also be obtained over a blood vessel in an arm or leg to see how effectively the labeled gas passes into the blood through the alveolar membrane.

Gut, Liver and Kidneys

Because most of the activity in the alimentary canal, liver, and kidneys is chemical, the techniques used for testing these functions are essentially carried out in laboratories on sample specimens. Tests made on the blood, stomach juices, urine, and feces cannot, however, locate the actual site of a disorder; they can only tell us that a given organ is or is not performing well.

If the trouble is in the lungs, stomach, duodenum

Most types of endoscope are used mainly for observation. The operating *cystoscope*, however, is a more complex device that allows surgeons to perform certain internal operations without opening the patient's skin. A cystoscope can be introduced up through the urethra into the bladder and used to treat tumors with a high-frequency electrical current; or in testing kidney function it can be used to pass a catheter into each ureter to analyze the products of each kidney separately. It is also used to fish out kidney stones.

If the alimentary canal is to be visualized doctors still rely in the first place on X-rays. The patient, starved for six hours to clear the intestines, eats a "meal" of emulsified barium sulfate, which is radio-opaque. At various times over the following three to six hours the progress of this meal is photographed on X-ray film. The large intestine can also be ex-

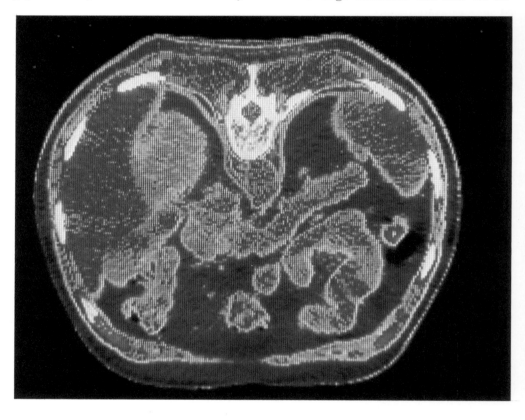

A cross-sectional X-ray through the middle of the abdomen. A thin X-ray beam is projected through the patient's body. A computer combines the series of pictures taken, so that a view can be taken at any angle, and presents different tissues in different colors.

or urinary tract, doctors can actually locate it without opening the patient. The device used is called an *endoscope*, a lighted flexible tube used to peer directly into the affected organ. Modern medical endoscopes are a modification of the industrial endoscope, designed initially for inspecting jet engines without dismantling them. Some are based on the principles of fiber optics – bundles of fine glass rods that, however bent or twisted, transmit light along their length. In most endoscopes based on these principles, there are two fiber-optic systems, one for carrying the field illumination into the patient, the other for carrying a picture out again. A *bronchoscope* is the instrument used for examining the interior of the lungs, a *gastroscope* for viewing the stomach.

amined by injecting barium through the anus in an enema. The kidneys themselves lie beyond the reach of any endoscope. The performance of the kidneys can be similarly recorded by injecting radio-opaque chemicals intravenously and seeing how and where they are excreted. A variation of this technique is to give the patient a drink or injection containing a radioactive isotope of some nontoxic chemical. For testing the kidneys, iodine-labeled hippuran, a sugar, is used. Some minutes after being drunk, by which time the kidney should be excreting the labeled hippuran, a scintillation counter is moved backward and forward over the area of the kidney. Where the activity is too weak or too strong the kidney is either failing or overactive.

It is possible to monitor chemical activity in the

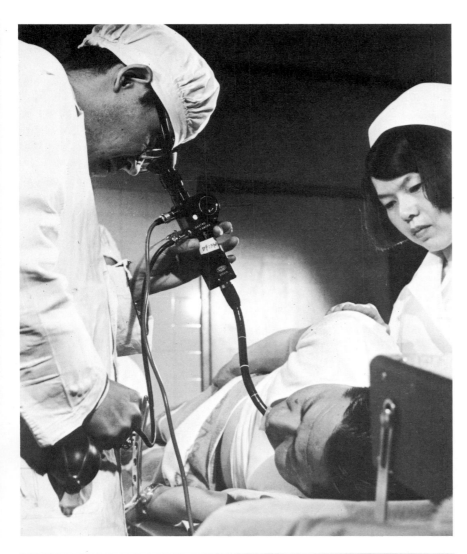

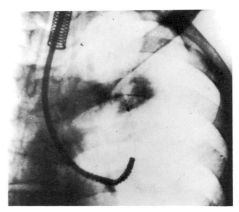

Left: the gastrocamera, which was developed in Japan, uses a flexible fiberscope to take photographs of the interior of the stomach. It has proved to be a valuable aid to the accurate diagnosis of gastric diseases, particularly in detecting stomach cancer in its early stages.

Below: X-ray photograph showing how a flexible fiberscope is used to take bronchial photographs.

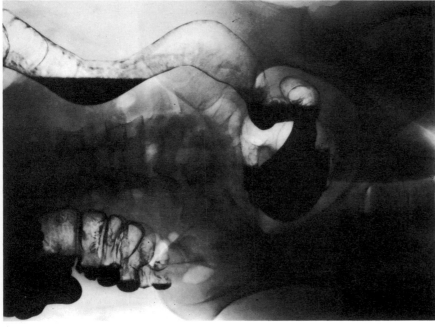

Left: X-ray negative of the large bowel. The patient's bowel was enema-injected with barium and then evacuated. The bowel was then partly filled with air, revealing where the barium has formed in pools. The convoluted bowel in the lower part of the picture is normal; the smoothed bowel at the top is diseased.

intestines by sucking out samples from a tube, which can occasionally be connected to an instrument that gives pressure readings. However, the readings obtained in this way will rarely bear any real relationship to the normal behavior of the intestines. To get more representative readings radio pills are used.

Some types contain a battery-powered radio transmitter and are sensitive to pressure; others can be used to record chemical reactions and temperature. Smaller pills have been made without a battery but containing a tuned radio circuit that can transmit information about intestinal activity.

251

The Facts about Diabetes

One of the chemical tests carried out during a routine checkup will be for sugar in the urine. The presence of sugar in the urine, a condition known as *glycosuria*, is a symptom of a number of diseases, including goiter and certain pituitary gland disorders, but it most commonly indicates diabetes.

Of course sugar in the urine is not something that a person would be aware of, but there are other symptoms of diabetes which will eventually cause a sufferer to see the doctor. These include a thirst so severe that the diabetic may be drinking between 10 and 12 pints of water a day, even waking up at night to quench it. The thirst may be associated with an unpleasant taste in the mouth. Frequent passing of large quantities of urine is another symptom. Loss of weight will also occur. However, this type of weight loss is dangerous because it is not only fat that is burnt away but muscle as well.

There are a number of other symptoms which if severe enough will prompt someone to seek treatment. For example there may be a profound tiredness, possibly accompanied by *amenorrhea* (cessation of periods) in women, and impotence in men. There may be blurring of vision, tingling in the fingers and

A pocket blood-glucose meter enables the diabetic to monitor his or her sugar levels. A spot of blood is placed on a test stick and the meter displays the blood-glucose value.

feet, muscular cramps and boils.

There are, in fact, two distinct types of diabetes. The juvenile form, so-called because it starts during childhood or young adulthood, is far more severe. Maturity-onset diabetes is more common and is often precipitated by overeating. There may be no symptoms other than a general lassitude, but it still requires treatment. Regular checkups are the best way of detecting maturity-onset diabetes.

If these symptoms are reported and diabetes suspected the doctor will order a *glucose-tolerance test*, in which the patient's blood sugar level is monitored before and after a glucose drink. However, symptoms of diabetes may develop gradually and the diabetic may get accustomed to them or consider that they are not worth troubling their doctor about. Meanwhile the patient's general health deteriorates and he or she may eventually end up in hospital in a *diabetic coma*. An illness or infection will often precipitate a diabetic coma in a person with an unsuspected case of the disease.

The body's chief source of energy is glucose, which it obtains from breaking down food, principally carbohydrates. But glucose cannot enter a cell by simple diffusion; it needs the hormone insulin to "help" it across the cell membrane. Diabetes is the result of an insulin deficiency. The diabetic may be unable to produce any or enough insulin or cannot use it properly, or may have factors in the blood which counteract it, for example antibodies or an excess of a hormone with an opposing action.

As a result glucose accumulates in the blood and has to be flushed out through the kidneys. Because of this large amounts of water have to be consumed. This in itself is nowhere near as serious as the other effects of diabetes on the body chemistry. The body still needs energy, so it burns fat, but cannot burn it completely because the complex metabolism of fat requires some glucose to be present. So poisonous intermediate products—ketones—accumulate. These account for the unpleasant taste; they also cause the blood to become acid (*acidosis*) and eventually a diabetic coma which may be fatal. Other possible complications are blindness and gangrene.

Diabetes is not as serious a disease as it used to be now that insulin is available for treatment. The important point to grasp is that although the condition is irreversible, diabetics are able to lead normal lives as long as they take the prescribed medication and readjust their diet, in particular the intake of carbohydrate. The patient learns the calorific values and fiber content of the carbohydrates he or she is likely to eat and regulates their eating habits accordingly. Doctors and diabetic clinics always bear in mind the diabetic's normal eating habits, preferences and cultural upbringing, and will not prescribe an unsuitable or unpalatable regime. Sugar is usually forbidden because it is a refined food which is absorbed immediately and makes demands on the body that a diabetic's inadequate insulin levels cannot cope with.

For diabetics who have a sweet tooth proprietary diabetic products are available which are made with artificial sweeteners. Overeating is dangerous for a diabetic because a deficient pancreas cannot meet the insulin requirement of the excess food. Diabetics are therefore told to lose weight immediately.

Many maturity-onset diabetics manage simply by regulating their diet. Tablets which lower the blood-sugar level can also be prescribed. Severe diabetes requires a daily intake of insulin. Since this hormone is digested in the stomach, it cannot be taken orally but has to be injected. Because the dose has to be precise, and the insulin requirements of the body vary according to the carbohydrate eaten, monitoring

lishment of a correct dose of insulin, is the possibility of a *hypoglycemic coma*. Unlike a diabetic coma, this is the result of too low a level of sugar in the blood. If too much insulin is injected, a meal is skipped or the patient undergoes a vigorous bout of exercise, the blood-sugar levels may be depleted to well below normal level with adverse effects on the brain. The diabetic begins to experience symptoms of weakness, trembling, sweating or slurring of speech. Two sugar lumps, glucose tablets or a heavily

Left: diabetic children learning how to inject themselves.

Below: a home kit for monitoring the urine sugar level.

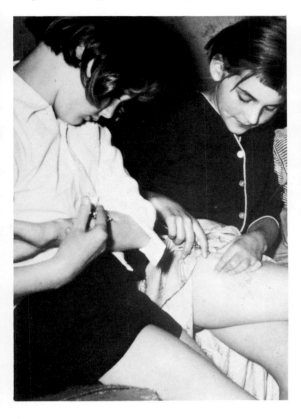

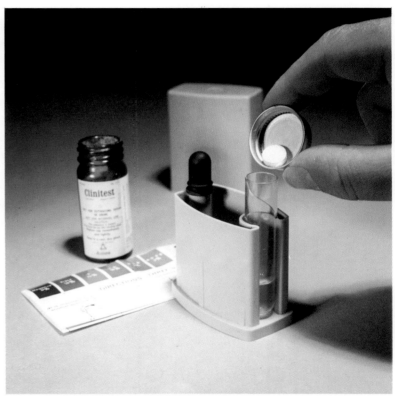

of food intake is especially crucial. It is far more practicable and safer to standardize the carbohydrate intake and keep to a fixed dosage of insulin than eat as one liked and have to work out the appropriate dose of insulin each day.

Various types of insulin are available. Soluble insulin is injected into the subcutaneous tissues and although its activity is relatively short-lived, its effect is predictable. Long-lived insulin, which needs to be injected only once a day, is available for patients whose work or lifestyle make numerous injections impossible. In general the diabetic is not tied to a doctor's surgery or diabetic clinic once he or she has learnt to cope with the problem, although regular visits are advisable, especially if an illness strikes. Monitoring of sugar level in the urine do not require laboratory facilities because kits are available for patients to perform their own analyses at home.

Diabetes, therefore, is a matter of control. The main problem that a diabetic faces beyond the estab-

sweetened drink will elevate the sugar level back to normal. Otherwise a coma may follow. An unconscious diabetic may be given an intravenous injection of sugar solution. All diabetics on insulin treatment carry sugar around with them so that it is easily available in case of an emergency. The possibility of a hypoglycemic coma is the only major factor which could affect a normal life. Once again it is up to the patient rather than the physician to cope with the situation. A diabetic soon learns how to recognize the symptoms and also when to anticipate them. Patients who have recently developed the disease are advised not to drive until they have learnt to cope with this particular problem. Educating one's family and friends, and carrying some form of notification of one's diabetic condition are also wise precautions as a hypoglycemic coma can often be mistaken for simple fainting or drunkenness. Alcohol is not banned from a diabetic's diet, provided he or she knows its carbohydrate content.

253

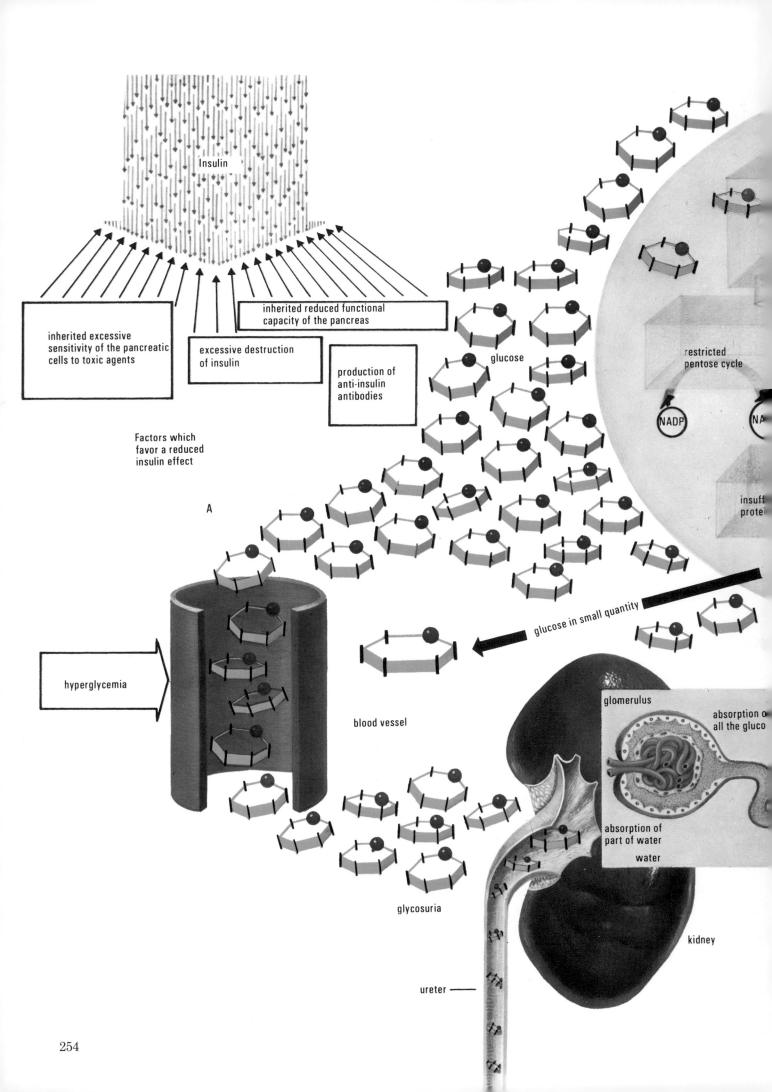

Insulin

inherited reduced functional
capacity of the pancreas

inherited excessive
sensitivity of the pancreatic
cells to toxic agents

excessive destruction
of insulin

production of
anti-insulin
antibodies

Factors which
favor a reduced
insulin effect

A

glucose

restricted
pentose cycle

NADP

NA

insuff
prote

glucose in small quantity

hyperglycemia

blood vessel

glomerulus

absorption o
all the gluco

absorption of
part of water

water

glycosuria

kidney

ureter

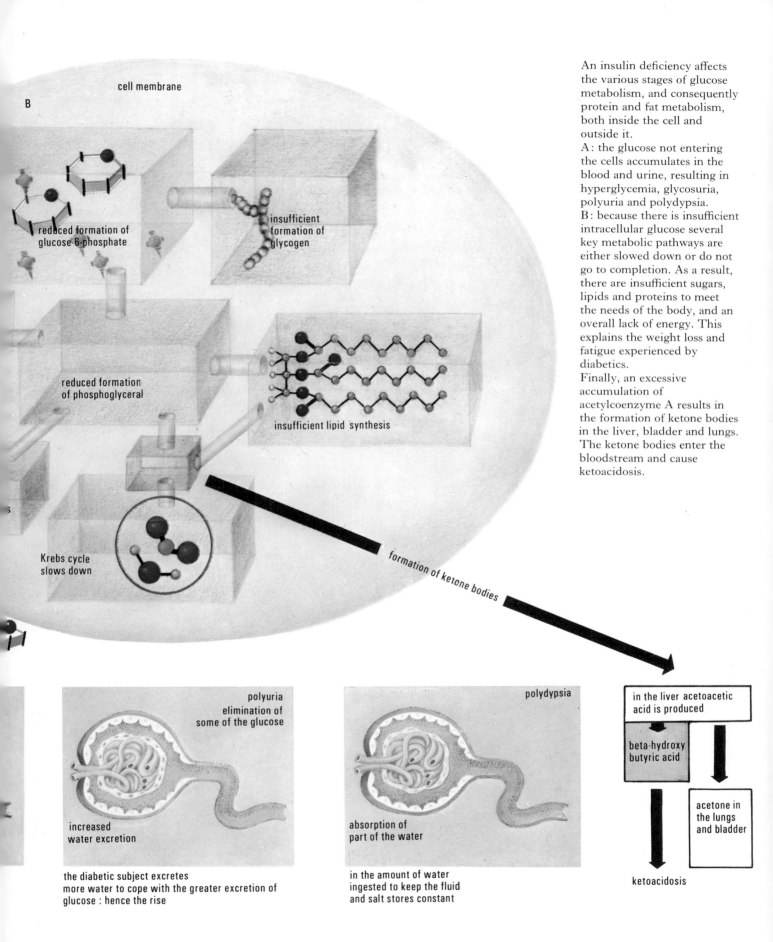

cell membrane

B

reduced formation of
glucose-6-phosphate

insufficient
formation of
glycogen

reduced formation
of phosphoglyceral

insufficient lipid synthesis

Krebs cycle
slows down

formation of ketone bodies

An insulin deficiency affects
the various stages of glucose
metabolism, and consequently
protein and fat metabolism,
both inside the cell and
outside it.
A: the glucose not entering
the cells accumulates in the
blood and urine, resulting in
hyperglycemia, glycosuria,
polyuria and polydypsia.
B: because there is insufficient
intracellular glucose several
key metabolic pathways are
either slowed down or do not
go to completion. As a result,
there are insufficient sugars,
lipids and proteins to meet
the needs of the body, and an
overall lack of energy. This
explains the weight loss and
fatigue experienced by
diabetics.
Finally, an excessive
accumulation of
acetylcoenzyme A results in
the formation of ketone bodies
in the liver, bladder and lungs.
The ketone bodies enter the
bloodstream and cause
ketoacidosis.

polyuria
elimination of
some of the glucose

increased
water excretion

the diabetic subject excretes
more water to cope with the greater excretion of
glucose : hence the rise

polydypsia

absorption of
part of the water

in the amount of water
ingested to keep the fluid
and salt stores constant

in the liver acetoacetic
acid is produced

beta-hydroxy
butyric acid

acetone in
the lungs
and bladder

ketoacidosis

Chemical Analysis

The body is such a finely balanced system that even minor disorders can quickly upset its chemical equilibrium. Our bodies maintain a critical balance between proteins, electrolytes, and other solutes in the body fluids and no single center in the body regulates all these components. The hundreds of thousands of chemical tests that doctors annually carry out on their patients are only rarely aimed at detecting traces of abnormal substances; their purpose, rather, is to find abnormal quantities of quite normal body chemicals, such as enzymes, proteins, metabolites, ions, dissolved gases, and waste products. The obvious place to find these chemicals is in the blood, although sometimes it is not necessary to tap the blood itself. Instead exhaled breath, which has been in near contact with the blood, can be analyzed; or urine, which is derived wholly from blood.

There are two basic approaches used to determine the quantities of the blood's various constituents: direct and indirect measurements. The presence of a substance in a mixture can be measured directly by shining a light of a known wavelength on or through the mixture and measuring the changes in intensity of the beams. These are known as *photometric* methods. Or the presence of a substance can be measured indirectly by allowing it to react with another chemical and then measuring the reaction.

Oxygen content in the blood stream does not exist in a simple solution but in loose combination with hemoglobin, forming oxyhemoglobin. All photometric methods for determining the oxygen tension of the blood depend on the different light reflection characteristics of these two substances. Some calculations are necessary in the first place so that the machine readings can be interpreted in terms of the oxygen concentration of the blood. But once the photometer is set up, the operator does not have to go through these calculations for each reading – the machine does the work. Having calibrated the instrument the light can be filtered and the deflections at these wavelengths can be interpreted directly as oxygen tension readings.

An instrument called a *spectrophotometer* similarly uses the properties of light as a basis of measurement.

An absorption spectrophotometer for determining the concentration of solutions such as blood or urine. Light of a predetermined wavelength is passed through the sample, and a photocell connected to a meter records the degree of absorption. This is compared with a standard control solution.

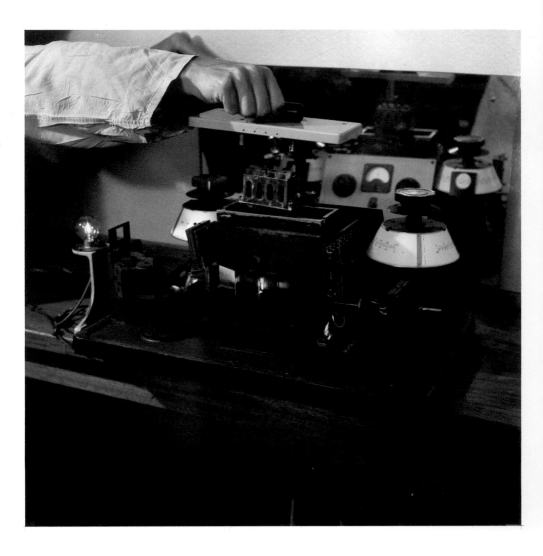

Individual elements and simple ions, if heated, will emit light of characteristic wavelengths: the intensity of the light depends on the temperature and on the concentration of the element in question. The most common machine operating on this principle is the *flame photometer*, which is used for measuring the amounts of sodium, potassium, and calcium in the body. If, however, the element in question is present

sulting spectrum, doctors can determine which elements are present.

A chemical variable that can be easily measured and that has great diagnostic value is the acidity or

Typing of blood groups by reacting the sample with serums containing specific antibodies. Group A blood is agglutinated by anti-A serum, group B by anti-B serum, group AB by both and group O by neither.

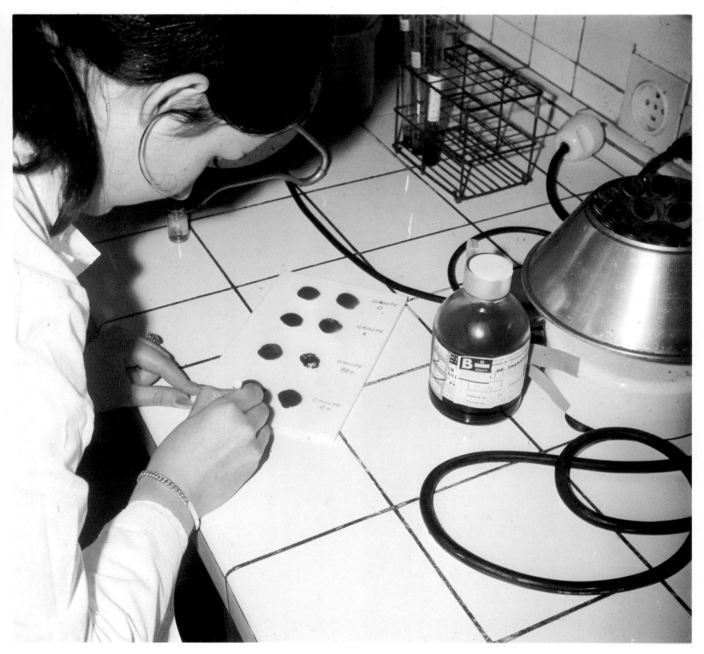

in the body only in minute traces (such as are chromium, magnesium, cobalt and copper), its emission may be too faint to measure accurately. But gaseous elements will absorb light of the same frequency as they emit; if the incoming light is powerful, absorption is easy to measure. Thus if a strong white light from a high-temperature source is shone through a lower-temperature flame containing certain elements, the light that emerges from the gas will be relatively deficient in certain wavelengths, and these will show as dark lines in the spectrum. By studying the re-

alkalinity of the blood or urine. These properties depend on the concentration of hydrogen ions and are measured on a scale of values called pH. The pH measurement is made with a *glass electrode*, which basically is a tubular membrane of a special glass that develops voltage when the pH outside differs from the pH inside. Only a tiny amount of blood has to be taken from the patient when this and other chemical tests are carried out – an important consideration if the patient cannot tolerate much blood loss, or happens to be a small child.

257

X-Rays in Diagnosis

X-rays, because of a very high frequency – which means a very short wavelength – penetrate dense bodies and create an image on a photographic plate as well as on a fluorescent screen. It is these two properties, penetration and photographic effect, that make them so useful. Simple X-rays provide doctors with information about cracked bones or hidden tooth problems. Also some inner organs, such as the heart and lungs, show up well. The heart's outline is clearly formed on the X-ray negative against the darker background of the air-filled lungs. The outline of the heart can be highly informative: an en-

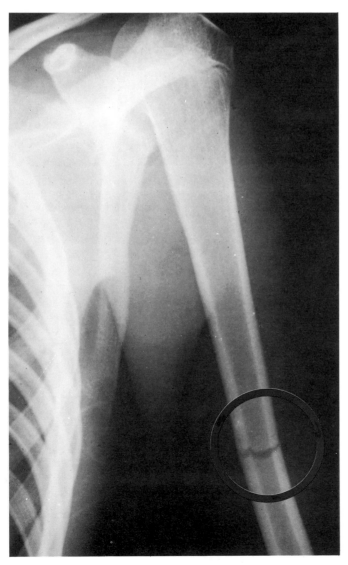

X-ray of a fracture in the arm. The fracture is simple, that is, it is not in direct communication with the wound, unlike a compound fracture.

larged heart may indicate high blood pressure, disease of the heart valves, or a disease of the heart muscle.

Tuberculosis, cancer, and other disorders of the lungs, often produce shadows of unusual appearances which can be seen on the X-ray photograph, and thus can sometimes be diagnosed accurately. Outside the chest, plain X-rays are used to pinpoint fractures, to identify gall and kidney stones and to locate metal objects such as pins that have been swallowed.

To overcome the problem of how to make soft tissues opaque to X-rays, radiologists use substances to create a contrast. To reveal the outline of the stomach, a patient is fed a barium meal, which absorbs X-rays and so reveals the alimentary canal. To investigate the respiratory system iodized oil is introduced through the trachea to the bronchi. Such contrast media are introduced into other systems: into the ureter or bladder to delineate the contor of these organs, into other body cavities, or ducts, such as salivary ducts and Fallopian tubes. The circulatory system can be put to use with advantage in this technique: an organic dye can be injected into the blood stream and carried into the kidneys or urinary tract. But X-raying the arteries or veins themselves presents a much greater problem.

Even spaces in the body not in direct contact with the circulatory system or the external atmosphere can be shown up on X-ray photography by using special techniques. Air, oxygen, or iodized oil can be injected, for example, into a joint, or into parts of the brain, or into the abdominal cavity, or any other cavities, cysts or abscesses. All these techniques are based on the fact that some materials absorb much more or much less X-ray energy than their surroundings.

Because a barium meal is gradually dispersed as it passes through the digestive system a special technique is used to examine the lower part of the system, the colon and the rectum. Water and barium are pumped into the colon as a barium enema. The barium lines the colon and any irregularities are shown up on the X-ray. This procedure is somewhat uncomfortable but it gives most reliable results and is daily helping to save the lives of many people with early cancer of the intestines. Today catheters are designed to release dye into the heart so that X-rays will reveal the blood's flow and turbulence.

A new and rewarding method is called *body scan radiography*. Special scanning cameras, sensitive to radioactivity, move to and fro across the body, leaving pictures behind them as they do so. Chemical elements with radioactive properties, called radioisotopes, are used to prepare the body for study by the scanning camera. These isotopes, if put in a patient's drink or injected into the bloodstream, will concentrate themselves in specific parts of the body. Radioactive iodine, for example, will collect in the thyroid gland. The scanning camera, which consists

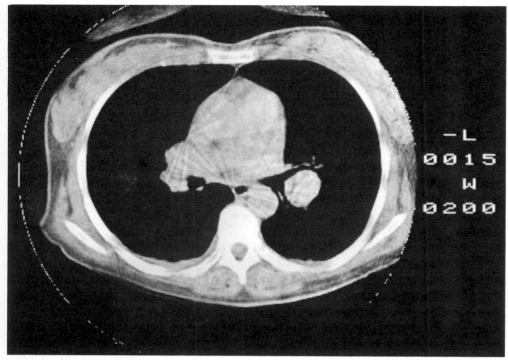

-L
0015
W
0200

This X-ray scanner enables the doctor to examine any clear cross section of the body, including soft tissue. It produces a series of readings which are combined by a computer to produce a televized image.

of a bank of radioactivity receptors, is set up in front of the person and moved across. If the thyroid is to be examined the camera will be placed near the neck. The scanner can "read" the radioactivity streaming out from the patient, and produces a "map" of the organ where the radioactive substance is concentrated. In a refinement of this technique, thermography, the scanner is connected, via a computer, to a photographic plate or color television screen, on which "hot" or radioactive spots are shown in red, "cold" ones in blue. It is possible for a doctor to assess the size and shape of a tumor simply by studying the resulting image.

Because radioisotopes carry with them the possibility of damage from ionizing radiation, techniques have been developed which intensify, either electrically or photographically, the image produced. Image intensifying techniques enable information to be obtained with the use of extremely small doses of radiation.

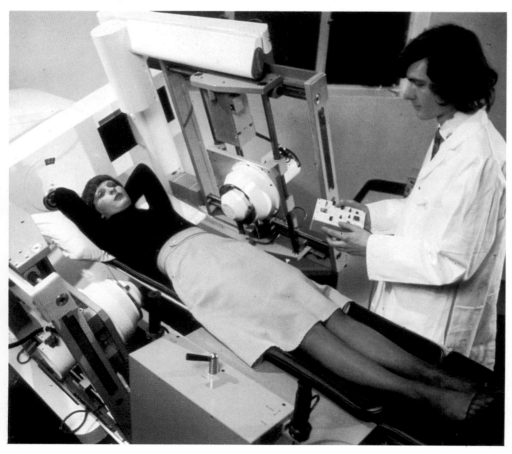

Tomoscanning the body, a "slice" at a time. First the patient has a radioisotope injected into the blood stream. Then the intensity of radiation is scanned, and fed into the computer as a series of "slices" which can then be intergrated to produce a composite picture of the whole body.

259

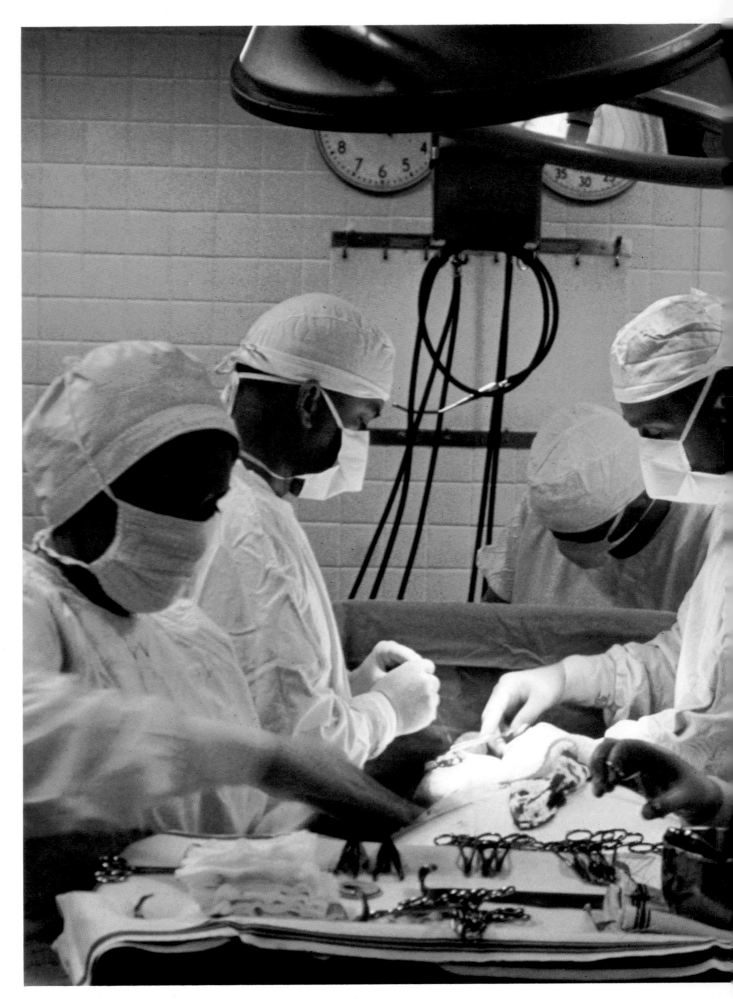

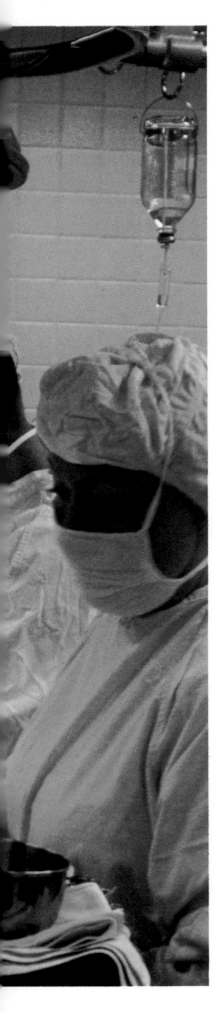

Chapter 14

Undergoing an Operation

Surgery on the human body is probably as old as civilization itself. Thousands of years ago primitive surgeons were removing pieces of skull to let the "evil spirits" out and operating on cataracts. The ancient Romans cut open women's abdomens and brought out babies that could not be born normally. But despite its long history it was not until the 20th century that having an operation became a relatively safe procedure. And now surgical technology has reached a stage where "spare part" surgery is commonplace and even heart transplants rarely make the headlines. However, these specialized operations represent only a tiny fraction of the life-saving surgery carried out in our hospitals every day.

Opposite: the rapid and dramatic advances in surgery have enabled many lives to be saved or made functional again. Yet many still fear the possibility of undergoing a surgical operation.

A Case History

Joseph Cussack had suffered an acute inflammation of the appendix in his late twenties, but as the pain in the middle of the abdomen had subsided in a few days, and later returned only very rarely, he forgot about it. He became used to living with his inflamed appendix. Then suddenly, when he was just over 70 years old, he woke one morning earlier than usual because of a sudden, severe, general abdominal pain, most marked near the navel. This was soon followed by nausea and vomiting. Six or eight hours later the pain shifted from the middle of the abdomen to the right lower part and Joseph noticed that the area was becoming completely rigid at an alarming rate. He took his own temperature but it was normal and this comforted him for some time. During the day he was able to carry out all his usual activities, but as he lived alone, he telephoned his son to tell him about his trouble. His son suggested that Joseph should call a doctor but he refused, because he was "not one of those people constantly going to the doctor and spending their time in waiting rooms." Later during the day the pain became more sporadic and Joseph was pleased to find what he felt sure was his condition in an old medical book, under the heading "Unruly stomach."

But that night the pain returned and Joseph could not sleep at all. The next morning he felt that something was still wrong with him because the pain in the abdomen was dull but constant. He decided to stay in bed for the day. He still did not have a temperature and he had stopped vomiting. But now he could ño longer tell exactly where his abdomen was painful. Then he remembered that in the past he could deal with his "appendix" with plain aspirin. So he took a couple, and to his relief it worked. During the whole day he felt much better, but he had to act with caution, because whenever he tried to move quickly the pain returned.

The next morning he was still in pain – so he took some more aspirin. But by now he realized that something was very wrong. During the morning his son Michael came to see him and the young man was quite shaken: his father was extremely pale and it was obvious that he had lost weight. He suggested that a doctor should now be called in, but Joseph was adamant, saying that an old man must "learn to live with his body," and everything would be alright.

Surgical suturing of a wound. Two types of material are used: absorbable catgut, and nonabsorbable materials such as nylon, silk and steel wire, the latter used for long-term strength.

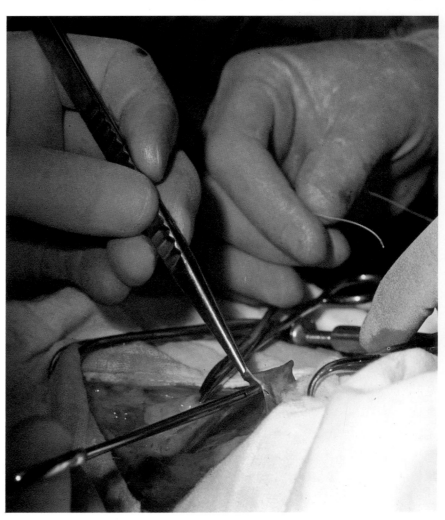

Mention of going to a hospital made Joseph furious and he refused even to talk about it.

Michael left his father, but he was worried. He decided to visit his own doctor and ask his advice. After hearing the story, Michael's doctor immediately went to see Joseph and after a brief examination he ordered his immediate transfer to the hospital. By this time Joseph was in no condition to object. He was operated on only four hours after being admitted.

Joseph had an *appendectomy* (removal of the appendix), and it was only just in time: the appendix was inflamed with adhesions on all sides. An abscess with an extremely thin wall was found on its lower part. It was obvious that the abscess would have perforated very shortly if the appendix had not been removed. This would have caused severe complications which, even today, despite the advances in the surgical treatment of this common disease, are extremely dangerous – and for Joseph would probably have proved fatal.

The operation was a complete success. The wound healed quickly, the pain disappeared, and Joseph felt better than he had done for many years. Although many times in the past Joseph had boasted that he had "never needed a doctor in his life," on this occasion he had to admit that without the surgeon's skill he would have undoubtedly come to an unpleasant end.

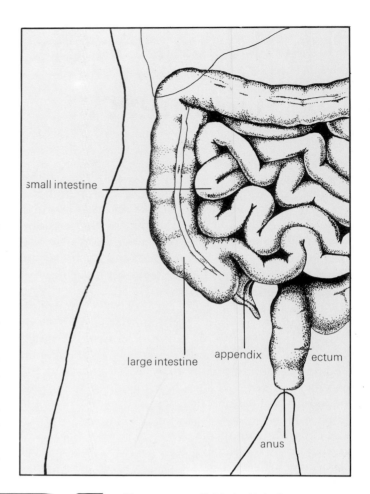

Above: appendicitis is the inflammation of the appendix, a 3-inch long blindended protrusion of the large intestine. In the human being it no longer serves any function.

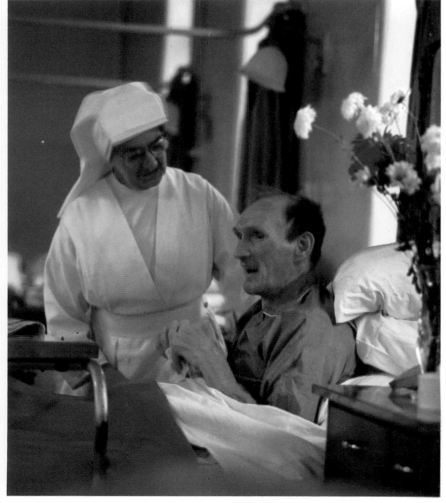

Left: for many patients surgical operations are a worrying experience. At this stage the nursing staff plays a valuable role, reassuring the patient and explaining forthcoming procedures.

263

The Development of Surgery

From ancient times surgery has held a universal fascination – more so now than ever before. This is due partly to general curiosity – the hypnotism of the drama of the operating theater – with the knowledge that many of us will become "players" in this drama at some time in our lives, and partly to the excitement of the ever-increasing sophistication of surgical techniques and the men and women who use them. It is possible that the first heart transplant, performed by Doctor Christian Barnard in Cape Town, South Africa, in 1967, produced as much worldwide interest as man's first step on the Moon.

The overcoming of pain by anesthetics and the conquest of surgical infection has opened up new possibilities of surgical progress undreamed of by the great surgeons of past centuries. In the past surgeons were superb technicians – they were only successful if they were extremely fast. Indeed, the manual dexterity of these surgeons was probably just as good as the well-trained operator of today. But, despite

their skills, infection and *suppuration* (the formation of pus) invariably followed any surgery. Therefore operations on the body's cavities – the brain, chest and abdomen – were rarely carried out since fatal infections were inevitable. In fact death following almost any kind of operation was common.

The conquest of infection still continues since the pioneering work of Ignaz Semmelweis, Louis Pasteur, Joseph Lister and others in the 19th century. Similarly, advances in anesthesia have, with both an increasing knowledge of lung function and the actions of a wide variety of anesthetics, taken place at an incredible speed.

In a modern operating theater the procedures have become safe and comfortable even for patients who are severely ill or of an advanced age, or even for infants. Aseptic surroundings have reduced the chance of wounds becoming infected and antibiotics have given surgeons a potent weapon against the dangers of spreading infection.

The enormous advances that have been made in the fundamental knowledge of disease processes have allowed surgeons to plan their treatment on a rational, scientific basis. And surgeons have taken advantage of the rapid development of other sciences – physics and electronics, chemistry and engineering – in order to solve their own problems with startling rapidity. From the engineer the surgeon has learned how to construct the pumps, oxygenators, and filters

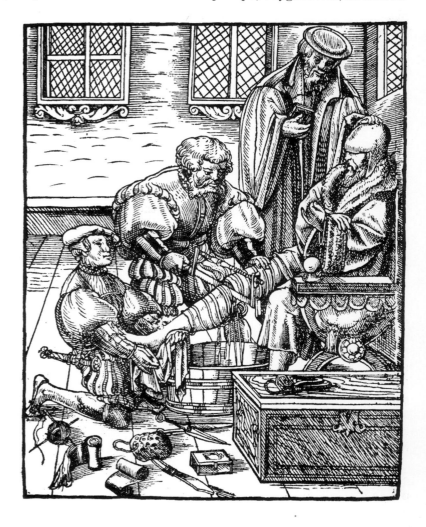

An amputation performed in the Middle Ages. The chances of the patient surviving the operation were very slim. With no anesthetics available, death from shock was common, but in any case, because antiseptics and antibiotics were nonexistent, a fatal infection was almost inevitable.

264

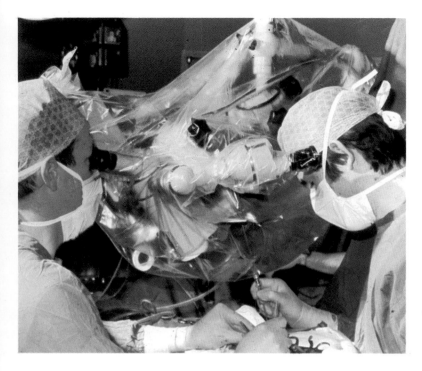

Left: microsurgery being used to remove a blood clot from the brain. Small tools, coated with a nonreflecting material, are manipulated under a magnification of ×20. This technique has cut the mortality rate due to brain hemorrhages by 50 percent.

Below: this British mobile operating enclosure provides completely sterile and infection-free conditions for surgical operations. It consists of a clear plastic box attached to an airconditioning system which pumps in sterilized air.

needed to produce efficient heart-lung machines that can take over the function of the heart while it is arrested and its damaged valves or narrowed ducts are repaired. From the chemist the surgeon has been given synthetic tubes to replace or by-pass arteries. The metallurgist has developed materials used as internal splints for fractures or complete joint replacements. From the field of electronics have evolved pacemakers to stimulate the flagging heart muscles. The laser beam, ultrasonics, radioactive scanning devices and machines that produce intense local cold temperature have been applied to surgical diagnosis and treatment.

The role of the surgeon has undergone a more subtle change. Today the operating room depends on the team effort of doctors, nurses and scientists, each member having the same objectives: to insure that the patient's disease will be diagnosed accurately, that the operation will be safe and without pain, and that the recovery will be a smooth one.

A general surgeon can perform most types of common operations, including appendectomy, hernia operations, removal of tumors, ulcer and gall bladder operations, and many more. Specialists or consultants include brain surgeons, eye surgeons, urological surgeons (who deal with the urinary tract and male organs of reproduction), and ear, nose and throat surgeons, who perform the common removal of the tonsils. Orthopedic surgeons perform operations on bones, joints and muscles. Obstetric and gynecology surgeons deal with special problems of pregnancy and childbirth, Caesarean sections, and also with disorders of the female organs of reproduction, such as removal of the womb (known as a hysterectomy).

Surgery involves teamwork: the surgeon, assistant and house surgeons, anesthetist and nurses. Nurses play an important part in the teamwork of both the

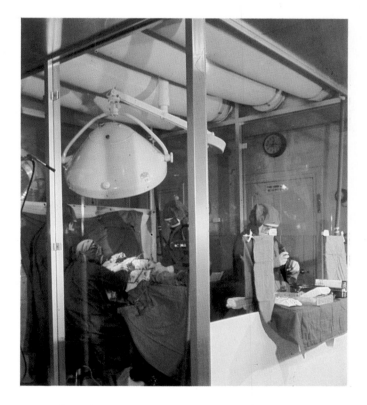

operating theater and the ward; they assist the surgeon and are a source of comfort to the patient. The surgical duties of the nurse concern those aspects of the nursing care of the patient which take place before and after the operation, including taking of patient's temperature, pulse and respiration rate.

Before the surgeon arrives in the theater nurses prepare the operating table and may swing the powerful lights into position. The surgical team "scrubs up" and puts on sterilized gowns, caps, and gloves. Everything possible is done to minimize the risk of infection. The operating team is now ready for the patient.

Preparing for Surgery

Many people who are about to have an operation – however minor – approach the event with a great deal of apprehension. This is usually because they have little idea of what is going to happen to them. A basic knowledge of what is involved, especially where preparation is concerned, will help to allay the patient's fears.

Even before the patient enters the hospital it is highly recommended that he or she smokes as little as possible for a few days. This will lead to a smoother anesthesia and reduce the chances of postoperative complications such as coughing, inflammation of the trachea, or lung congestion. The same warning applies to alcohol: it is wise not to drink heavily for a few days before surgery. Excessive drinking affects digestion and most of all the liver, and it is important that the inner organs' functions are not impaired when major surgery is to be performed.

After arrival at the hospital several routine procedures will be carried out to make sure that the patient is ready for surgery. As a primary precaution there will be a careful examination to insure that the patient is fit enough to be operated on. As the bowels may not move for several days after surgery, an enema is usually given the night before most operations, but this is not done where there is acute inflammation in the intestinal tract or abdomen. The patient usually has no food or drink for about six hours before the operation. This is because there is a danger that such food could be vomited and inhaled into the lungs.

Before the operation special attention is paid to the wound area. A wide area around the operative site is shaved. This is done to prevent infection and insure surgical sterility. For a chest operation the entire chest is shaved, and an entire limb may be shaved for surgery on an arm or leg. For an abdominal operation the pubic hair and all the hair on the abdomen and upper thighs is removed. The skin is then washed with ether soap, thoroughly rinsed with sterile water, and painted with an antiseptic.

Nowadays, surgical operations are carried out under aseptic (as opposed to antiseptic) conditions. All equipment, dressings, tools and materials, as well as the entire operating area, are sterilized beforehand.

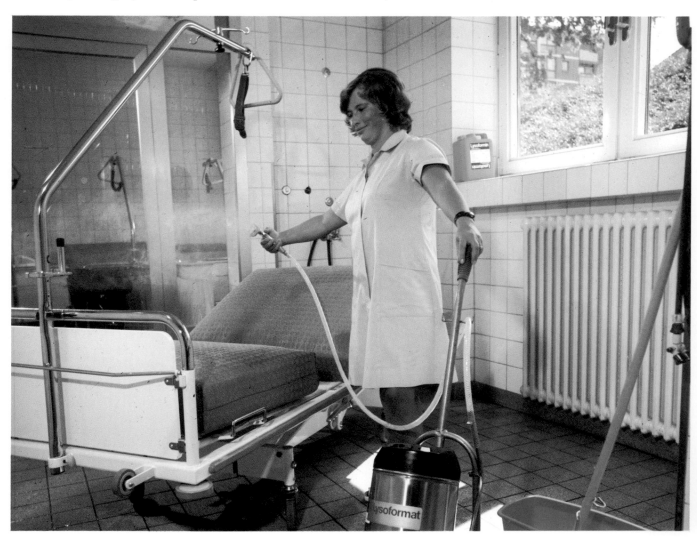

266

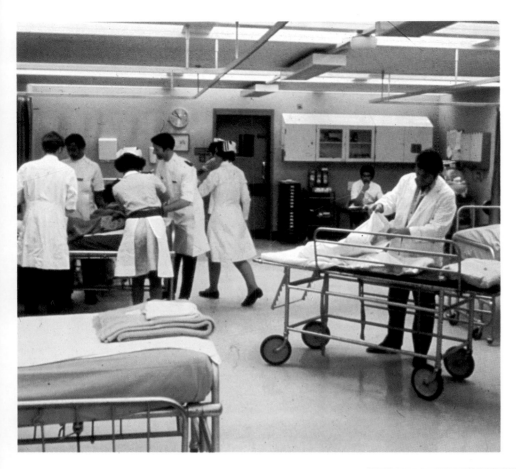

Left: a casualty patient being wheeled in for an emergency operation.

Below: all members of the opearting team spend about 10 minutes scrubbing up. Even so, because it is impossible to rid the skin entirely of bacteria, sterilized rubber gloves have to be worn.

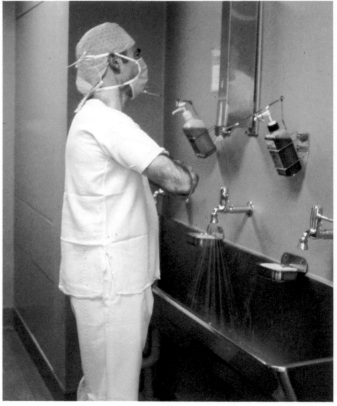

All dentures are removed from a patient's mouth so that they are not dislodged during anesthesia. If the patient has a loose tooth, the surgeon should be informed so that this may be attended to before the operation.

Sometimes a patient's water balance has to be regulated. Dehydrated patients may be given intravenous injections of nutrient liquids, and also vitamins, proteins, sugars, or antibiotic drugs. Patients who have already lost blood or are severely anemic will be given a blood transfusion.

For certain kinds of abdominal operations, particularly those performed upon the digestive system, the stomach must be completely empty. A rubber tube is therefore inserted through the nose into the stomach and attached to a suction apparatus. This may be done the night before, or early on the morning of surgery. These tubes are often left in place throughout the operative procedure and for a few days after. Patients will be much more comfortable after the operation if their bladder is empty. To insure this, a catheter is sometimes inserted into the bladder before the patient goes to the operating theater.

No matter how minor the operative procedure and no matter how limited the area to be subjected to surgery, all the patient's clothes are removed before he or she goes to the operating theater and replaced with a special gown.

It is natural that most patients, and particularly those having major surgery, will be worried and nervous. Therefore a good night's rest is insured before the operation with an appropriate dose of sleeping pills. Also, about one hour before surgery the patient is given a "pre-med" injection that induces a calm, semiconscious state. Relaxed and suitably prepared, the patient is wheeled into the operating theater by nurses and orderlies.

267

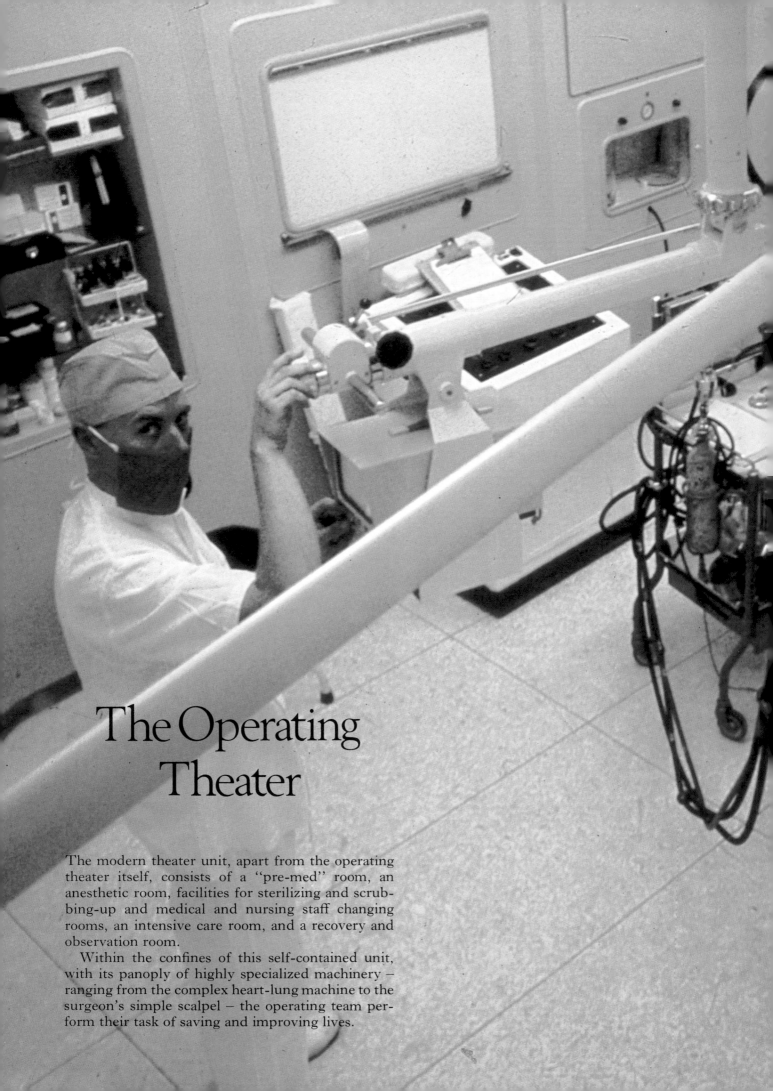

The Operating Theater

The modern theater unit, apart from the operating theater itself, consists of a "pre-med" room, an anesthetic room, facilities for sterilizing and scrubbing-up and medical and nursing staff changing rooms, an intensive care room, and a recovery and observation room.

Within the confines of this self-contained unit, with its panoply of highly specialized machinery – ranging from the complex heart-lung machine to the surgeon's simple scalpel – the operating team perform their task of saving and improving lives.

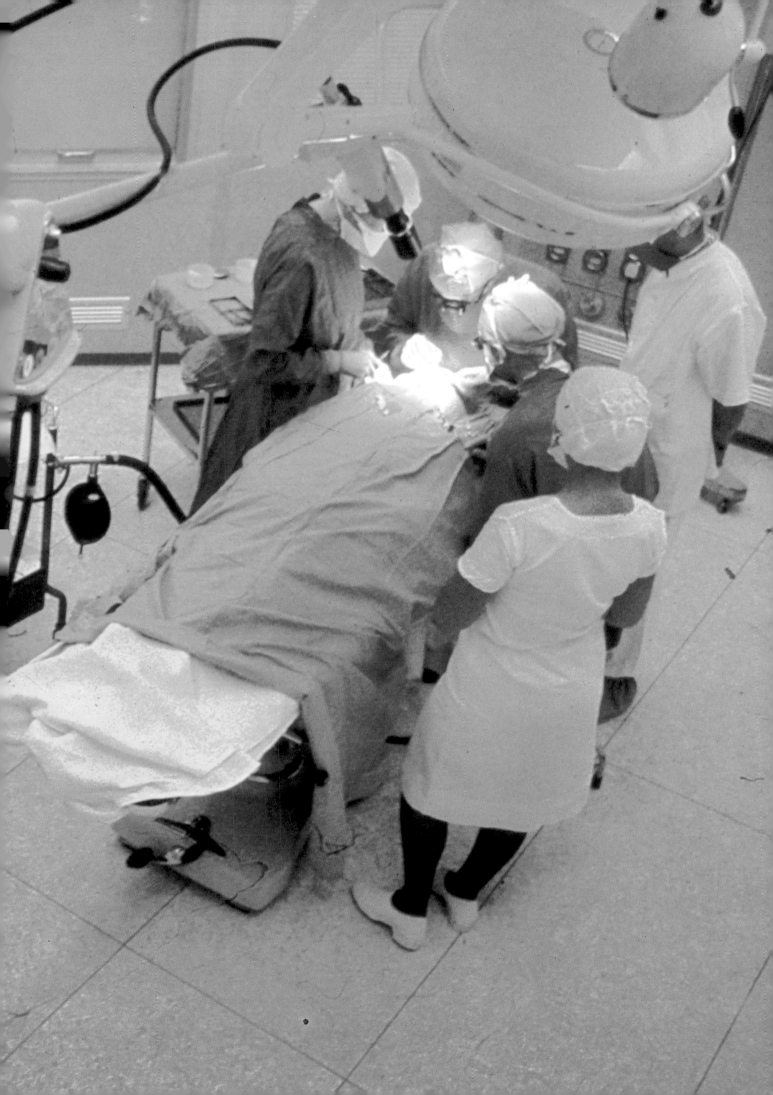

Anesthetizing the Patient

The anesthetist is a highly skilled doctor and technician, without whom most modern operative techniques would be impossible. He or she puts the patient to sleep and throughout the operation controls and monitors the complex machinery of anesthesia. Before the operation the anesthetist studies the patient's medical record to determine the most suitable type of anesthetics. If there is any doubt about the patient coming safely through the anesthesia and surgery, the anesthetist will recommend to the surgeon that the operation should be postponed – or possibly cancelled.

The anesthetist administers the general anesthetic that puts the patient to sleep, so that any type of operation may be performed. Usually, a general anesthetic is injected straight into a vein – with very rapid results – followed by the inhalation of gases such as nitrous oxide, halothane, or trichlorethylene. Almost every function of the body is modified in some way by a general anesthetic, and this is why the anesthetist must select the best possible drug for each individual patient and each operation.

After the patient has been put to sleep the anesthetist will often place an *endotracheal* tube in the windpipe. The patient will breathe through this throughout the operation. It has the advantage of protecting the respiratory tract from secretions or vomit.

In certain operations large doses of muscle relax-ants, such as curare, are given to paralyze the respiratory muscles. The patient will then be put on a machine called an intermittent positive pressure ventilator which will gauge the correct rate of respiration mixture and the amount of gases and oxygen forced into the lungs with each breath from a rubber bag. This technique is invariably combined with the insertion by the anesthetist of the *endotracheal* tube mentioned previously. The method is always used in chest surgery, and frequently employed in abdominal surgery. The tube can also be placed in the bronchus leading from the trachea to one of the lungs, thus isolating the lung that is being operated upon. Heart surgery was virtually impossible before the advent of endotracheal anesthesia, which enables the anesthetist to keep the lungs oxygenated when a pleural cavity is opened and its contained lungs collapsed. At first it proved possible, with endotracheal anesthesia, to repair wounds of the heart, later to remedy congenital defects outside the heart, and with further advances to remedy constriction of the passage between the heart's chambers.

Hospital anesthetists are on call 24 hours a day. With their unique experience in applied physiology and techniques of resuscitation they are often summoned to assist in the emergency treatment of patients who are gravely ill. As anesthesia becomes more sophisticated so more patients are anesthetized who would, in the past, have been considered too ill for it. As the number of these patients increases, so the amount of monitoring equipment used in operating theaters proliferates. But the day when the machines will take over the task of the anesthetist is still a long way off. Only years of training and experience can equip a doctor to interpret the patient's responses and maintain the body's vital systems while undergoing surgery.

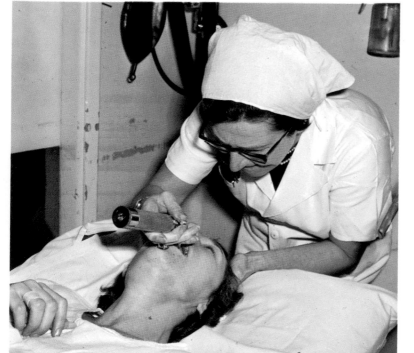

Left: endotracheal anesthesia. A tube inserted in the trachea during thoracic operations keeps the lungs, which would normally collapse, inflated with oxygen. The endotracheal tube also supplies anesthetic gas to the patient.

Opposite: general anesthetic equipment. As no one single chemical provides all the necessary requirements, several types of medications are given in combination to produce the overall desired effect. A premed relaxes the patient beforehand, and a saliva-inhibiting drug is also given to prevent inhalation of saliva. Usually one agent is administered to induce unconsciousness, and another produces the analgesic effect. In addition curare is injected as a muscle relaxant.

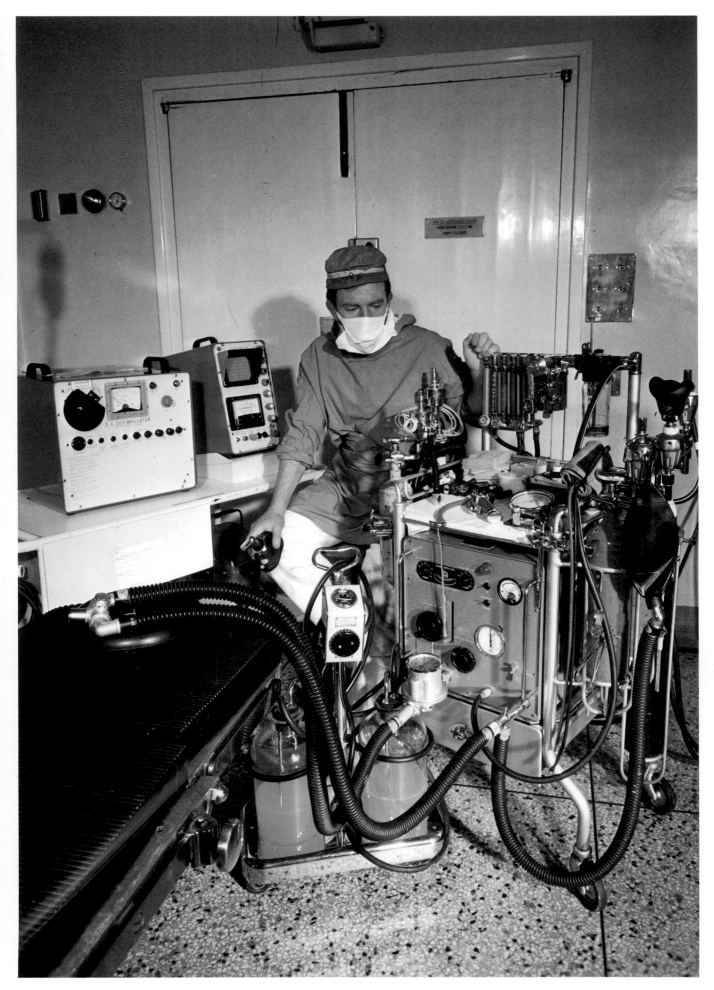

Postoperative Care

Once the operation has been completed, the aim of the hospital staff is to insure that the patient has a speedy and comfortable recovery and convalescence. If the patient is taken back to the ward immediately after an operation, he or she is placed in a warmed bed. However, in many hospitals it is usual after major surgery to transfer the patient to a specialized intensive care unit which contains various types of apparatus necessary to combat any possible post-operative complications — all manned by highly experienced personnel. Intensive care is necessary for patients who have undergone open heart surgery or other major operations, or are suffering from severe

shock. Unfit patients, particularly those with heart or respiratory weaknesses undergoing more minor operations, also benefit from a stay in the intensive care unit. However, patients are not usually kept in intensive care for more than a few days. Once out of danger they are returned to the ordinary ward.

Modern medicine advocates that the patient gets out of bed as soon as possible after surgery. On his 42nd birthday Paul Rainer experienced a severe attack of gall stones. After a major operation, in which four horny, half-inch thick stones were removed from his gall bladder, he was out of bed 24 hours after the operation. Some 30 years ago this would not have been thought possible. There are, however, a small number of patients who must remain in bed for a week or longer after an operation.

Immediately after patients have recovered from the effects of the anesthetic, they are urged to change their position frequently and to move their limbs

Following an operation, a patient may be kept in an intensive care unit. If the person has had a heart attack or stroke, resuscitation equipment is kept at hand.

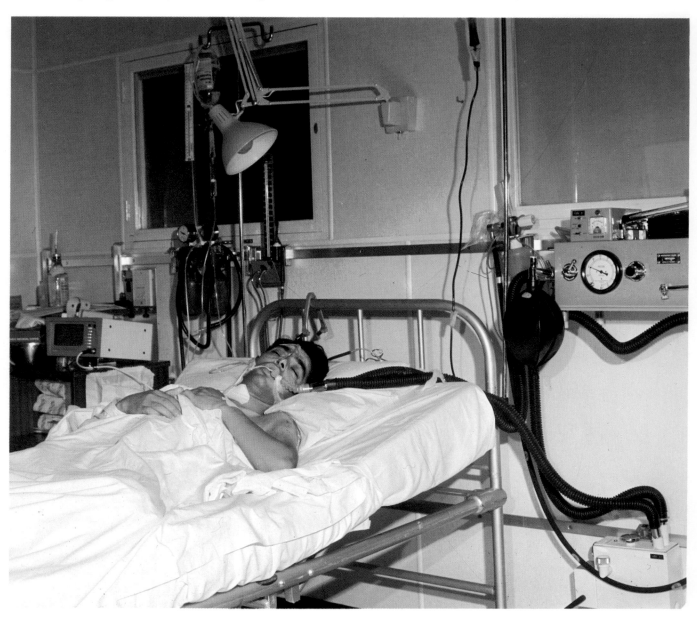

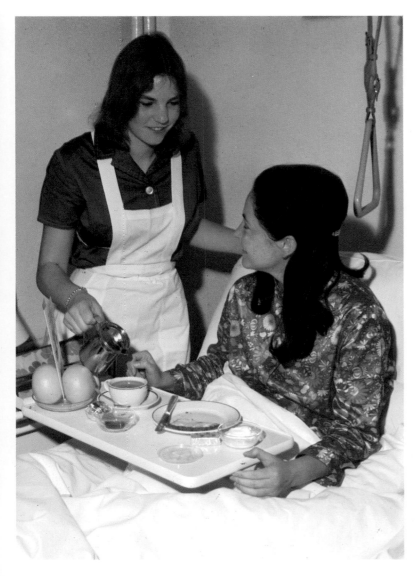

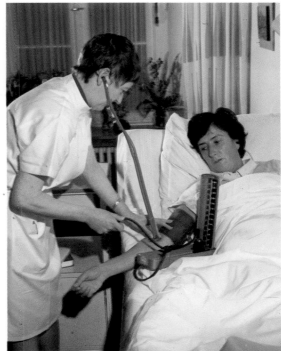

Above: after a surgical operation, a constant check is kept on a patient's temperature, blood pressure and pulse. Any complications that arise can be dealt with immediately.

Left: all patients fast before a surgical operation, and few feel like eating much after the event. Subsequently light, bland meals are given. In some cases the stomach becomes severely distended and the patient will be fitted with a rubber tube to deflate it.

about in bed. This stimulates circulation, thus reducing the danger of blood clots forming in the veins of the arms or legs.

Distension of the stomach after an operation is a common occurrence which can cause great distress and discomfort. To avoid this a rubber tube is sometimes passed through the nose into the stomach and allowed to remain there for a day or two. In order to make sure that the stomach remains deflated, this rubber tube is sometimes attached to a suction apparatus.

Most patients are extremely thirsty after their operation, particularly when they have had nothing to drink for hours before surgery. Small amounts of water or tea are often given within a few hours of the patient being returned to the ward. On the following day they usually take small amounts of soft, bland food and may be eating normally within a week. After some operations patients are not allowed to drink or eat for two to three days and have to be given intravenous fluids.

Since all people will have varying degrees of pain following surgery, pain-relieving drugs and sedatives are given, if necessary every few hours for the first day or two. Fear of drug addiction can be discounted because once postoperative pain disappears, the patient no longer needs relief.

Every major operation involves a certain amount of blood loss, and if large quantities are involved the surgeon will order a transfusion. So it should not be thought that the patient's condition is precarious merely because blood is being given. The inability to have a bowel movement after surgery is also no cause for alarm: the bowels often do not function very satisfactorily at first after abdominal surgery.

The realization of the dangers of exposing operative wounds in the ward has led to the practice of interfering with them as little as possible. Once they have been dressed and covered in the operating theater, surgical wounds are often sealed with flexible adhesive plaster and are not disturbed until the stitches are removed.

With most minor operations, if there are no complications the patient will be up and about within a day or two and will be discharged very quickly. The recovery period for major surgery may be longer and involve further hospital treatment. Once the patient has been discharged he or she will only return to the hospital for a final examination by the surgeon who performed the operation.

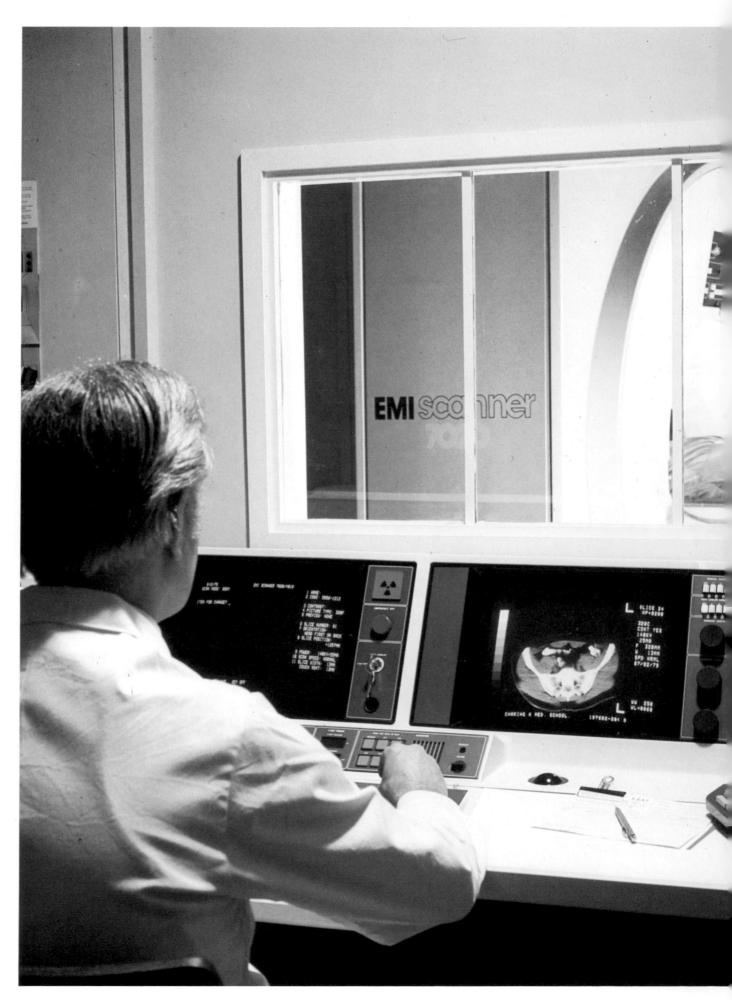

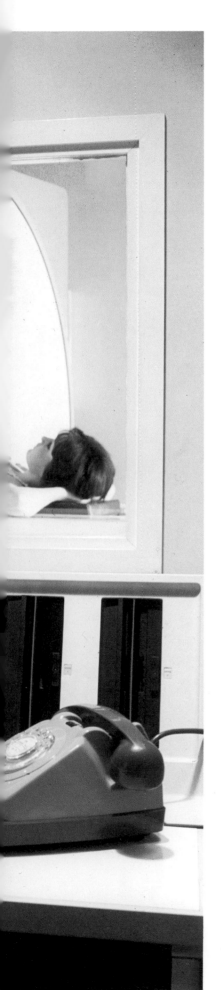

Chapter 15

Serious Illnesses

Fear of the unknown is very understandable. And fear of serious illness is probably the most common form that this fear takes. We are frightened of cancer; we dread the thought of having a stroke; and our attitude to mental illness is full of apprehension. Although we are often ignorant of the processes of serious illness, we know that it involves pain and suffering – and this increases our fear. But a wise man once said: "A man who fears suffering is already suffering from what he fears." And if people can achieve a better understanding of what serious illness is all about, and how medical science is fighting – and winning – the battle against pain and suffering, this will give them the courage to face any future illness, armed with the weapons of knowledge and understanding.

Opposite: the computerized tomography scanner. It displays cross sections of the body on a television screen, and unlike conventional X-rays, enables soft tissue to be visualized as well as bone.

Fear of Discovery

The attitude of the average person on visiting the doctor is nearly always tinged, for the most part unconsciously, with anxiety and fear. Many people ignore investigating major symptoms for fear of being told that they have an incurable disease, while others, convinced that death is imminent, worry their doctor at the slightest excuse.

Illness constitutes a threat not only to a person's physical integrity but also to their social status. When a grown person becomes ill, it often means an enforced return to a state of being dependent on others, a change usually accompanied by feelings of apprehension that sometimes leads to frank anxiety and depression. It is for these reasons that many adults in positions of responsibility feel a greater concern about the economic and social implications of their illness than about the illness itself. This explains a number of common psychologic defenses that such people may have against illness. They may refuse medical aid; or if they summon the courage to consult a physician, they may minimize or even fail to mention the very symptom about which they are most deeply concerned. On the other hand there are some people whose road to maturity has been tedious and uncertain, so that the dependency

Right: for some people, a stay in hospital is a bewildering and frightening experience. This is particularly so in large teaching hospitals, where the frequent visits by doctors and attendant staff lend an ominous gravity to the situation.

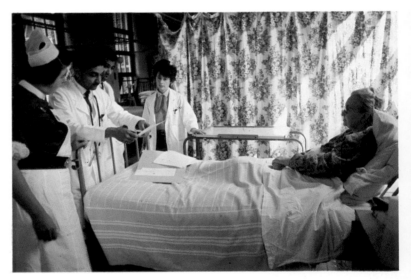

Below: many patients will need constant reassurance about their condition and the chances of recovery.

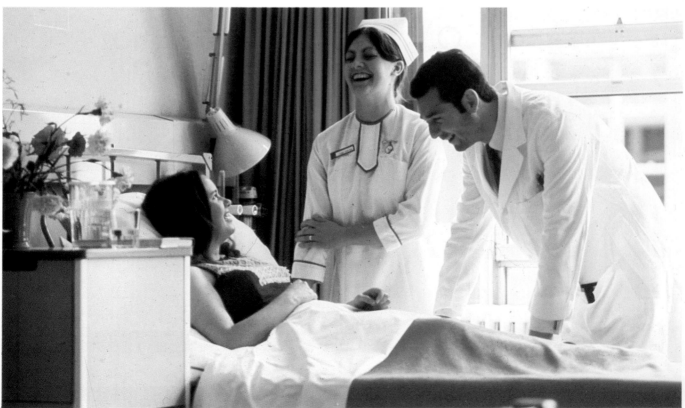

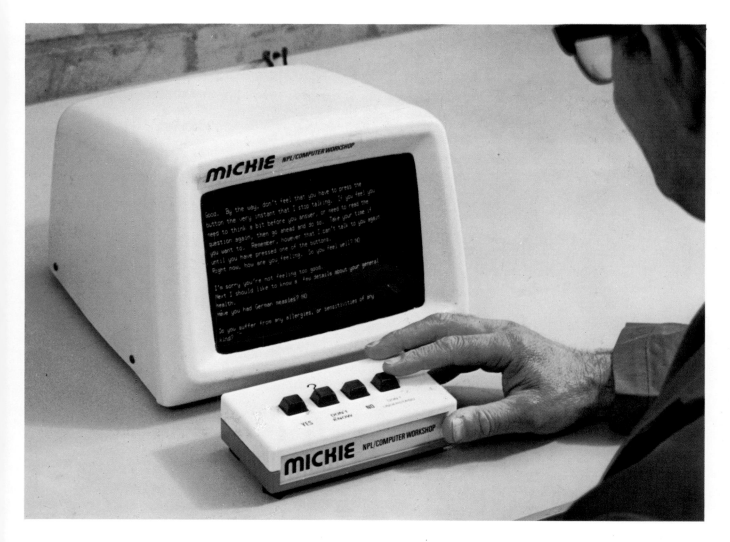

On the screen (partially legible):

> Good. By the way, don't feel that you have to press the
> button the very instant that I stop talking. If you feel you
> need to think a bit before you answer, or need to read the
> question again, then go ahead and do so. Take your time if
> you want to. Remember, however, that I can't talk to you again
> until you have pressed one of the buttons.
> Right now, how are you feeling. Do you feel well? NO
>
> I'm sorry you're not feeling too good.
> Next I should like to know a few details about your general
> health.
> Have you had German measles? NO
>
> Do you suffer from any allergies, or sensitivities of any
> kind?

forced on them by illness comes as a welcome relief from adult responsibility. They appear to enjoy their illness and to resent anything that menaces their state of "invalidism."

For the doctor it is not always easy to keep the above simple facts in mind when examining a patient in the relatively impersonal atmosphere of the hospital ward, or even in the private consulting room. The doctor has a special role in society and should be skilled as a psychologist in human behavior as well as an expert in human diseases. As well as bringing highly technical knowledge and abilities to bear upon a patient's bodily functioning, the good doctor should also inspire a confidence and security based upon the conviction that no effort will be spared to effect a cure. The doctor should try to make the patients feel that their unique individualities are recognized and appreciated and that their life's problems are meaningful. This approach is just as important in patients with well-defined organic diseases as it is in those with "stress" symptoms brought on largely by emotional pressures expressed through the body.

Today there are signs that the doctor-patient relationship is in danger of deteriorating because of the changing setting in which medicine is increasingly practiced. In many cases the handling of one individual patient requires the active participation

Above: medical interviewing computers have proved extremely acceptable to patients. With no intellectual or social barrier to overcome, and no feeling of "wasting the doctor's time," patients give more honest and accurate answers.

of a variety of trained professional personnel — not only doctors but also nurses, dietitians, biochemists, psychologists, and physiotherapists, as well as para-medical personnel. The patient can benefit greatly from such collaboration, but should know that a qualified and concerned doctor is retaining responsibility for the crucial decisions concerning diagnosis and treatment.

Changes in the setup of medical practice is also altering previously existing doctor-patient relationships. An increasing number of people are being cared for by groups of doctors, by clinics, and by hospitals, rather than by the single independent practitioner. There are many advantages in the use of such organized medical groups composed of a number of various specialists, but there are new hazards both to the patient and the doctor. The patient must be in no doubt as to the identity of the doctor who is primarily and continuously responsible for his or her care. And it is this doctor who must have an overview of the patient's illness and who must know all about the patient's reaction to illness, to drugs, and to the problems of daily living. This is specially important when a serious illness is involved.

Abnormal Blood Pressure

What is a normal blood pressure? This question is difficult to answer satisfactorily. One might as well ask what is normal height – for both show considerable variation. Blood pressure is even more difficult to deal with as it can vary quite markedly in the same person from minute to minute.

Medical science has good reason to be proud of its control of blood pressure disorders. We have come along a long way since 1733, when Stephen Hales became the first man to measure arterial blood pressure. He did this by inserting a small glass tube into a horse's leg artery. Using a goose's windpipe as tubing, he connected this to another very tall tube. Arterial pressure caused the blood to shoot up to a level of nine feet, then oscillate steadily with each heart's beat.

Systolic pressure is the pressure where the heart is contracting. *Diastolic* pressure is the pressure in between heartbeats. Blood pressure is measured with a *sphygmomanometer*. In infants blood pressure averages 90 systolic; in children 60 to 100 systolic; and in adults 95–150 systolic and 60–90 diastolic. Over the age of 50, blood pressure usually rises; although some tribes show no rise in blood pressure with advancing age. Young women have a slightly lower blood pressure than young men, although the pressure of older women is slightly greater than that of men of a similar age. In several conditions pressure can reach values as high as 300/160 (300 systolic; 160 diastolic), although this is fairly unusual.

Life insurance statistics have provided a great deal of information about the dangers of high blood pressure, called *hypertension*. If we take a figure of say 140/90 as the boundary between normal blood pressure and hypertension, then we know that a young man with a pressure higher than this has a shorter life expectancy than average. The young

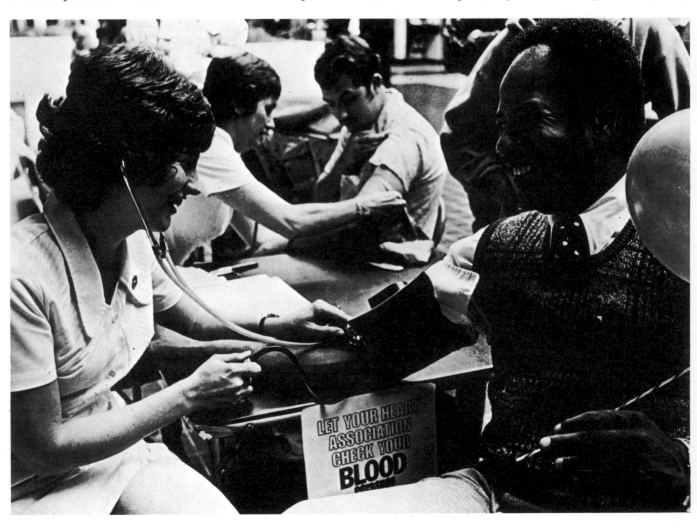

The American Heart Association has sponsored a community program of regular blood-pressure screening in order to identify adults and children with abnormal hypertension. The screenings are held in shopping centers, business premises and fairs.

man's life expectancy improves, say the insurance companies, the lower his blood pressure falls. This is oversimplifying a complex subject, but there is considerable support for believing that hypertension is a

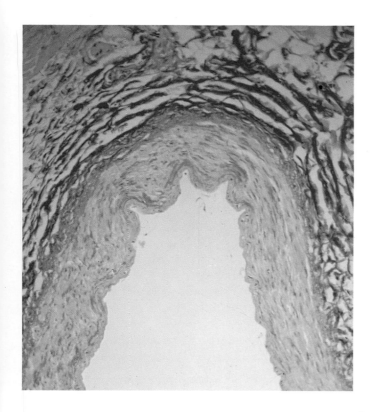

about what causes hypertension is almost within their grasp. The majority feel that the key lies in the small arteries, although some doctors think that abnormalities of the heart are linked to hypertension. Others believe that changes in the behavior of the kidneys are involved. Time alone will reveal who is right – if indeed there is one answer.

Under certain conditions a low blood pressure, called *hypotension*, can be dangerous. If the heart cannot pump the blood at a greater pressure than 70 millimetres of mercury, kidneys are damaged within an hour or two. This situation occurs quite often after a severe blood loss or coronary thrombosis. Certain diseases can lower the blood pressure by attacking and involving the nervous pathways that control the heart and the blood vessels. But this

Left: hypertension aggravates the condition of unhealthy, diseased arteries, and increases the risks of coronary thrombosis and strokes.

Below: biofeedback used to reduce hypertension, a condition usually connected with sweat glands. As the skin emits more sweat, the attached machine emits a loud noise which can be consciously reduced by the patient relaxing.

real disorder. For example it is known that several diseases give rise to hypertension, particularly kidney diseases. But there are still cases, where there is no apparent cause – so-called "essential hypertension." Diet can also play a part in producing hypertension. Obese people tend to have a higher blood pressure than average for their age and sex, although doctors allow for the fact that the padding on a fat arm tends to make the blood pressure reading artificially high. What there is no doubt about at all is that serious hypertension can cause heart failure and apoplexy (stroke).

A question that is often asked is whether there is any relationship between high blood pressure and stress. There is good reason to believe that relaxation helps to lower blood pressure. For instance during sleep or after taking sedatives the blood pressure can fall from, say 120/80 to 90/60. During strenuous activity or anxiety, it can rise to 140/90 or above in many people. Some people seem to become hypertensive at times of stress. These people usually have blood vessels that constrict excessively in response to pain or cold. And with the individuals who are probably destined to develop sustained hypertension in a few years time, it seems likely that if they had not been exposed to a stressful life they would not have eventually developed high blood pressure.

Except for surgically remediable causes such as tumors and kidney disease, the treatment of hypertension is generally far from satisfactory. Sometimes vigorous treatment produces symptoms worse than the disease itself. Treatment may include reassurance, weight reduction, encouragement of relaxation, and the use of mild sedatives and tranquilizers, or the prescription of specific antihypertensive drugs.

However, many scientists believe that the truth

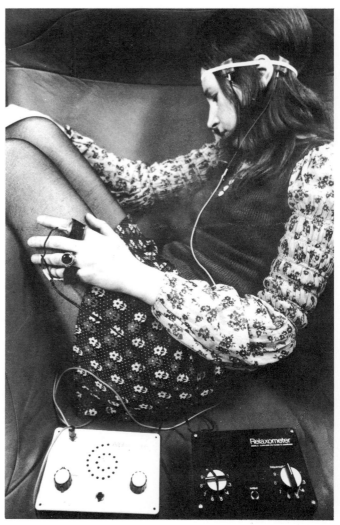

happens rarely and most people with a blood pressure below the average for their age and sex should consider themselves lucky, since their life expectancy is, at least statistically, better than average.

What is a Stroke?

A stroke is one of the most commonly occurring disabilities. The correct medical term is *cerebro-vascular accident*, and refers to a condition in which part of the circulation of the brain is interfered with. Because nerve cells can survive for only a short time without oxygen and blood, they generally die and the result is some form of permanent damage.

Strokes vary in intensity and severity. Some cause almost no symptoms while at the other extreme there are fatal strokes. The stroke victim generally, but not always, loses consciousness and all power of voluntary motion. A slow pulse, flushed cheeks, pupils of unequal size, and breathing which sounds like snoring are other symptoms. *Hemiplegia* – paralysis down one or the other side – also occurs. There may also be loss of speech and incontinence. Most cases of apoplexy are quite sudden – the victim is literally struck down. Occasionally, however, there may be warning signs such as numbness on one side, headaches, giddiness, vomiting and ringing in the ears.

Most strokes victims are elderly, and the disease is most common in those suffering from some form of cardiovascular disease; hardened or fatty arteries, a diseased heart, or clots in the leg or lung, and high blood pressure can all make a person more susceptible to a stroke, as can any factor which aggravates these conditions. Smoking, obesity or exertion can all precipitate a stroke. In children a stroke sometimes follows whooping cough.

A stroke may occur as the result of *thrombosis*, in which a diseased artery in the brain gradually gets blocked up by a clot. The cause may be an *embolism*

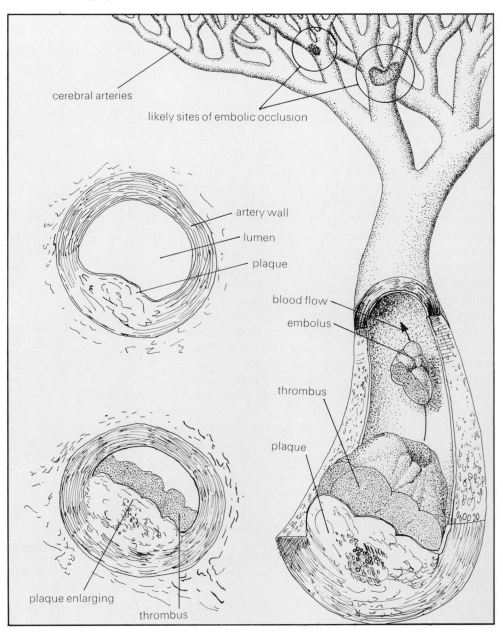

cerebral arteries

likely sites of embolic occlusion

artery wall

lumen

plaque

blood flow

embolus

thrombus

plaque

plaque enlarging

thrombus

A stroke may be the result of a clot forming in a cerebral artery and blocking it up (thrombosis) or a portion of a clot elsewhere breaking off and lodging in the brain (embolism). The clot or thrombus itself is the result of blood platelets congealing in a mass on the fatty lining of a diseased artery.

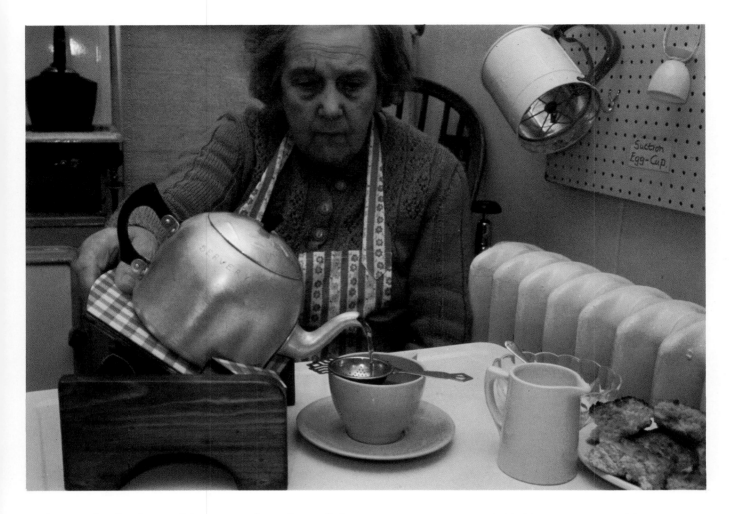

Many ordinary household objects present a problem to a hemiplegic. This stroke victim, paralyzed on her left side, is using a specially designed holder for her teapot.

such as a clot in the cavities or on the valves of the heart breaking off and being carried to the brain where it plugs up an artery. The most serious type of stroke is due to a *cerebral hemorrhage*. This is caused by a blood vessel in the brain rupturing. The damage done and the chances of recovery depend on the size and location of the rupture, and the fate of the blood afterward.

Recovery after a stroke depends on the age and general health of the victim, as well as on the severity of the attack. The victim may die within a few hours of the stroke, or two or three weeks afterward if the hemorrhage increases or restarts. On the other hand, if the patient survives the first two weeks the chances of subsequent recovery are good.

Patients take a long time to recover from a stroke, and the emphasis during treatment is on nursing and physiotherapy, with subsequent rehabilitation. Little can be done for stroke patients while they are unconscious, except keeping their blood pressure from rising. Skilled nursing and physiotherapy are essential to avoid permanent future disabilities. The muscles and joints must be manipulated in such a way as to prevent stiffness and contraction, while on the other hand avoiding tearing and damage. As the patient starts to recover efforts are concentrated on overcoming the hemiplegia. Patients are encouraged to regain independent movement. First there are simple exercises such as sitting down and standing up. While the paralyzed arm is usually supported in a sling to prevent it from swelling, it is also exercised to avoid future stiffness. Gradually the patient is encouraged to walk, first with the help of splints, walking bars and frames, and eventually with walking sticks. The physiotherapist will teach the patient how to use other muscles to overcome disabilities in movement. One of the problems that a hemiplegic victim faces at this point is muscle spasm, which can be counteracted using ice on the affected muscles, splints and sometimes drug therapy. In addition to hemiplegia, the stroke victim often suffers from *aphasia* (loss of speech) and speech therapy will be essential.

Eventually a stroke victim will return home. Depending on the extent of the paralysis certain changes of habit may be necessary, however. For example, clothing may have to be adjusted to make independent dressing and undressing possible. The home may have to be rearranged to enable the victim to carry out such activities as bathing, going to the lavatory and cooking. As well as professional help from the medical staff, physiotherapists and occupational therapists, members of the family can prove invaluable. Their help, patience, and active participation in the patient's therapy can be a major contribution to a stroke victim's rehabilitation toward a normal life.

The Facts about Cancer

Cells in the body of a person in good health behave like the population of a civilized and harmonious community. Every cell has its distinctive role and maintains its rightful place and everything happens in a spirit of cooperation. Occasionally however law and order breaks down and is replaced by an aggressive form of anarchy in some parts of the body. Cells begin to multiply and produce an abnormal growth – this is cancer. In many cases the cancer cells spread to other parts of the body, where they form colonies, called *metastases*.

The basic nature and origin of cancer are still unknown but research so far has shown that more than 110 viruses and 1000 chemicals are capable of producing cancer in animals. The vagaries (departures from an expected course) manifestations and courses of the disease and its prognosis are countless. Unlike other cells cancer cells have no growth control; they continue multiplying, forming tumors which interfere with the workings of other organs. If left unchecked their proliferation will ultimately result in the death of the organism. Not satisfied with uncontrolled growth cancerous cells can penetrate the blood and lymph streams and get carried along to other sites in the body where they form secondary tumors. This is another crucial difference between the cancer cell and its normal counterpart: cancer cells lose their functional specialization and are not particular as to which part of the body they can take root in. And having no physiological function, all they can do is grow and multiply.

The first indication that anything is amiss may be the appearance of a swelling or lump, in the breast, for example, which on further examination will be found composed of abnormal cancer cells. These changes may occur in any tissue of the body. Yet not all abnormal growths in the body are cancerous. There are also benign tumors. These are often quite harmless and they do not produce the secondary tumors (metastases) that are commonly found in cancer.

The prevalence of different forms of cancer varies considerably in different parts of the world. Cancer of the stomach is particularly prevalent in Japan, accounting for nearly one half of all cancers. Yet this form of cancer is almost totally absent among the Javanese and is very rare in Southeast Asia and Africa. On the other hand, liver cancer is remarkably common in Africa.

Different factors determine which types of cancer are common in different areas of the world. The cause of the high incidence of thyroid cancer in Switzerland, for example, is probably due to the low iodine content of the drinking water. Similarly the increased incidence of skin cancer in parts of Australia is thought to be due to excessive exposure of pale skins to sun. Several forms of cancer are now known to be occupational diseases, associated with materials used in particular industries. Cancer of the scrotum was at one time common among chimney sweeps. Similarly an increased frequency of lung cancer has been reported in men working with asbestos.

Clearly there is a strong association between smoking and lung cancer, and few experts still question whether it is a direct cause. The genetic pattern of any given individual may possibly determine whether he will be susceptible to cigarette smoke. Some scientists believe that a person's particular constitution creates his craving or noncraving for tobacco and

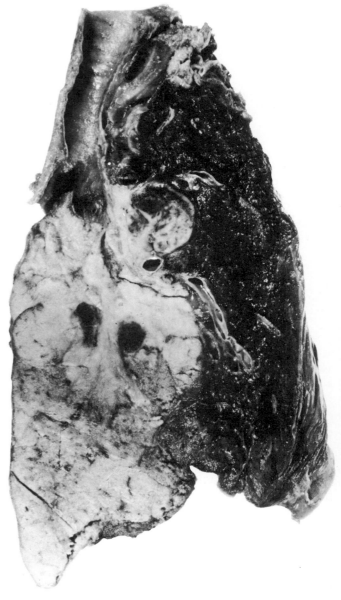

The lung of a heavy, long-term smoker. The left side is almost totally invaded by cancer. In its curable stage, lung cancer usually presents no symptoms.

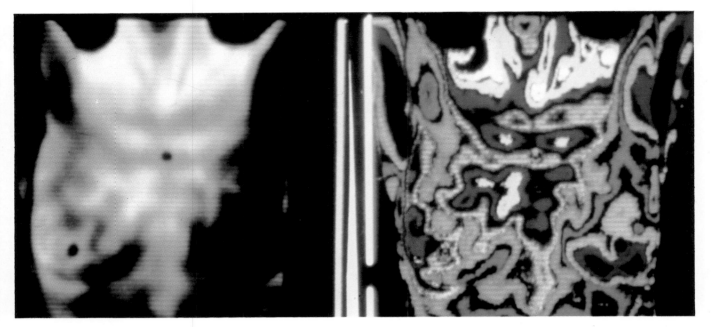

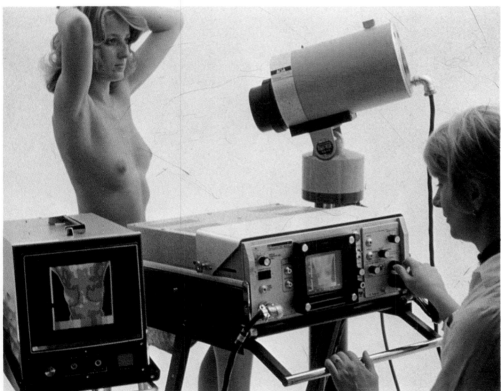

Above: thermography is used for preliminary screening of breast cancer, and can indicate which breast should be investigated further, even before a palpable lump has formed. The left picture is a graded monochrome image, showing a cancer in the right breast. The right picture is a color-coded version which gives accurate contour lines for each temperature. The cancer growth is warmer than the surrounding tissue.

Left: screening for breast cancer.

that some people's bodily chemistry makes them more receptive than others to lung cancer. A substance in tobacco smoke called benzpyrene, which also occurs in industrial smoke, can cause cancer in animals and is thought to be at least one of the culprits in causing human lung cancer. Benzpyrene is only one of the thousands of chemical now known to induce cancer. These chemicals are called *carcinogens.* The Institute for Cancer Research, Lyons, France, sponsored by the World Health Organization, has produced a list of chemicals, each of which is produced yearly in quantities of more than 100,000 tons, and all of which are carcinogenic.

X-rays and some other forms of radiation can cause tumors when administered in large doses, or in small doses over a long period of time. Many cases occurred when X-rays were first used in medicine, before safe procedures had been worked out. Leukemia, a cancer of the bone marrow that produces the blood cells, was, and still is, common among the Japanese survivors of the atomic bomb attacks on Hiroshima and Nagasaki.

No human cancer has yet been shown to be related to a virus, except possibly a tumor called Burkitt's lymphoma, which primarily affects the jaws and is common in parts of Africa. Viruses related to human herpes viruses have been found in tissue taken from patients with this tumor, but absolute proof that these cause the disease is still lacking. It may be caused by some unknown biological agent.

Screening for Cancer

The natural history of cancer suggests that the best way of containing it would be firstly to prevent it, and secondly to provide for early diagnosis and appropriate treatment. Many detection clinics have been set up, but the desirable goal of universal prevention by early detection is still a long way in the future – even in the world's most developed countries.

In the first stages of cancer there is an interaction between some inciting stimuli (chemical, physical, nutritional or biological) and the person's body. This is a dormant period, when nothing seems to be wrong. Then a change appears in the tissue of a localized site and this is called cancer *in situ*. At this stage the

Below: before the type of treatment is decided upon, oncologists have to evaluate the type and size of the cancer, and the extent of its spread. For most cancers surgery and radiation therapy are the common forms of treatment. A certain number respond to chemotherapy – treatment using drugs or hormones.

tissue changes are easy to identify, but unfortunately the patient has no symptoms of illness. Finally the cancer is localized in a particular organ and signs and symptoms can be identified: the person is ill. At this time the cancer may begin to spread and finally remote metastases appear: the person now has chronic cancer with death as the likely outcome if he or she is not treated or if the treatment comes too late.

At the present time there is no simple general screening test for cancer and the search must be painstaking and on an organ-to-organ basis. Lung-cancer detection requires a complete X-ray of the chest; early cervical cancer cannot be revealed without a cervical smear (Pap test); early detection of cancer of the rectum or colon makes use of a protoscope or sigmoidoscope; and early cancer of the larynx is difficult to detect without a laryngeal mirror. The Pap test is simple, and the majority of doctors perform it as a routine but other tests require examination by specialists.

The establishment of centers for cancer screening in every community is essential for the early detection of malignant diseases. But as this is still very much in the future, every man and woman should know the warning signals of cancer:

1. unusual bleeding or discharge from any body orifice
2. a sore that does not heal
3. a change in bowel and bladder habits

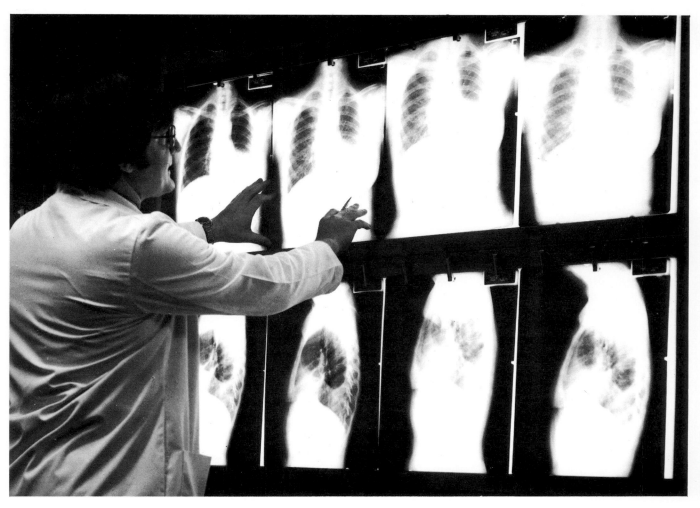

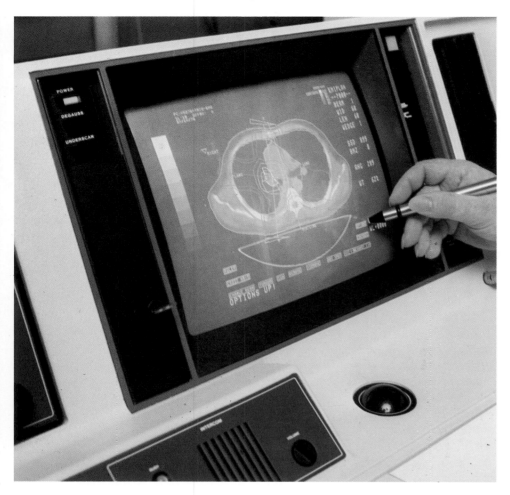

Left: the anatomical cross-section scanner can accurately diagnose a tumor even in its very early stages.

Below: cervical cancer has been found to develop from invasive cancerous cells in the surface epithelium of the cervix. The Pap test takes advantage of this by examining smears from the tip of the cervix.

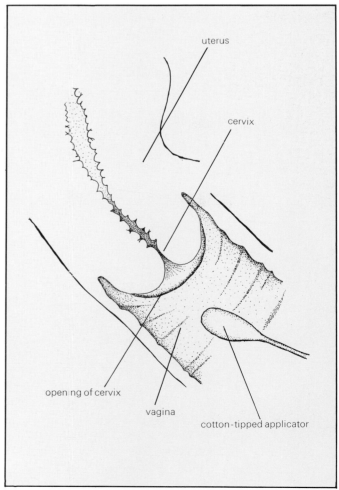

uterus

cervix

opening of cervix

vagina

cotton-tipped applicator

4. a lump or thickening in the breast or elsewhere
5. persistent hoarsness, cough or blood spitting
6. indigestion or difficulties in swallowing
7. a change in a wart or a mole.

The importance of being aware of these early signals and acting on them is illustrated in the results of breast self-examination which has been well publicized through the mass media. Ninety percent of breast cancers are detected by women themselves while examining their breasts for lumps with their own eyes and fingers. Whatever the cause – and it is obvious that not every lump, sore, or other change indicates the presence of cancer – all these symptoms need medical attention.

Mass screening programs are still the hope of the future. The goal is to bring the patient to the doctor in time, and no matter how difficult it may be to organize such programs, the rewards – social and economic as well as medical – are so great that no effort should be spared to make them a reality. At the moment mass screening techniques are tedious, excessively time-consuming for patients and doctors alike, and extremely expensive. But much of this is because of shortcomings in the existing structure of health care. The emphasis is still on the treatment rather than on the prevention of illness. The necessary change of emphasis from treatment to prevention cannot be the work of doctors alone.

The conquest of cancer is responsibility of society as a whole.

285

Incidences
of Cancer

It is not often realized that many cases of cancer have an excellent chance of being arrested. One and a half million people who had cancer five or more years ago have had it stopped. Yet every sixth death in Europe is caused by the disease. It is estimated that about half of the deaths occurring as a result of cancer could be prevented by earlier detection and appropriate treatment. And if some two dozen carcinogenic compounds produced today could be excluded from the environment the toll payed to cancer could be reduced still further.

Statistics of incidences of the various types of cancer are being collected from all over the world to help cancer researchers find the initial causes of the disease. Data collected in United States show that the cancer death rate is definitely rising. In 1900 only 3.7 percent of all deaths were attributed to cancer, in contrast to 16 percent in 1965. The majority of people who die of cancer are between the ages of 45 and 64. Among the most common cancers are those of the breast, the cervix (narrow end of the womb), lungs, colon and stomach. Leukemia is responsible for about 50 percent of deaths in children under 15.

Changing trends of cancer among adults are not always understood; for example the rate of cancer of the pancreas is rising for unknown reasons. But cancer of the stomach, which is becoming less frequent, may be linked to nutritional factors early in life. The Japanese, who have a high incidence of stomach cancer in their native country, see the risk diminished when they have emigrated to the United States and partially changed their eating habits. For reasons that are not clear, people who live in urban areas are more likely to develop cancer of the colon and the rectum than residents of rural areas. Leukemia is frequent in Israel, Denmark, the United States, and Japan, and its rising incidence is linked to radiation exposure. Whether or not leukemia is caused by relatively low doses of medical X-rays, radiation from natural sources or atomic radiation is not clear.

One of the most striking changes in the pattern of cancer is the increase in lung cancer (23 percent of cancer deaths in men, 5 percent in women). Current

Ionizing radiation has been shown to cause various cancers. The radiation does not have to be particularly intense, as the dosage accumulates. Consequently, prolonged exposure to low doses, a problem faced by personnel working with radioactive materials, is still dangerous.

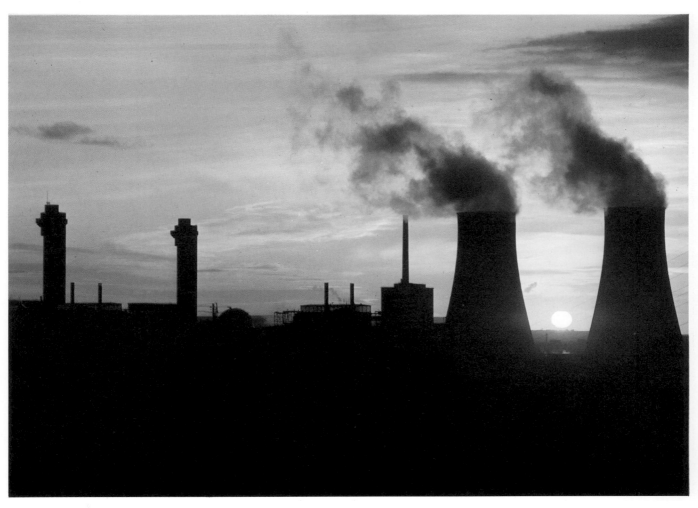

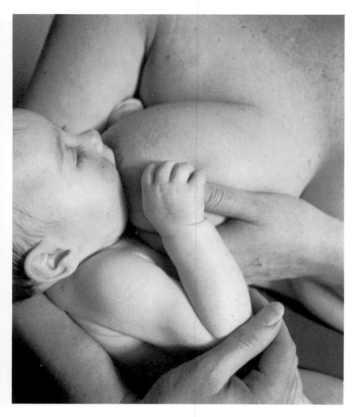

evidence indicates a very strong relationship between cigarette smoking and lung cancer – so great that it far outweighs other possibilities, such as air pollution, living in cities, family history and occupational hazards.

Although breast cancer is the single most important cancer among women, its rates of survival and death have been stationary for a number of years. It has been found that there is a tendency in women with breast cancer to undergo the natural menopause at a later age, which suggests that the menopause acts as a protection against breast cancer. Japanese women, who have in general a longer lifetime experience of breast feeding than European women (as well as an earlier menopause), have a lower death rate from breast cancer.

The gathering and interpretation of statistical information on cancer involves an enormous investment of manpower, time, and money – but the results are worth the effort and expense. Although the fight against cancer is long and hard, statistical evidence is proving to be an important weapon in providing vital information for all those involved in the struggle.

Above: it has been found that Japanese women, who breast-feed for a longer period and in larger numbers than European women, have a lower incidence of breast cancer. An earlier menopause has also been shown to protect against breast cancer.

Below: certain cancers are far more prevalent in some geographical regions than others. By isolating the environmental factors responsible, scientists have been able to learn more about the development and prevention of this malignant disease.

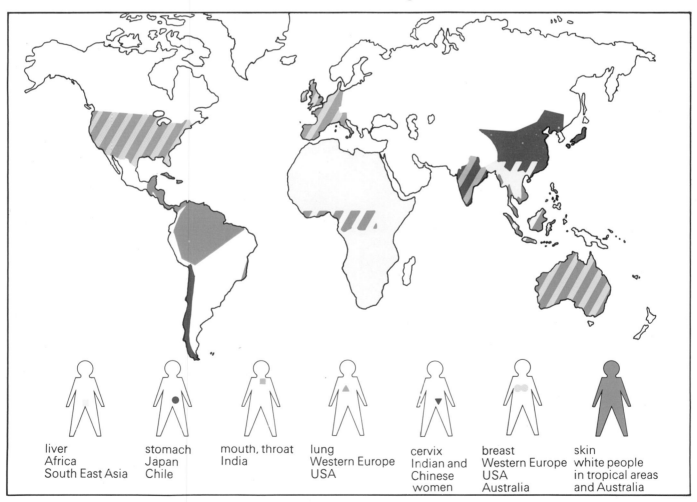

liver	stomach	mouth, throat	lung	cervix	breast	skin
Africa	Japan	India	Western Europe	Indian and	Western Europe	white people
South East Asia	Chile		USA	Chinese	USA	in tropical areas
				women	Australia	and Australia

Successful Treatment

The surest method of treating any malignant tumor is removal by surgery at as early a stage as possible. In many cases the result is a complete cure. With lung cancer, doctors can sometimes completely remove an affected lung if diagnosis has been made early enough. The fundamental justification for the use of surgery as the cure of cancer rests on the argument that an operation can remove every last surviving cancer cell from the patient. Such a premise is questionable as blood-borne metastases are beyond surgical control. But this is not necessarily true for metastases carried by the lymph stream. Lymph nodes in the vicinity of cancer sites, the regional lymph nodes, may filter out the cancer cells reaching them and can almost invariably be removed by modern surgical techniques with little detriment to the patient.

Radiotherapy also offers hope. X-rays or other forms of radiation are focused on the cancerous cells in such a way as to destroy them without harming normal tissues. Since the 1950s the introduction of highly sophisticated apparatus has meant that high-energy radiations can be used to great effect. Among the newer machines are telecobalt units, and linear and cyclic accelerators such as the cyclotron and betatron. Telecobalt units have many advantages, but their main disadvantage is a "shadow effect" requiring the use of a larger field in order to get an even dose of rays into the tumor. Both linear and cyclic accelerators have a high output that makes the administration of a good depth with a minimum skin dose possible. The use of electron beams allows healthy tissues beyond the target to be spared as these electrons have a limited depth of penetration in the tissues. Electron therapy is particularly effective in the treatment of surface cancers in contrast to the high-energy X-ray therapy which is also possible with the accelerators and which is especially suited for the treatment of deep-seated cancers. Accelerators, however, are expensive machines, requiring complicated maintenance.

Another form of radiotherapy is the use of radioisotopes. These disintegrate and emit radiation which will destroy the cell into which the isotope has been absorbed. They are chosen on the basis that they will be selectively absorbed by the tumor. For example radioactive iodine is used in the treatment of thyroid cancer.

Radiotherapy can sometimes cure a cancer, or when this is impossible reduce its size and rate of growth. Unfortunately, irradiation affects normal tissues as well as tumor tissues, so that the total dose for the tumor must be balanced against the tolerance of normal tissue. In large doses irradiation adversely affects the body as a whole. However, radiotherapy remains the best treatment for a wide variety of cancers, particularly the lymphomas, cancer of the cervix and the central nervous system and esophageal cancer. It is also often used as an invaluable additional

This cyclotron is being used to treat cancer. It accelerates neutrons to high energy, and these are used to bombard deep seated tumors in the stomach and bowel without damaging surrounding tissues. A steerable beam enables the particles to be focussed on the target from any angle.

As radiation can destroy healthy tissue as well as cancerous cells, the dose must be chosen carefully and the beams focussed with great accuracy. In most modern medical physics departments computers are used to assess the correct dosage for therapy.

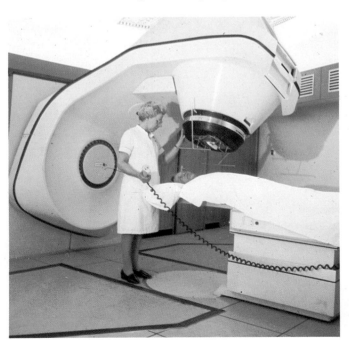

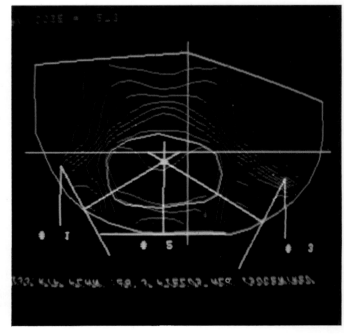

treatment for those people who have first had surgical treatment of their cancers.

The treatment of a disease by drugs is called *chemotherapy*. Many cancers can be retarded in their growth by the use of cytotoxic chemotherapeutic agents, and drug therapy is used in the treatment of leukemia and Hodgkin's disease (cancer of the lymphatic system).

Since modern methods of treatment are still unable to cure many cancers, some experts believe that the human body's own natural mechanisms used for its own protection and defense should be taken advantage of. Immunological defense accounts not only for the regression of certain cancers, but also for the variability in the course of a similar tumor in different people. The most exciting and promising aspect of all recent work is the attempt to bring into action against cancer cells various *cytolytic* (cell destroying) agents and *interferons* (proteins produced by cells attacked by viruses and similar agents).

Thus future cancer therapy may well involve a combination of the eradication of the bulk of the tumors by surgery, irradiation or chemotherapy, combined with the destruction of the last few remaining tumor cells by induced immunological reactions. However it is important to remember that many cancers would not occur if the initial stimuli (from excessive ultraviolet light, cigarette smoking, exposure to poisonous compounds, and so on) could be controlled.

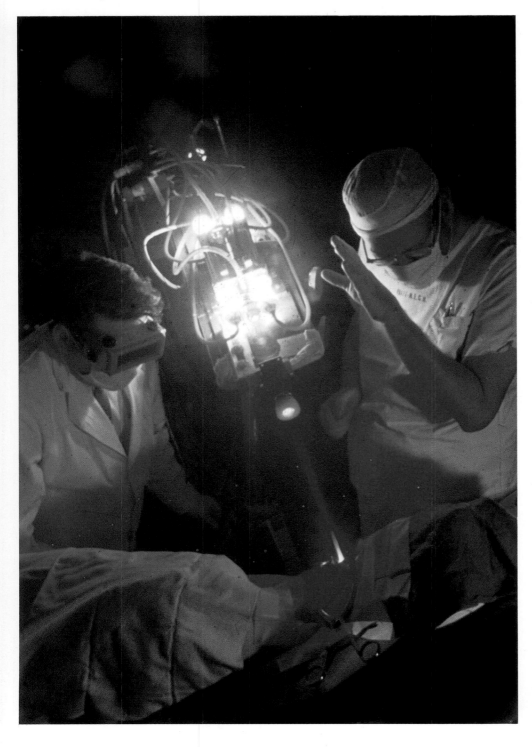

A surgeon using a laser beam instead of a knife in a skin-cancer operation.

What is Pain?

Pain, it has been said, is one of "Nature's earliest signs of illness." Few will deny that it is the most important sensory experience that indicates the existence of disease within themselves – and is therefore an important protective device. There are relatively few illnesses that do not have their painful phases.

Pain *receptors* are fine, freely branching nerve endings, which form an intricate network throughout the body. A single primary pain *neurone* subdivides into small peripheral branches to supply an area of skin. Every spot of skin is within the domain of from two to four sensory neurones. Various stimuli acting on free nerve engings in the skin muscles, blood vessels and inner organs, give rise to impulses which are transmitted, first to the spinal cord and then through special pathways to the brain – and pain (or some other sensation) is experienced.

There are distinct differences between the pain arising in the skin and that originating in the viscera (within the body). Pain in the skin and other outer areas may be caused by mechanical, thermal, chemical, or electrical stimuli. At their lowest levels these stimuli may evoke sensations of touch, pressure, warmth, or cold. Only when they reach a certain intensity, usually approaching tissue destruction, does pain develop. Pain thresholds vary from person to person. Neurotic or mentally ill people in general have the same pain threshold as normal people, but their reaction to the pain may be excessive or abnormal.

Pain arising in the skin has a pricking or burning quality and can be localized with a high degree of precision. Visceral pain is mostly dull and lacking in quality; it is poorly localized and its borders are only

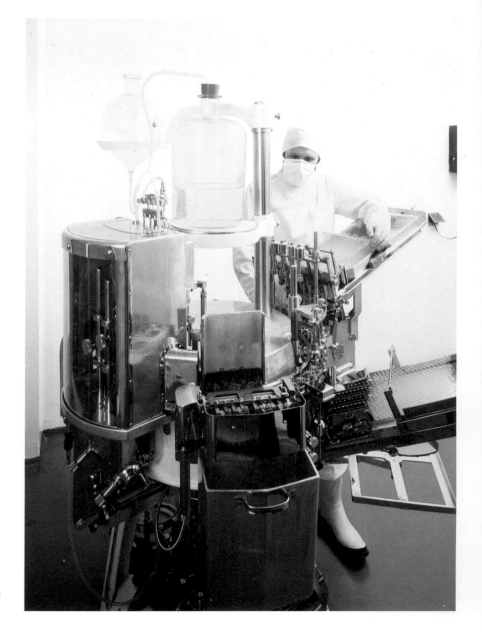

Production of buprenorphine. This highly effective analgesic differs from other opiate derivatives in that it is nonaddictive.

vaguely defined. The existence of visceral pain was long disputed, but it is now generally accepted that pain arising from inner organs does occur, provided that the stimuli are adequate. The same applies to deep skeletal pain.

Referred pain may occur in one part of the body while having its origins in a totally different site. A typical example is the pain experienced in the arm because of cardiac trouble. This pain is due to the anatomic fact that the first thoracic segment of the spinal cord supplies the inner surface of the arm as well as the chest and heart. Thus it is just as natural for heart pain to appear in the characteristic location in the left arm as it is in the chest.

As visceral pain and deep skeletal pain originate from a common deep sensory system, it is not surprising that their characteristics should be similar and that on occasion it is extremely difficult to differentiate between the two. Thus a small tear or injury in a lumbar muscle or ligament may give rise to a pain whose quality and localization, including radiation into the groin and scrotum, are indistin-

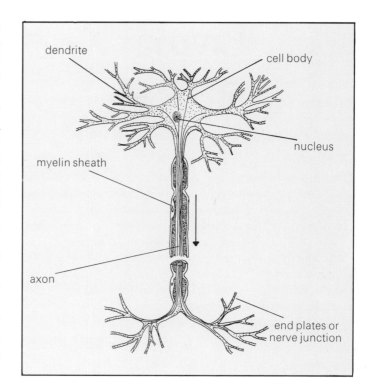

Above: pain is transmitted by specialized nerve fibers. Two types have been postulated: fast-conducting fibers which result in a sharp sensation, and slow fibers which cause an aching feeling.

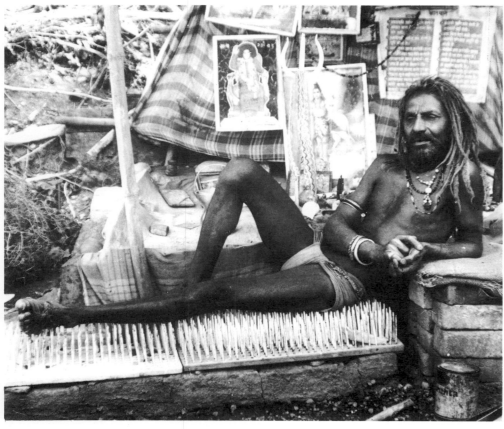

Left: The pain threshold is a highly individual characteristic. The Eastern mystics, for example, are legendary for their resistance to pain.

guishable from those of pain caused by renal colic. A similar injury in the right upper muscles of the abdominal wall may cause gall bladder colic pain; and an injury to a muscle or ligament deep in the chest wall may cause pain which radiates to the left arm, producing the same symptoms as angina.

The concept of pain is closely tied in with psychological factors and there is no reliable way of measuring the various pain thresholds. The influence of emotional states and the importance of racial, cultural and religious factors on the response to pain cannot be overestimated. It is well known that some individuals, by virtue of training, habit or phlegmatic character, are relatively stoical and that others are excessively responsive to pain. An athlete may suffer an extremely painful injury during a race, but not be aware of it until the race is over. Men are supposedly much more sensitive to pain than women. But one rarely encounters people who are totally incapable of experiencing pain throughout their lifetime.

Living with Pain

Chronic pain can have a devastating effect on the entire nervous system. There is increased irritability, fatigue, troubled sleep, poor appetite and loss of emotional stability. Sufferers may become irrational about illness and make unreasonable demands on their family and doctor. A person in this state, which is called *pain shock*, requires delicate but firm management, and the effect of pain-killing drugs often complicates the situation.

For the pain of cancer, diseases of the brain, and other incurable diseases, the doctor must decide whether it is better to operate or to resort to the controlled use of drugs. The age of the person, life expectancy, and mental state are all of importance in selecting the form of treatment. Too often nowadays an operation on the spinal cord or brain is chosen in preference to the controlled use of drugs. The fact is perhaps forgotten that many people with cancer were at one time kept relatively comfortable and active by judicious use of morphine and similar drugs and were never subjected to costly operations or rarely deprived of any of those qualities of mind and character which are so treasured by their families.

Superficial skin pain rarely presents a problem. Aspirin or paracetomol taken every four hours is usually effective, and when combined with caffeine is useful for overcoming central nervous system depression. Adequate rest and relief of muscle tension will also help ease pain. The application of heat, especially moist heat, is also beneficial. Occasionally cold applications are used; but with the exception of cooling packs applied to inflamed, burning skin or to a *causalgia* (a constant, burning pain resulting from injury to a peripheral nerve), cold is more likely to aggravate than to sooth a painful condition.

Occasionally skin and deep pain of skeletal structures is so severe as to require more powerful

Research into backache. The subject wears rods on her back which, in conjunction with overhead mirrors and a calibrated floor and wall, assess the angle of the spine and the degree of flexing and extension. Signals emitted by a radio transmitter previously swallowed by the subject record the abdominal pressure during lifting, pushing and pulling.

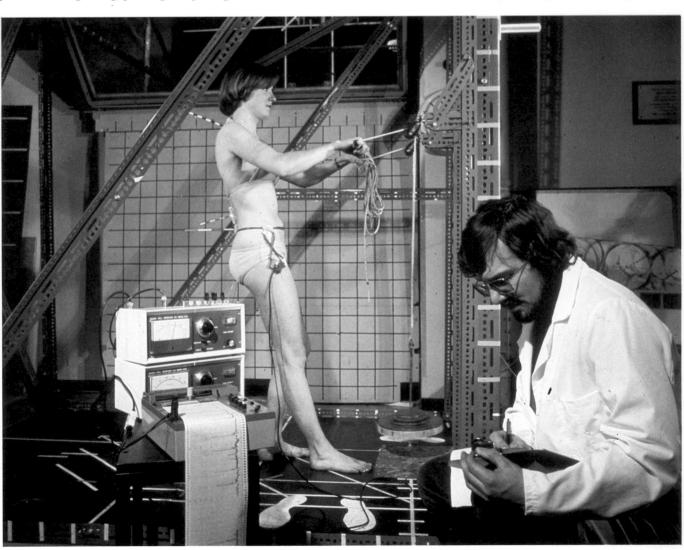

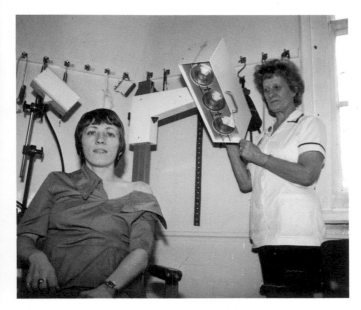

Above: this patient is receiving infrared heat treatment for a painful stiff shoulder to relieve pain and restore normal movement. Other patients find that heat worsens the problem, and have ice therapy instead.

Below: cryoanalgesia, a technique for relieving pain by freezing the nerves with an ice probe. The probe is guided by an image intensifier linked to a television screen. The operation is carried out under local anesthetic.

analgesics. When the pain is unusually severe, some degree of sedation is necessary, and morphine is the ideal drug. Minute doses will often relieve pain without causing undesirable nausea and vomiting. If the dose is too small, a second dose of the same size is often given. This divided dose is less likely to induce nausea and vomiting than a larger single dose. Morphine and related analgesics occasionally produce itching and therefore are used with care in people with skin irritability.

Visceral pain originating in the stomach, gall bladder, intestines or heart is usually very poorly controlled by mild analgesics, and along with intractible pain due to diseases such as cancer is one of the most difficult problems that patients have to face. Strong analgesics relieve the pain but mask the state of the patient, and the opium derivatives such as morphine are also addictive. As a rule doctors resort to such drugs because otherwise the patient's pain would be unbearable, and addiction is accepted as the lesser of two evils. A possible alternative is pain-relieving surgery, which has advantages in certain cases over the continuous use of drugs. This involves either the removal of certain nerves arising from the spinal cord or directing electrodes onto the brain.

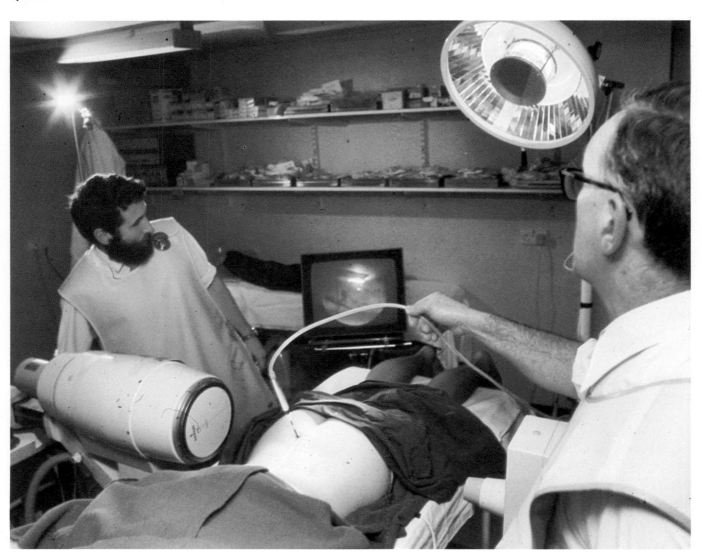

Defining Mental Illness

Psychiatrists seldom discuss mental illness with the same confident assurance about causes, symptoms, and treatment that doctors have when they talk about physical illness. Such uncertainty is hardly surprising. There is still no general agreement, for instance, about whether certain abnormal states are really "illnesses" at all. Also different societies have different standards in defining mental states. In general we can say that when someone is unable to lead a useful life in society – when he fails to adjust to himself, to others, and to his environment – he can be considered as mentally ill.

It is difficult to say to what extent inherited characteristics influence mental illness. Expert opinion is widely divided, but there is a general agreement that a few diseases producing physical defects run in families according to the laws of heredity. An example is the rare disease called Huntington's chorea; roughly half the children of a parent whose genes carry this disease will get it. It does not show itself until middle age, when a brain deterioration begins to affect the mind. Some psychiatrists maintain that in a similar way people may inherit tendencies or predispositions to certain kinds of mental illness along with various physical defects, glandular imbalances, or food allergies.

But even if this is true, other experts point out that a predisposition does not necessarily lead to actual mental illness. Such illness is usually triggered off by environmental stresses. In general it would appear that the role of heredity in directly determining mental disorder is relatively small. More certain is the fact that some forms of mental defects are congenital, that is they may result from a harmful drug taken by a mother during pregnancy, from a disease (such as German measles), or from birth injuries.

Psychiatrists believe that many mental disorders are predominantly reactions of the mind to stress. Some of these reactions, called *functional psychoses*, are so serious that their victims are unable to lead useful purposeful lives. The milder disorders are called *neuroses*, and are far more common; hardly any of us avoid neurotic behavior altogether. The typical neurotic tries to cope with reality by relying too much on defensive mechanisms (anxieties, compulsions, imaginary illnesses, and so on), learned early in life. Though most of us fall back on some form of defense mechanism from time to time, they seldom help us come to terms with the problems of maturity.

Between "normality" and neurosis there is no hard and fast dividing line. A harassed mother, for example, may complain of constant "nervous" tension and fatigue and many people admit to panicky feelings in elevators or subway trains, but psychiatrists hesitate to label such people as neurotics. We might do better to think of a neurosis not as a disease in itself, but as a symptom.

A psychiatrist can treat typical neurotic symptoms only by helping his patient discover the truth about his basic personality. Anxiety symptoms, for example, are likely to be disguises for deeply rooted fears and feelings of inadequacy. It can take shape as a disproportionate fear (a phobia) of being shut in, of heights, of cats, or snakes, or it can consist simply of a vague sense of impending disaster.

Hysteria is another type of neurosis; it can result in loss of memory or in various physical symptoms. A hysterical neurotic avoids a distressing situation simply by dissociating from the rest of his or her personality a disturbing memory or a threat posed symbolically by one of the senses. Hysterically

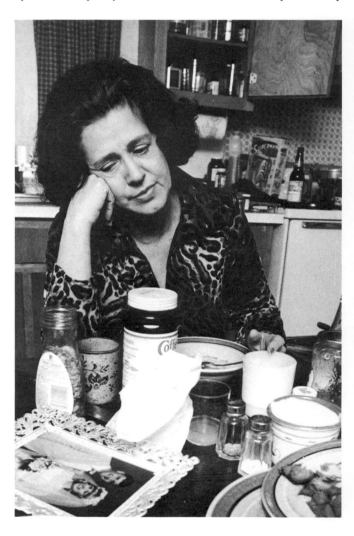

Depression is a very prevalent illness even though in many cases it is not recognized as such. It affects adults far more so than children, is more common in younger men than women, but in middle age, women are more prone than men. The depressive lacks motivation, which sometimes goes as far as a lack of the will to live. Another characteristic of depression is the extreme self-criticism, even self-hatred, experienced by the sufferer.

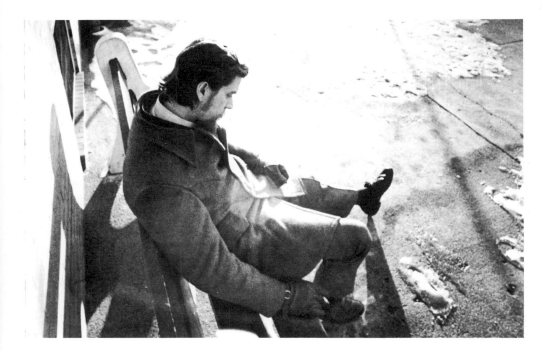

Left: for many depression is aggravated by loneliness. This is especially so in urban societies, where family ties are broken quickly. Often the person feels inadequate and inferior, and this prevents him or her from making friends and acquaintances.

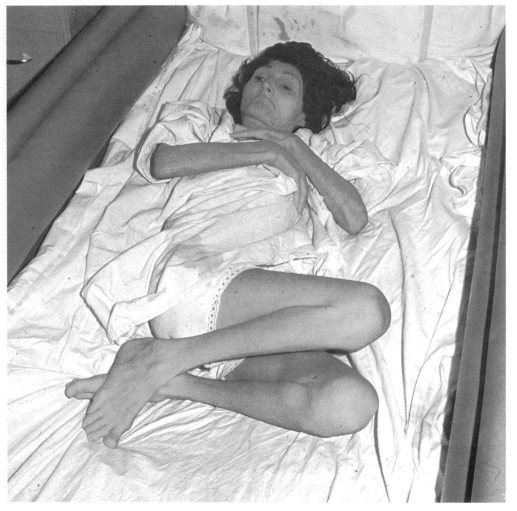

Left: a victim of Huntington's chorea. The onset of this rare hereditary disease does not appear until middle age. Muscular spasms become progressively more debilitating, and the disease is invariably fatal.

induced blindness, for example, shuts the victim out of a world he or she is afraid to face.

Common obsessive states are exaggerated forms of such persistent ideas – familiar to everyone – as the notion that you have not set your alarm clock or locked the front door – you may know this is unreasonable but you feel compelled to check. But neurotic obsessions are far more troublesome. An idea that the world is full of dangerous germs, for instance, may compel certain types of neurotics to wash their hands constantly. But this compulsive act fails to get rid of their obsession since it does not cope with the real danger – perhaps an unconscious concern with sexual guilt, or with aggressive feelings.

The Types of Psychoses

The most serious mental diseases are labeled psychoses. Psychotic patients are severely disturbed, totally disabled, by their illness. The symptoms are obvious – thought and behavior are disordered – but the causes are not so clear. There are two sorts of psychosis: disorders of organic origin (arising from changes or deterioration of the brain and nervous system) and disorders of purely psychological origin (psychiatrists call these functional psychoses).

Many patients in mental hospitals today suffer from organic psychoses and in most cases the advance of these diseases is irreversible. They may lead to a progressive deterioration that treatment can only alleviate. For example chronic alcoholism can cause damage to brain cells and result in erratic memory and confusion about time and place. The deterioration that accompanies senility or arteriosclerosis can lead to organic psychoses. Similar psychoses can be caused by carbon monoxide poisoning and other toxic conditions brought on by infection (such as sleeping sickness and syphilis), stroke, and even by severe vitamin deficiencies.

Among the functional psychoses *schizophrenia*, literally "split mind," can start early in adolescence as a deterioration of the intellect. It can culminate in a state of complete withdrawal from the world or in regressive infantile behavior. The earlier the onset, the darker is the outlook for a schizophrenic. One type of schizophrenic believes that he is being persecuted in sinister ways – for example by atomic devices known only to his persecutor. These are called *paranoid* or *paraphrenic* states. A typical paranoid case is that of George Schulmann, who went to the United States from Europe in the 1930s. He returned to his brother's widow after 35 years as poor as he left. Immediately after his return he started unending procedures to regain the money that "a conspiracy took away from him". His relatives made many attempts to help him and were surprised at the negative answers from the bank managers who according to George had promised to send him his money. He visited an ear specialist and asked him to remove a hidden listening device that he was convinced had been planted in his middle ear. *Hebephrenics* react in a more obviously deranged way. They grimace and giggle in inappropriate situations, and become increasingly out of touch with

Right: the title of this painting is *Loneliness*. The artist, a schizophrenic, has attempted to express graphically her profound sense of isolation.

Below: art therapy is used to treat psychotically disturbed patients. It can provide a release of feelings and give clues as to the cause of the illness.

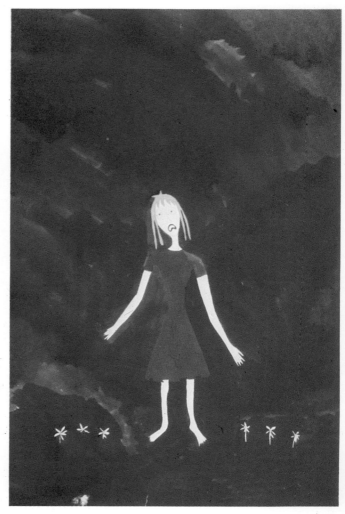

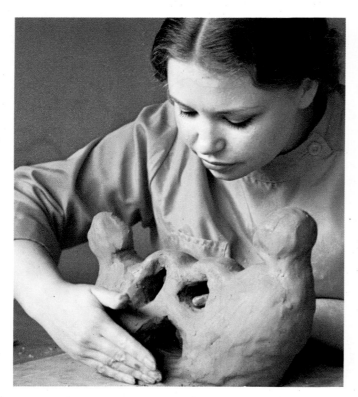

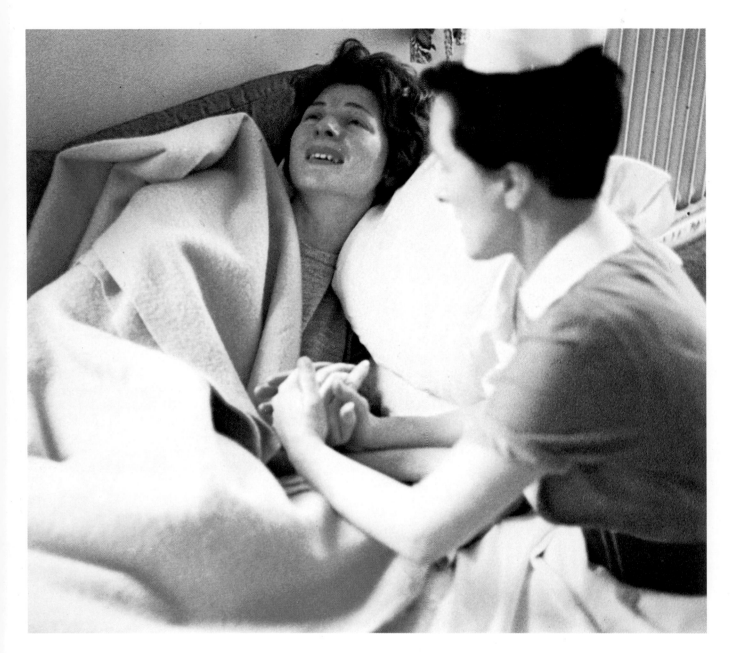

anyone who tries to help them. Their speech is illogical and rambling, and they frequently talk to themselves.

A *catatonic* is withdrawn, hostile and has a generally inhibited negative attitude to society. A catatonic patient may retreat into rigid postures and hold them for hours while remaining alert and hostile – observing his or her "enemies." But suddenly he or she may run berserk, committing acts as violently destructive as murder.

Organic depressive psychosis presents a different picture. For one thing, the person had usually led a reasonably well-adjusted life before the onset of the illness, though there may have been a record of moodiness. This particular type of psychotic may have had periodic attacks of depression alternating with cheerfulness; in fact the cheerfulness may have been of the kind that other people find a little wearing. Such an illness simply exaggerates these traits. Periods of intense excitement follow periods of the deepest depression. Psychiatrists call this excitement

Drugs and psychiatric therapy are commonly used in the treatment of phycoses. However, the release of traumatic experiences, bottled up for so long, can be extremely frightening for the patient, and skilled nursing staff will be needed close at hand.

mania. Mania can be relatively harmless or so uncontrolled that physical restraint or tranquilizing drugs are necessary. Periods of depression may be either mild or so severe that the patient speaks to nobody except to admit some "unforgivable" sin. This, of course is a delusion, but a logical one in the context of the depression.

Typical manic-depressive conditions are less common than isolated attacks of depression that require treatment perhaps only once in a lifetime. Or a period of depression may occur with mild, hardly noticeable periods of elation between. Men and women eminently successful in their everyday lives may disappear into a hospital or nursing home once in a while for "a rest" without any of their friends realizing the true nature of their illness.

The Modern Approach

In the year 1800, an English Quaker, William Tuke, established a "Retreat" at York for mental patients, where "a milder and more appropriate system of treatment than that usually practiced might be adopted." His milder system meant that patients were not physically restrained and lived as normally as possible in the pleasant surroundings of the Retreat. Unfortunately, any widespread humanitarian treatment of the mentally ill did not take place for a hundred years. One 20th-century advance (really a return to humanity shown by Tuke) was the unlocking of wards. Patients had the freedom to move about, and later psychiatrists came to realize that they could carry out treatment of selected cases even more effectively in nonhospital environments.

Although separate mental hospitals are still common today, psychiatric departments have become a part of an increasing number of general hospitals and sufferers are sometimes treated as outpatients, or they share hospital wards with the physically ill. These changes came about partly as the result of new methods of treatment, such as psychotherapy (basically involving verbal encounters between the patient and the therapist) and the use of drugs, and partly as a result of changes in public attitudes to mental illness. In "day" hospitals patients receive treatment in the day time and go home at night. Or they spend weekends in the hospital and work on regular jobs during the week.

Electroconvulsive (shock) treatment mysteriously returns some mentally ill people to "sanity" and makes them receptive to supportive therapy after they emerge from convulsions and coma. It is carried out by applying two electrodes to the sedated patient's head and passing an electric current between them. This method is most beneficial for the treatment of severe suicidal and other depressive states.

Despite the little that we really know about their effects on the entire body, drugs remain one of psychiatry's best hopes. In the relatively short period since their introduction, the number of violent patients has been reduced, the course of acute mental illness shortened, and in many cases psychological

Right: for a severely disturbed patient, a stay in the psychiatric ward of a hospital may be the only solution. This is particularly so where the the patient may present a danger to himself and to others.

Below: in cases of severe depression, electro-convulsive therapy still offers the best chance of a cure. During the treatment a protective gag is placed in the patient's mouth to prevent his damaging his teeth or biting his tongue.

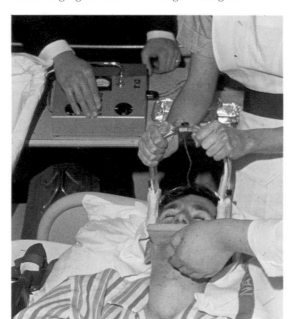

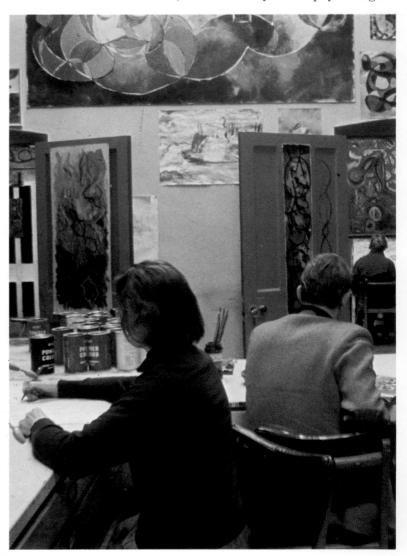

A severely withdrawn patient
may need months of patient
therapy and rehabilitation
from professional staff.

deterioration prevented. Drugs include tranquilizers, antidepressants, sedatives, stimulants, and hallucinogenics.

Tranquilizers help to relax some mentally disturbed people, and others help violently disturbed schizophrenic patients to become manageable and sometimes remove psychotic symptoms entirely.

Advances involving the use of drugs are showing promising results and a severely ill person's stay in hospital can be considerably shortened. The patient is admitted and put under continuous sleep treatment; or a combination of electroconvulsive treatment and drugs may be given. When the patient is brought out of sleep he or she is often completely cured, and there is no memory of the treatment period.

Another recent advance is even more exciting. It is now generally recognized all over the world that a single mineral, lithium carbonate, stops or greatly modifies manic-depressive psychoses. How such a simple mineral works is not known. Many schizophrenics have attacks of excitement, but with added delusional ideas and hallucinations, and then periods of illness when they are deeply depressed. Such patients were often kept permanently in chronic wards. But now they may be given lower doses of tranquilizers, with a therapeutic dose of lithium, and possibly also an antidepressant drug. The patient will often emerge from chronic schizophrenia into normality, and is able to return into the community.

Antianxiety drugs have virtually replaced the surgical operation once performed on those suffering from severe obsessional states and some psychoses. This operation, called *lobotomy*, in which some of the nerve fibers connecting the emotional centers of the thalamus with the cortex are severed, lessens emotional fears and drives. But there is some loss of general mental ability and emotional stability, as well as other, not always predictable, personality changes.

Rheumatism and Arthritis

Among the major chronic diseases, rheumatic illnesses cripples most and kill least. The terms used for abnormal conditions of the joints are numerous and often confusing. *Rheumatism* is a general term used for a group of diseases characterized by pain, stiffness, or often disabling deformity of the joints, muscles and related structures. The rheumatic diseases include a large group of disorders causing alterations in joint capsules, cartilage and bone, or in connective tissue surrounding the joints. Many of these disorders can accompany connective tissue diseases. The term *arthritis* is used to describe inflammation of the joints.

Public health surveys show that more than 3.5 million people in West Germany suffer from some form of rheumatism, which makes it the country's most prominent chronic disease causing disability.

Of these 3.5 million people, 45 percent have arthritis, over 10 percent are partially disabled, and almost 2 percent are completely disabled. More than half the disabled are under 45 years of age. In other countries the toll from rheumatic disease is even greater. In the United Kingdom, for example, 7 percent of the population are incapacitated for at least one day each year by rheumatism and it accounts for 16 percent of all absences from work. Age is no barrier: much disability occurs in young people.

Joint disorders have many causes. A number of infections can cause arthritis, such as tuberculosis and syphilis. Arthritis can follow a specific infection, the best known being rheumatic fever. On rare occasions people develop arthritis because of a hypersensitivity to drugs, or metabolic or endocrine disorders.

Rheumatoid arthritis is the most severe form of the disease, occurring most frequently in middle-aged women. It causes deformities, especially swellings of the hands and wrists, and is frequently severely disabling. *Osteoarthritis* is a chronic and painfull disorder, commonly affecting the ankles, knees, and hip. There are a number of different kinds of osteoarthritis and it very often develops with advancing age.

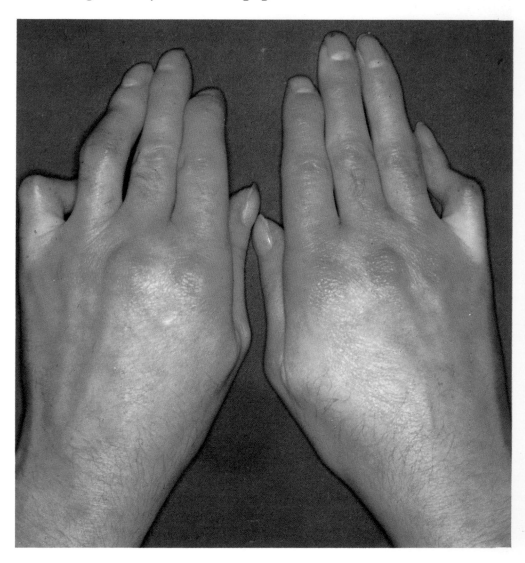

Rheumatoid arthritis affects the connective tissue under the skin, in particular the knuckle joints and wrists. The tissue becomes inflamed and forms tender, painful nodules.

Many people complaining of rheumatism often have symptoms resulting from malfunctioning tissue around the joints, for instance tendons, *bursae* (closed sacs filled with a serous fluid which reduce friction in joints), bones muscles, nerves, and fatty tissue. This group of disorders is responsible for more mild rheumatic complaints than any of the joint disorders proper. Approximately 30 percent of people attending arthritis clinics have this "nonarticular rheumatism."

Fibrositis is a term used to cover many forms of nonarticular rheumatism. In addition to stiffness and soreness, the affected parts are often tender and movement can be extremely difficult. Pain attacks the lower part of the back, the neck, shoulders, and chest.

Other forms of nonarticular rheumatism include *bursitis* – inflammation of one or more of the 140 or so bursae in the body. A familiar form is "housemaid's knee," or water on the knee, and apart from the knees it causes pain and stiffness in the shoulders and elbows.

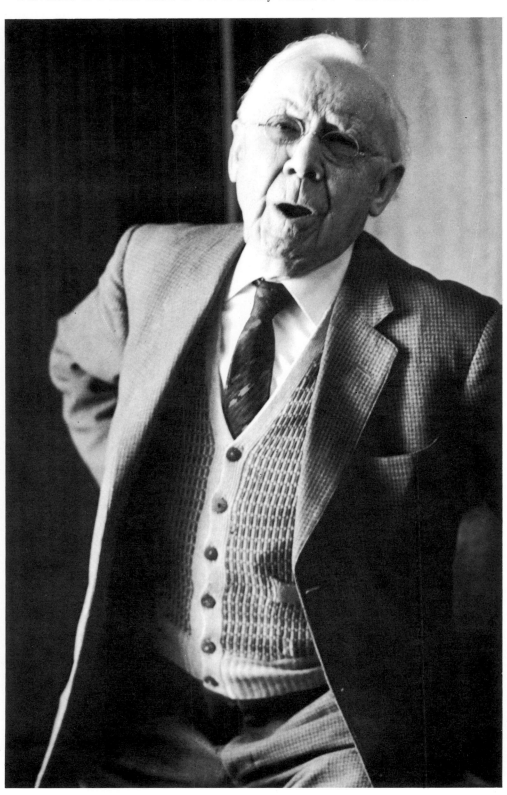

Fibrositis or muscular rheumatism is a common cause of backache. Faulty posture and tension are frequently the causes.

Treatment of Arthritis

Today's therapy for rheumatic diseases is more effective than that of even a decade ago. In this relatively short period remarkable progress has been made in relieving pain and improving function in these potentially crippling diseases. The disease is being fought in three main ways: with drugs, with physical therapy, and through sophisticated surgery.

Pain must be relieved before active physical therapy can be begun, and drugs such as aspirin are frequently tried first. Aspirin is one of the most effective drugs, even for dealing with the pain caused by severe arthritis.

Following treatment, a patient may be referred to an occupational therapist, who will evaluate the movement of the limb and its limitations, and devise a rehabilitative program.

A wide range of drugs are available for treating the pain caused by arthritis. Indomethacin can be of striking benefit to many people suffering from rheumatoid arthritis, often giving dramatic relief of pain and disability. Phenylbutazone is highly effective in most of the so-called benign rheumatic diseases, including osteoarthritis, gout, bursitis, and fibrositis. In advanced cases corticosteroids and immunosuppressive drugs may be used. When cortisone was first introduced, it was thought to be the greatest boon of all time for rheumatoid arthritis sufferers. But though still considered effective it is used with great caution.

Gold salts have been used in the treatment of rheumatoid arthritis for more than 40 years. This therapy offers, according to the majority of rheumatologists, a good chance for a true drug-induced relief of the disease. Its greatest disadvantage is that its favorable results take a long time to manifest themselves, and unpleasant side-effects may occur sometimes.

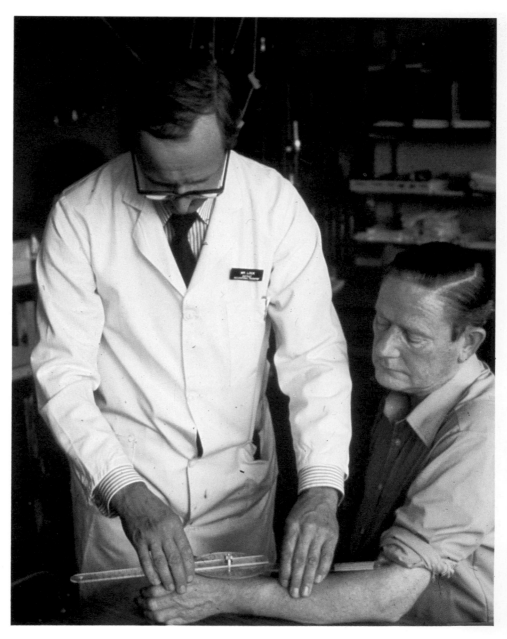

Physical treatment is often essential to relieve pain and restore the useful function in affected joints. Rest may be necessary: the more painful the condition, the more rest is required. Both heat and cold therapy can relieve pain, depending on the condition. Such treatment includes hot tubs and compresses, paraffin dips, swimming pools; and deep heat.

Exercise for the arthritic person is aimed at restoring mobility and strength without aggravating the disease. Exercises are designed to cause the least possible pain and to be repeated only as frequently as is considered essential to achieve some benefit. They usually consist of daily nontiring movements to carry the joints through their normal range of motion.

Prevention of deformities is of utmost importance, especially where a person's position in bed and

Below: for certain arthritic joints, surgery is the most successful form of treatment. This may involve the replacement of the diseased joint with an artificial one (arthoplasty), for example in the hip or elbow.

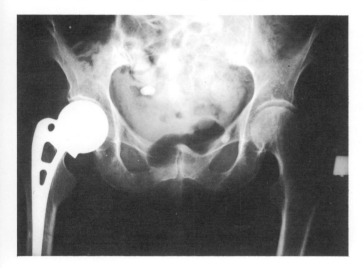

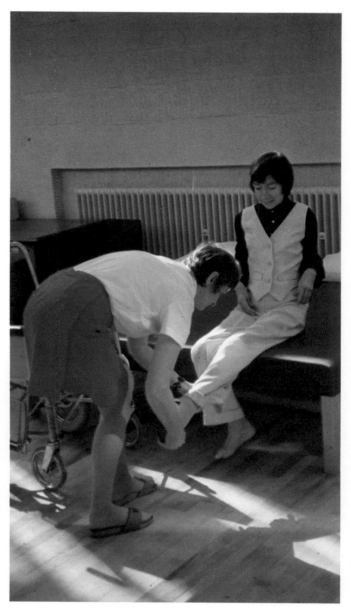

Above: treatment of severe rheumatoid arthritis may involve a combination of rest, drug therapy and physical exercise. The victim may have to be equipped with orthopedic appliances to correct the deformities. Physical therapy is of particular importance in rehabilitating disused or diseased limbs, especially after surgery.

posture in general are concerned. Sufferers are encouraged to lie flat on their back when resting or sleeping, to use as small a pillow as possible under the head and neck, and to avoid altogether using pillows under the knees. Therapists also train arthritics to increase their capacity in performing the normal activities of daily life. In addition, specially designed aids, such as a long-handled shoehorn, a bathtub seat, and a built-up knife and fork, can help a person to remain self-sufficient. Splints and braces can be used effectively to prevent permanently crippled limbs.

Surgery for the arthritic serves two purposes: relief of pain and correction of deformity, both of which can help to restore normal functioning. Only a few of the available techniques can be mentioned here, but for the most part surgery is aimed at salvaging joints that have been partially or completely destroyed by the disease.

Degenerative changes at the hip, wrist, and knee can be helped with an operation called *arthrodesis*, which involves immobilizing a joint by removing the

cartilaginous surfaces so that the bones grow solidly together. *Arthroplasty*, the making of an artificial joint to replace a diseased one, or the reconstruction of a new joint from one that has fused, has proved of great benefit and hip joint replacements are now common. *Osteotomy*, cutting and realigning the bone, and *meniscectomy*, the removal of a meniscus (a cartilaginous disc) from the knee joint, are other surgical techniques in use.

Surgery for arthritis is often successful, but usually involves a fairly vigorous program of rehabilitation after the operation, including the taking of drugs and a great deal of physiotherapy and exercise. Therefore anyone contemplating such an operation should be given a clear understanding of all the processes involved.

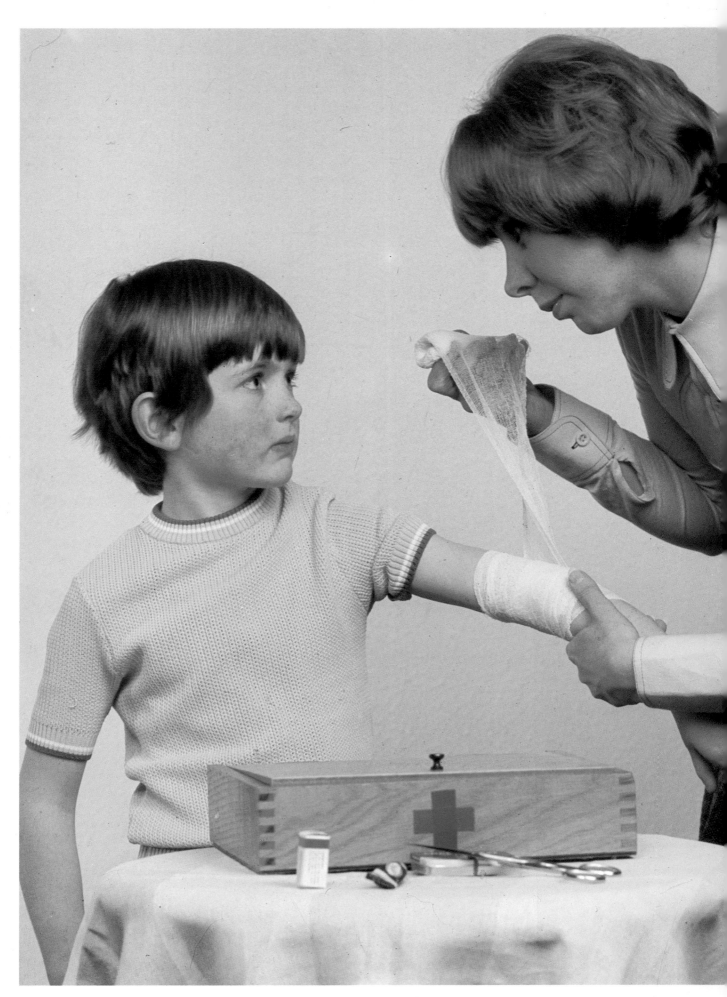

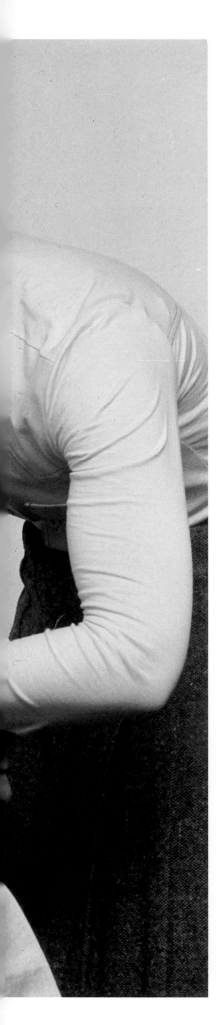

Chapter 16

First Aid Section

Your child has swallowed some aspirin. How can you tell if he or she is seriously ill? What should you do? Call a doctor, or wait to see what happens, or make the child vomit? Your husband develops severe pain in his chest. Is it a heart attack? Should you bundle him into the car and rush him to a hospital? On the road you see an accident has just happened and there is an unconscious person lying on his back. Could he die if you leave him in this position? You will find the answers to these – and other questions – on the following pages. In the short time it will take you to read them, you could learn how to save a life – perhaps the life of someone very close to you.

Opposite: a well stocked medicine chest should be one of the priorities in your home. So should a knowledge of First Aid. One day you may be the only person at hand in an emergency.

Know your First Aid

When a serious accident or sudden illness happens, you must know what to do at once. There is no time to thumb frantically through a first aid manual. There may not even be time to call for medical help. You have to act instantly – and you have to do the right thing. That means knowing in advance the kind of action to take. The following pages will help to give you that advance knowledge in such a way that you will not find it difficult to remember. Here you will find straightforward, practical advice on how to handle some of the most common and dangerous emergencies that any of us might have to face at some time, usually suddenly and quite un-expectedly, or just at a time when you are occupied with so many other things. These emergencies in-clude bleeding, shock, breathing failures, falls, fractures and head injuries, burns and scalds, poisoning, unconsciousness and fainting, heart attack and stroke.

Perhaps you think that reading about first aid will be of little use when you are put to the test. Maybe you feel you are bound to forget all you ever read in a crisis as panic would immobilize you completely. Can just reading about first aid really help you to cope with the unexpected in an emergency? Yes it can – provided the information tells you *why* to do things as well as *how*. The advice you will read here includes explanations of the whys and wherefores of any action to be taken. You will easily remember the main symptoms you will see when someone suffers an accident and is in a state of acute shock. You will understand what those symptoms mean, know the specific dangers entailed, and how, because of this, you should deal with them. You will be able to apply these basic rules in any emergency – and these pages will only take you 15 minutes to read.

There are a number of rules that must be observed at any emergency. First you must do your best to remain calm. If you demonstrate quite clearly that you are in total command of the situation, then the casualty will feel much more secure and any other people present will be ready to help you. The second rule is that you must always act carefully – not to cause unnecessary pain – but nevertheless, you must act immediately! Sometimes minutes are vital. All the symptoms and the extent of damage should be evaluated: very often a small wound can distract our attention from other much more serious symptoms. You should act deliberately, with calm and with purpose in your mind. Above all you must know what *not* to do to make matters worse.

If you are faced with an emergency, the first thing you must do is make sure of the basic facts and then make some quick decisions:

1. Can the patient, or the victim of an accident, be left in the position in which he or she was found, or would leaving the victim in this position make the condition more dangerous?

2. Is the patient conscious, breathing, can you detect any pulse? If the patient is not breathing, what sort of artificial respiration should be tried? Always start

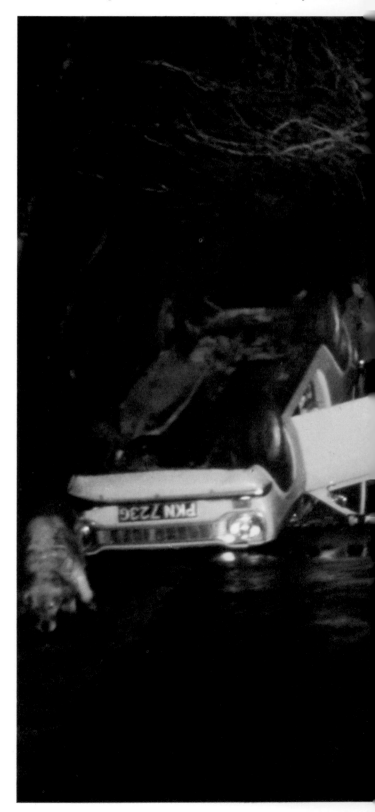

artificial respiration, even if you doubt that it will be of any good.

3. Because of patient's general condition, is it necessary to arrange for immediate transportation to hospital? Or can you wait for the patient's condition to improve and help with first aid. Never let the victim's appearance deceive you into thinking too fast instead of waiting calmly for the ambulance to arrive. Improvized transportation is usually harmful and sometimes even fatal.

4. Can the patient or the victim be given anything to drink or to eat, or would this aggravate his state? A general rule to remember is that a drink is allowed to anybody who is able to bring a glass to their lips.

Once you are satisfied that you are in command of the situation and have carried out the basic fundamentals as described above, you can then continue with the appropriate first aid treatment.

Do not move a car-accident victim. Wait for the ambulance.

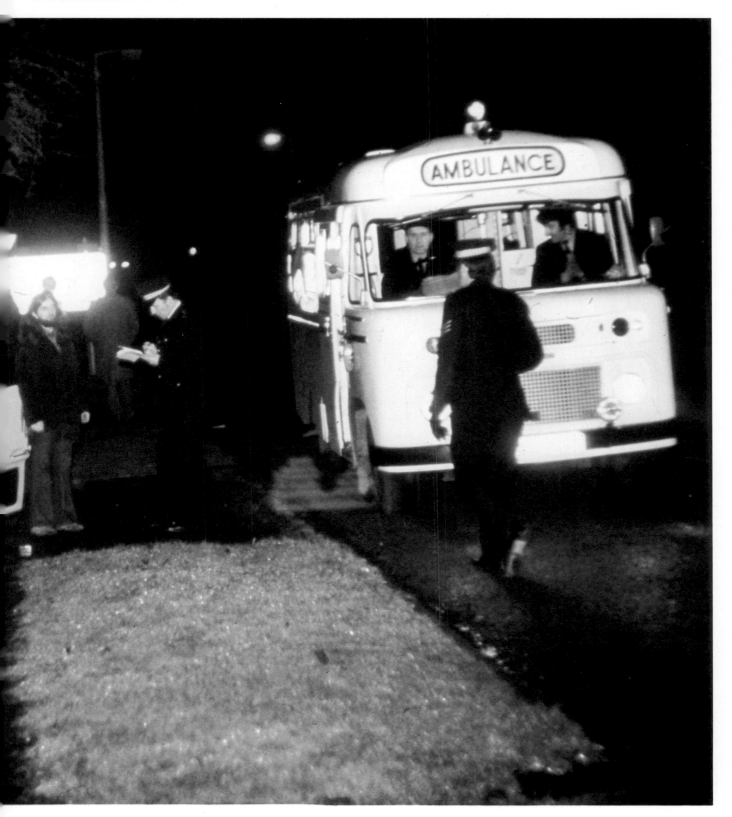

Bleeding

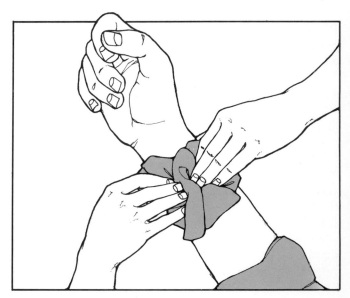

The average adult has about five to six quarts of blood being pumped round the whole body. The exact amount of blood depends on a person's body-weight – a big person has more blood than a small one. Overweight people should not forget that their bodies must build an extra mile of blood vessels! The average person can lose a pint of blood without any danger, and this is the usual amount given by a blood donor. However the loss of blood from a wound should always be taken seriously. In the case of accidental bleeding, not only is it difficult to judge the amount of blood lost, but there is the added risk of infection. It has been shown that the body can lose a third of its blood supply without apparent serious effects, but the loss of half the body's blood is almost always fatal and even the loss of two pints will always produce shock.

What should be done if the bleeding is severe? First the bleeding must be stopped. If someone else can call the ambulance while you deal with the bleeding, immediately make the victim lie still and press your fingers or the palm of your hand directly on the bleeding area, using a clean cloth if possible. Press the edges of the wound firmly together if you can, but continue pressing with your hand until the bleeding has abated. Do not waste time looking for bandages. Grab the cleanest material at hand – a towel, a clean handkerchief, a shirt – to use as a pad. If you have no material of any kind, just press on the wound with your bare hand. The hospital will be able to take care of cleaning the wound later. While maintaining firm and constant pressure on the wound, seat or lay the casualty down, preferable with the legs raised, and raise the bleeding part, if possible, to reduce the flow of blood. When blood soaks through the original pad, do not remove it, but just cover it as fast as possible with new layers of material. When the bleeding ceases, secure the pad firmly with a bandage until you can get medical help. Even the most severe and profuse bleeding can almost always be stopped by direct, continued pressure.

A constrictive bandage (tourniquet) stops bleeding by cutting off the blood supply to an injured arm or leg, but if it is put on too tightly and not loosened often enough, it may cause the entire limb to die. A tourniquet should therefore never be used except by a trained person, and even then is rarely necessary.

Internal bleeding may occur in the chest, abdomen, or skull, following a fall, blow, crash, or injury from a stab wound or a bullet. It can also happen in some chest and abdominal illnesses. The bleeding may in these cases remain unseen, or blood may escape from the body some time after the injury. Symptoms of internal bleeding may include shock, dizziness, loss of consciousness, pallor, rapid breathing, severe pain or swelling, collapse, and anxiety.

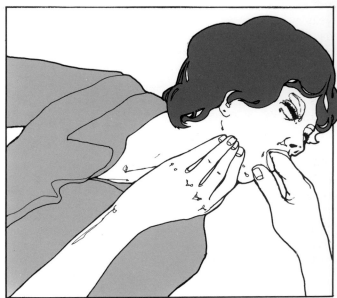

Above: for severe bleeding, press hard with a clean pad.
Center: correct position for a person who is also vomiting.
Below: for a nosebleed, seat the victim over a bowl.

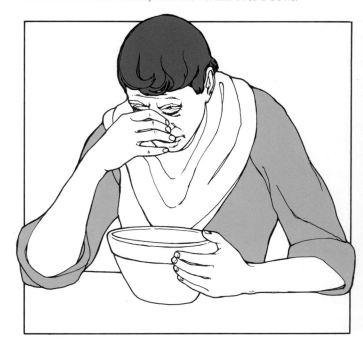

If you suspect internal bleeding, do not move the patient. Keep him lying down, warmly covered, with head low, and send for urgent medical help.

Sometimes the victim may be vomiting. In this case lay him on his side with his head turned to one side and the arm and leg of that side drawn up and loosen all tight clothing.

Small cuts or scratches do not require such drastic treatment. Just wash the cut under cold running water and cleanse the surrounding skin with soap and water. Antiseptics are not necessary except if the wound was very dirty, but do not forget to cover it with a small bandage to prevent infection.

Puncture wounds are more dangerous even if they do not look so on the outside. A rusty nail, or a dog bite, which can cause little bleeding but go deep under the skin, must be treated promptly. As children are immunized against tetanus during their first year and every few years thereafter, no special precautions are necessary. If however you or your child suffers a puncture wound from an object that has been lying in the dirt or even worse on a field, you should ask your doctor to administer a booster injection if this has not been done so for over a year. If the victim is an adult, ask the doctor whether an antitetanus inoculation is necessary.

On occasion a nosebleed may become a problem. The best way to handle it is to sit the victim with the head forward and over a bowl. The nostrils should then be held firmly together for up to 10 minutes. By that time in the majority of cases the bleeding will stop. If it does not, pinch the nostrils again for another five minutes. If the victim loses more than one pint of blood, a doctor should be consulted.

Shock

Shock is a dangerous state of collapse, which, if not controlled, can be fatal. Shock occurs when the supply of blood to the brain is reduced to such an extent that the brain cannot operate properly, and the vital body functions that it controls are disrupted. Shock may therefore arise in any condition that upsets the circulation of the blood, such as heavy loss of blood or body fluids (as in serious injuries, large fractures, and serious burns); internal bleeding from a burst appendix or perforated ulcer; heart attack or stroke. If the blood supply is cut off from the brain, the brain cannot survive for long and the victim will die.

A person who goes into shock feels giddy and nauseous, may grow extremely pale, and sweat profusely. The skin may become cold and clammy, vision blurred, and breathing rapid but shallow. A shock victim may complain of thirst, become restless and anxious, and possibly lose consciousness. However, the vital point to remember is that shock is likely to occur in any serious medical emergency and should be treated urgently without waiting for specific symptoms to appear.

Stop any bleeding by direct pressure and obtain medical help. Remember, shock is caused by a shortage of blood to the brain, and without blood the brain cannot function for long. Treatment must therefore be directed toward restoring the blood supply to the brain as quickly as possible. In the case of heavy bleeding or loss of body fluid, medical treatment will probably involve a transfusion to replace the blood or fluid lost. That is why it is vital to get the victim to hospital as fast as possible – even when bleeding has been stopped. While waiting for an ambulance to arrive, keep the victim quiet, as comfortable as possible, and reassured. Keep the victim's head low so that blood can reach the brain more easily. Try and arrange the victim so that he is lying down with the legs raised and head turned to one side in case of vomiting. If the victim is un-

A shock victim should be laid feet higher than the head.

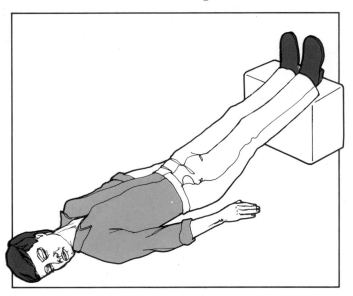

conscious, use the coma position (see page 314). Loosen any tight clothing and cover him with a blanket or coat. Give nothing to drink except to a *conscious* burned casualty.

True shock is always caused by a serious shortage of blood supply to the brain. However, severe fright, extreme pain, a horrifying sight, or other violently emotional experience can cause a kind of shock. This will often cause fainting, due to an impairment of the nervous system, but it may result in many of the symptoms of shock already described. The major difference between this kind of emotional shock and serious physical shock, however, is that it can almost always be quickly and simply relieved by treating the casualty for fainting (see page 314). In this case too it will do no harm to give the casualty a warm, sweetened drink – once he or she is conscious and has started to recover. However, it is vital to remember that these measures apply only where the cause of shock is purely emotional, and can be dangerously time-consuming if the casualty is suffering from true shock following some medical emergency.

Resuscitation

Anyone whose breathing has stopped needs immediate artificial respiration. Breathing can stop from one of many reasons: drowning, electric shock, poisoning, suffocation, or a sudden illness such as a heart attack.

The air we breathe supplies the oxygen that is vital to keep every part of the body alive. And the brain itself is the first to suffer from lack of oxygen. If no air is entering the lungs, the heart will continue to beat for a little longer, supplying blood to the brain and other parts of the body. But soon the supply of oxygen already in the blood will be used up. First the patient loses consciousness, because the brain is no longer getting sufficient oxygen to function. Then lack of oxygen in the heart causes it to stop beating.

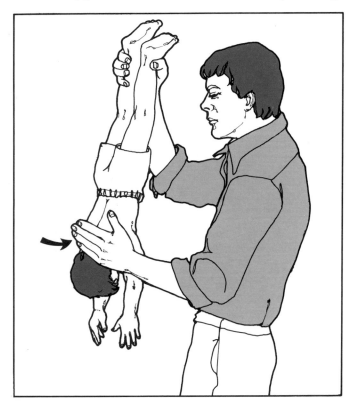

Without oxygen the brain can survive undamaged for only about four minutes. The heart may survive for as long as 12 minutes. But within six minutes, the person will almost certainly be dead.

To check whether a person is breathing, the best way is to put your ear close to his nose and mouth: you should be able to hear air passing in and out. Or you can put a mirror close to the victim's lips: if he is breathing, the mirror becomes misty.

If someone stops breathing your aim is to get air into his body as fast as possible and you have three priorities: make sure his air passages are clear; breathe air into his lungs; and stimulate his heart if it has stopped beating. In a baby or small child who has been choking or gasping for breath before becoming unconscious, the air passage is probably blocked by some object in his throat, so immediately hold the child up by the heels, or over your lap with his head down, and slap his back sharply several times. This alone will probably be enough to dislodge the object and enable breathing to start again. In an adult, clear the air passage by bending the patient's head back as far as it will go, pressing firmly on the forehead or pulling his hair. At the same time, push the lower jaw upward and forward until the teeth meet. In this position, the tongue cannot fall back and block the back of the throat and that may be the only reason why an unconscious person cannot breathe. He may now gasp and start breathing. If not, quickly check the inside of his mouth for any other obstruction – false or broken teeth, blood, vomit, or mucus – that may be blocking the air passage. If the victim is chocking immediately apply the Heimlich manouver. If he still does not start to breathe you must start mouth-to-mouth resuscitation immediately.

Keep the victim's head tilted right back as far as it will go, with the chin jutting up. Place one hand under the neck to lift and support. Open the victim's mouth. Take a deep breath, and place your mouth tightly over the victim's mouth. Pinch his nostrils firmly

Left: hold a choking child up by his heels and slap hard.
Below left: push chin up and back to free air passage.
Below: check that there are no obstructions in the mouth.

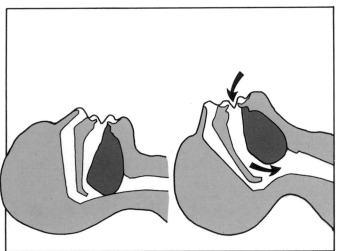

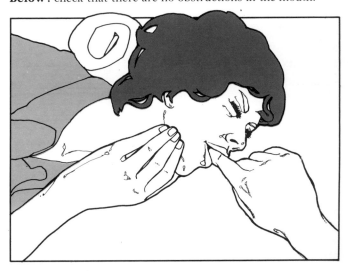

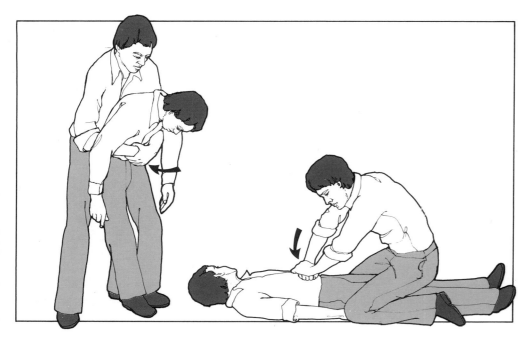

The Heimlich manouver. If victim is sitting or standing wrap your arms around his waist from behind. Grab your fist and place the thumb side of your fist against the victim's abdomen, slightly above the naval and below the rib cage. Press into the victim's abdomen with a quick upward thrust. Repeat if necessary. If the victim is prostrate, kneel astride him. With one hand on top of other, place heel of lower hand slightly above navel and below rib cage. Press with quick upward thrust. If victim is vomiting place his head to one side and wipe out mouth.

shut so that no air can escape. Blow slowly and deeply. His chest will rise as his lungs fill. Then take your mouth away and watch the patient's chest fall as the air comes out. By keeping your ear close to his mouth, you may also hear, or feel, the exhaled breath.

If the victim does not exhale after the first breath, quickly tilt the head further back and try again. As soon as the casualty has completed an exhaled breath, breathe into his mouth again. Blow again, allow the air to escape, then begin again. Give the first four breaths as rapidly as possible. After that continue at a steady, rhythmical rate, in time with the rise and fall of the victim's chest. This will probably mean giving about 10 or 12 breaths per minute. For babies and small children, cover both nose and mouth with your mouth, and blow gentle puffs of air – just sufficient to cause the chest to rise. The first 6 to 10 puffs should be given as rapidly as possible. After

Open the victim's mouth, pinch the nostrils, and blow until you see the chest rise. If the victim does not exhale, blow again, waiting each time for the air to escape.

that the child will need around 15 to 20 breaths per minute.

Continue mouth-to-mouth resuscitation until the casualty is able to breathe freely by himself or until professional help arrives. His breaths will be weak and shallow at first.

If the casualty does not start breathing in spite of your efforts, it may be because his or her heart has stopped beating. This is particularly likely in cases of severe electric shock. In this case continue to give mouth-to-mouth resuscitation, but between breaths, check that the heart is beating. Feel for the pulse to the side of, and behind, the Adam's apple. If you can feel no pulse, the heart has stopped. The patient will be blue-gray in color and the pupils will be dilated.

What can you do? Strike the chest smartly over the heart. This may be enough to start the beat. If not, quickly place the heel of one hand on the lower half of the breastbone and cover it with the heel of the other hand. Press down firmly on the lower part of the

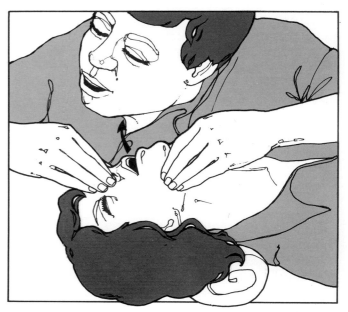

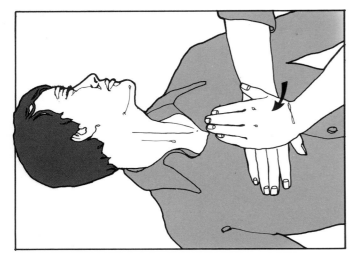

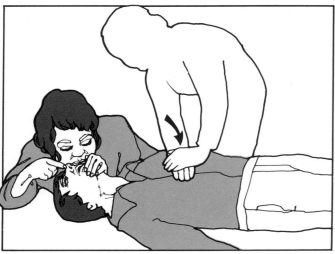

Press the heel of your lower hand over the lower part of the breastbone by rocking forward, arms straight. Alternate six heart compressions with your partner's two mouth-to-mouth resuscitations.

breastbone by rocking forward with your arms straight. Do this about once a second for an adult. For a child, use one hand only and press more rapidly – about 80 times a minute. For a baby use fingertips only and press 100 times a minute. Meanwhile, you must continue to give mouth-to-mouth resuscitation. If you are alone, alternate two inflations of the lungs by mouth-to-mouth breathing with 15 heart compressions. Counting aloud will help you. If you have help, one person should do mouth-to-mouth breathing only; the other should do the heart compressions. The two of you should not act simultaneously, but alternate one air inflation with six heart compressions.

If the heart has restarted, the patient's color will improve strikingly. The pulse will return and the pupils will become smaller. Continue pressing on the heart until this happens. Carry on giving mouth-to-mouth resuscitation until the casualty is able to breathe of his own accord. It may be necessary to continue lung-heart resuscitation, or mouth-to-mouth breathing alone, for an hour – or even considerably longer. Never give up until you can hand the victim over to a medical professional.

Falls and Fractures

Most falls can be avoided if the right precautions are taken. However, concussion or a bone fracture is not so rare and it may happen to you. Concussion is a shaking up and bruising of the brain following a knockout blow to the head. A victim of concussion will lose consciousness after the blow, but will often recover fairly quickly. However, there is a danger that the blow which knocked the victim out may also have damaged the brain and this may be serious if not treated. If this happens, the victim of concussion will slowly lose consciousness again – possibly not until several hours after the accident – and may not recover unless medical help is obtained. That is why it is vital for any one who blacks out, even momentarily, after a head injury, to be examined by a doctor. As long as this precaution is taken, concussion rarely causes any lasting damage.

Inability to move the injured part, pain, swelling, or misshapeness may indicate a fracture, or you may be able to see the end of a broken bone poking through the skin. Often, however, there are no symptoms beyond swelling and pain, and a fracture can easily be mistaken for a sprain or even a bad bruise. For this reason it is safest to treat any injury that causes pain or swelling around a bone as a fracture and keep any pressure off it until you can get medical advice.

In any situation where you suspect a fracture, do not move the injured person at all, even to make him more comfortable. If there is bleeding, stem the flow of blood, but do not try to push a protruding bone back into place. Cover any wound, place a blanket over the casualty and call a doctor or ambulance. On no account transport the patient yourself to the hospital. Moving the patient may make the injury much worse. If the person must be moved to get him out of danger, this should be done by two people. One should hold the injured limb in exactly the position it was found, while the other lifts the casualty onto a flat, hard surface that will support the injured part. If – and only if – it is essential to move the casualty any distance before medical aid can arrive, you must first prevent the injured limb from moving. This is best done by strapping the limb to the patient's body, in the case of a broken arm, strap it gently to the patient's side with scarves, belts, or any other available material. For an injured leg, tie both legs gently together. Always remember to tie above and below the suspected fracture, not over it. Under no account attempt to move a person who appears to have neck, spinal, or skull injuries (beyond getting him out of the path of immediate danger, in which case he must have something firm beneath his back to keep it straight). Incorrect moving could cause permanent damage, paralysis, or even death. Keep a fracture victim still, and warm, and keep a watch on breathing. Do not give anything to eat or drink, as the victim may need an anesthetic prior to having the bone set.

Burns and Scalds

Burns are classified according to the depth of damage they cause. In a first-degree burn, there is reddening of the skin caused by swelling of small blood vessels, but the skin remains unbroken. In a second-degree burn, fluid escapes from the swollen blood vessels into the skin and causes blisters. In a third-degree burn, the skin and some of the tissues beneath it are destroyed. More important than the depth of the burn, however, is its extent. An extensive burn that effects a large area of the body's surface is dangerous, regardless of its depth.

In burns the damage is due to the heat, which coagulates the proteins and produces a wound. Injury to the skin is the same whether caused by dry heat, as in a burn, or by moist heat, as in a scald, or corrosive chemicals such as sulfuric acid or caustic soda.

The chief danger of a burn lies in the loss of fluid through the damaged skin. This fluid, called *plasma*, comes from the bloodstream and contains a number of important chemicals. Its loss reduces the supply of blood to the brain and may thus cause a form of shock which could be fatal. The fluid lost from a small burn may not be more than a thimbleful and will cause no harm. But in a large burn, several pints of fluid may be lost, and the greater the surface affected, the more fluid will escape. In an extensive burn, therefore, it may be necessary to replace the lost fluid by a transfusion. Another possible cause of death from burns is infection. Here again, the larger the surface, the more germs are able to enter through the wound into the body.

Doctors estimate that when more than 15 percent of the skin area of the body is burned, the fluid loss becomes serious. The skin covering the back or the front of the trunk, or a leg, for example, represents about 18 percent of the body's total skin area. Anyone burned over the chest and abdomen, or the back, or the whole of one limb, should therefore receive urgent hospital treatment. Most doctors consider that if a burn is bigger than the victim's hand, then it needs hospital treatment.

In a severe burn, immediately cover the burned area with sterile gauze or clean sheeting, and get the victim to the hospital without delay. If you have no car available, call an ambulance. While waiting for an ambulance, give the injured person frequent small drinks of cold water, adding no more than a quarter teaspoon of salt and a quarter teaspoonful of bicarbonate of soda to each pint glass, to replace body fluids. Treat for shock (see page 309). Do not remove any burned clothing which has cooled, as this will already have been rendered sterile, and do not interefere with any blisters, for while the skin re-

mains intact over the blister, germs cannot enter.

Do not apply iodine, ointments, lotions, oils, or any antiseptic to a severe burn. The drugs in these may be absorbed into the body and cause dangerous reactions, or interfere with subsequent medical care.

If a burn or a scald is mild, immerse the burned area in cold running water, say under a shower, to cool it and to relieve pain. Allow the area to dry and cover it loosely with a sterile gauze bandage or a clean cloth. If possible use specially packaged gauze impregnated with a petroleum jelly.

This helps prevent any blisters from breaking and guards against infection. Remember not to tamper with blisters, and do not use any other cream – not even a burn ointment.

If the burn is caused by a chemical, immediately rinse the chemical off the person's skin with large amounts of cold water, under a shower if necessary. Cut away affected clothing. If an eye is affected, wash it immediately and thoroughly to remove all traces of the chemical. Turn the head so that the water does not pass from the affected eye into the other eye. Chemical burns are usually caused by a strong acid, such as sulfuric acid, or by an alkali such as caustic soda. They can cause serious damage.

Chemical powder burns are commonly caused by careless handling of fireworks, cap pistols or firearms. Remove any splinters and dirt from the wound and wash it with soap and water – but do not probe the wound. Apply a dry, sterile dressing.

Unconsciousness

Unconsciousness may vary from a brief fainting spell to a deep coma and it occurs when the brain is unable to function properly, either because it is not receiving enough oxygen or enough blood, or because it is injured by an accident or a disease. The main causes of unconsciousness are therefore blocked breathing, head or other injuries, heavy bleeding and shock, electric shock, lowering of blood sugar levels as in diabetes or insulin shock, heart attack, stroke, epilepsy, convulsions, or poisoning.

The vital first step is to make sure that the casualty can breathe. The greatest danger in unconsciousness is the risk of death by choking. Doctors report that more accident victims die from choking while unconscious than from their original injury. An unconscious person is unable to do anything to help himself. His tongue may fall backward and block his throat. False or knocked-out teeth may also block his breathing. Because he cannot cough, spit, or swallow, blood, vomit or even saliva may choke him. These risks are very much greater if the casualty is lying on his back. So, when you find someone unconscious, quickly check that his mouth is clear of anything that could block the air passage, lie him down and bend his head firmly backward as far as it will go. In this position the tongue cannot block the

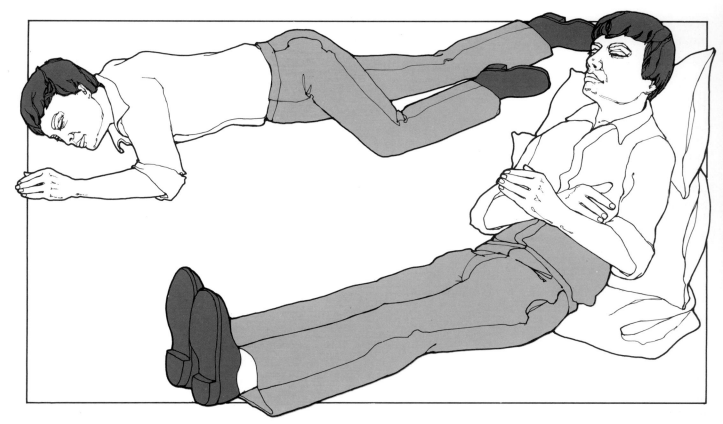

Above: coma position. **Below:** position if you feel faint.

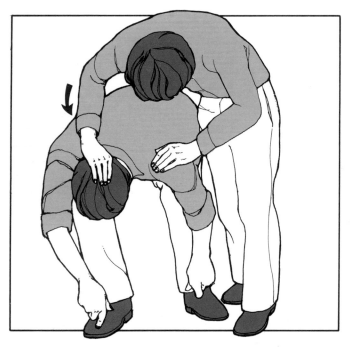

throat. If the casualty has stopped breathing, immediately start mouth-to-mouth resuscitation. Control any bleeding by direct pressure. Once you are sure that breathing has returned, place the casualty into the *coma* or *recovery* position.

This is a position that should be used for any casualty who is unconscious but breathing – unless serious injury prevents his being moved. Place the patient on his side, with the upper leg and arm bent in front of him so that he cannot roll back. In this position his head will be inclined downward. The jaw will sag forward so that the tongue cannot fall

back into the throat. Any blood, vomit, or fluid will also come forward and run safely out of his mouth. Cover the patient with a blanket or coat, and keep him in the coma position until medical help arrives. If the person cannot be moved because of injury, continue to keep the airways clear by bending the head as far back as it will go, and continue to watch the victim's breathing.

Unconsciousness that follows severe blood loss or serious injury is a sign of shock and should be treated as such (see page 309). If you are in any doubt at all about the reasons for a faint, use the same treatment as for unconsciousness. But if the cause of fainting is obvious – an emotional upset, getting up too soon after an illness, standing for too long in a crowded atmosphere, for example – simply lay the person down with his head turned to one side and his legs raised. Loosen any tight clothing and insure that he gets plenty of fresh air. As he revives, be calm and reassuring but firm in advising him to rest for a few minutes before getting up again. If he has not fully recovered within five minutes, call the doctor. Laying the patient down is always best, but if this is not possible, sit him down with his head between his knees until he recovers.

An unconscious person should never be given anything to drink. Remember, he cannot swallow. Any liquid you give him will pass into the lungs and may easily choke him.

What should you do if you find someone unconscious following an electric shock? Above all do not touch him, or you may receive the same shock. Instead immediately unplug the wire of the appliance involved, or shut off the house current switch. If this is impossible, stand on the nearest dry insulating material you can find (a thickly-folded newspaper, wood, or a large book) and drag the person away from the wire with a dry, nonconductive object, such as a broomstick, chair or shoe – do not use an umbrella, it has metal ribs. When the person is clear of the wire, you may need to begin mouth-to-mouth resuscitation and heart compression.

Sometimes a victim of a heart attack may lose consciousness. However, the majority of heart attacks are not fatal, but you must send for the doctor immediately. If he or she is not available, call an ambulance. Meanwhile, treat the patient for shock, but keep him in a sitting position, with his head and shoulders supported by pillows or cushions, so that he can breathe more easily. Try to keep him as calm as possible, reassuring him that medical help is on its way. Do not give him any medicine or drink. Watch him carefully and if he stops breathing, immediately start mouth-to-mouth resuscitation and heart compression.

A stroke causes headache, nausea, confusion, slurred speech, and sudden or gradual loss of consciousness. One side of the person's face or the limbs on one side might become paralyzed. Call an ambulance or a doctor immediately. Meanwhile make sure that the person is breathing. If not give mouth-to-mouth resuscitation until medical help arrives.

Poisoning

Dangerous poisons may include alcohol or other drugs that can be used safely in moderate doses, or substances that were never meant to be swallowed, such as corrosive chemicals, household cleansers, pesticides, poisonous berries, or bad food. The amount that causes harm varies. Ten or 12 aspirins gulped down in quick succession, could be fatal. So could nine or ten large whiskies. Less than a couple of ounces of some chemicals or poisonous fungi or berries may be highly dangerous. Children are more at risk than adults from poisoning. Four or five adult aspirin tablets (around sixteen junior aspirin) might endanger the life of a child. And even a single cigarette eaten by an infant could be fatal, as nicotine is a highly poisonous substance.

Many cases of poisoning could have been prevented. Never store poisons or corrosive chemicals in unlabeled bottles or within easy reach of children. The same applies to adult medicines which hold a fascination for many children. Keep them locked up securely in your medicine chest.

An overdose of drugs or alcohol affects the central nervous sytem. This may disrupt brain signals to the lungs until the victim stops breathing and his heart ceases to beat. Symptoms of an overdose of aspirin, tranquilizers, barbiturates (sleeping tablets), or heroin may include stomach pain and nausea, extreme sleepiness, unconsciousness, pinpointed pupils, sweating, blue skin, gasping and either deep

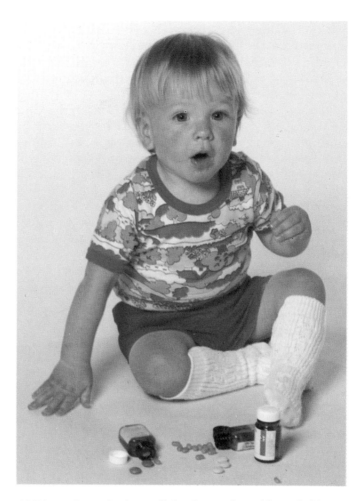

Children often mistake medicine for candy and household cleaning fluids for soft drinks. Keep all poisons clearly labeled and locked out of their way.

snoring or very rapid shallow breathing. Too much alcohol causes confusion, uncoordinated movements, enlarged pupils, and unconsciousness, and the victim will, of course, smell of drink. Remember, alcohol and barbiturates taken together are a particularly dangerous combination, each reinforcing the effect of the other. Corrosives, such as bleach, ammonia, disinfectants, and other strong acids or alkalis, burn the mouth, gullet, and stomach. Someone who has swallowed a corrosive is likely to complain of intense pain all the way down to his stomach. His lips and mouth may already be burned yellow, gray, or white, and you may be able to smell the substance on his breath. Poisonous plants and food may act directly on the food passage, causing vomiting, pain, and often diarrhea. They may also cause drowsiness or unconsciousness. Any of these symptoms should alert you to the possibility of poisoning.

Suppose you find your child playing with an open container of tablets or household chemicals. What should you do? Quickly remove any tablets that may still be in the child's mouth. If possible, calmly ask how many tablets the child has eaten. Check the container to see what he has swallowed. Then telephone your doctor or call the nearest poison control center (you should find out if there is one in your neighborhood). Remember to take the container with you to the telephone, so that you can read out the contents on the label. If you have a car, drive the child to the nearest hospital, being sure to take the container of tablets or chemicals with you, plus any vomit for analysis.

If you have to wait for medical help, then the kind of treatment you can give depends on the kind of poison that has been taken. That is why it is important to get advice from your doctor or poison control center and follow it exactly. Many of the poisons a child may swallow are not immediately harmful, and since being treated for poisoning can be very frightening, it is best left to a doctor whenever possible. However, if you have been advised to treat the child yourself, or if you have to wait as long as 10 or 15 minutes for an ambulance, you may have to take action on your own. This may mean making the child vomit, or doing all you can to prevent him vomiting, according to the substance he has swallowed.

Do not make a person vomit if he has swallowed a petroleum product or a corrosive substance (ammonia, bleach, disinfectant, drain cleaner, lye, oven cleaner, rust remover, any kind of strong acid or alkali, styptic pencil, toilet bowl cleaner, washing soda, or any other cleaning fluid, benzene, kerosene, lighter fuel, gasoline, metal or furniture polish, turpentine, spot remover, typewriter or gun cleaner, or wood preservative). Many pesticides, insecticides, and rat poisons also contain harsh acids or alkalis, so check the labels. Any of these substances burn the lining of the stomach and, if vomited, may cause further burning, or may be inhaled into the lungs with fatal results. The best way to counteract the harmful effect of these poisons is to dilute them by giving drinks of water – aim at three of four glasses, but only give the victim as much as he or she can manage. Do not try to give water if the victim is unconscious or having convulsions.

If – and only if – you are satisfied the victim has not been poisoned by a corrosive or petroleum product, try to make him vomit. This is specially advisable if he has taken aspirin, sleeping tablets, tranquilizers, or other drugs – unless he is already drowsy or unconscious. To induce vomiting, use syrup of ipecac: a bottle of this should always be in your medicine chest. Above all, do not use salt water as an emetic. If you have no ipecac, give the victim a drink of carbonated beverage, turn him over on his stomach with his head down, and put your fingers right to the back of his tongue and leave them there until he vomits. Have a basin ready, as the doctor will have to examine the vomit later. If medical help has still not arrived, repeat the process a couple more times.

If the victim is already unconscious, say from an overdose of drugs, first check to see if there is breathing. If not, give mouth-to-mouth resuscitation until medical help appears. If the victim is unconscious but still breathing, place him in the coma position, cover him with a blanket, and get him to hospital as fast as you can, together with any evidence that might identify the poison or drug taken. Do not attempt to give any fluids – these may choke and kill him. In many cases only hospital treatment will save someone who is unconscious as a result of taking an overdose of drugs.

Home Medicine Chest

A first aid kit is invaluable and every home should have one. It should be kept safely out of the reach of children, usually in a wall-mounted cupboard and in an airtight, locked box. It will be needed for minor injuries and one day may help to save a life.

Bandages. 1in wide (2 rolls); 2½in wide (2 rolls); 2in crepe (2 rolls); triangular (1).

Bandages are used for holding a dressing in position – but they should not be used without a dressing. If a wound is bleeding, the bandage should be tied tightly, but in most cases avoid bandaging so tightly that it restricts circulation.

For bandaging the foot and ankle, or the head, and for making an arm sling, triangular bandages or scarves are the most suitable. Crepe bandages will stretch to follow an artificial shape, and are used for holding a dressing, such as on the hand or foot.

Dressings. Gauze (2 packs); gauze pads (2); petroleum jelly gauze (1 pack); cottonwool (1 pack); cleansing tissues (6); assorted adhesive plasters; plaster strip (1 roll); scotch tape (1 roll).

An injury should first be cleansed with soap and water with the use of cottonwool or with cleansing tissue. Adhesive plaster is very useful to fix the free end of a bandage or to hold a dressing in place. Minor burns should be covered with petroleum jelly gauze dressings. Adhesive plaster dressings are used frequently, mostly to keep dirt out of minor cuts and scratches.

Instruments. Safety pins (6); bandage clips (3); splinter forceps; dressing scissors.

Use bandage clips or scotch tape to fix the end of a bandage without tying. Splinters are best removed with splinter forceps under a good light and possibly a magnifying glass. A triangular bandage or improvized arm sling is best fixed with safety pins. Bandages should be cut with scissors. If you are cutting off a dressing, keep the blunt-ended blade next to the skin.

Medicines. Aspirin; paracetamol; junior aspirin; travel sickness tablets; indigestion tablets or medicine; syrup of ipecac; antiseptic; calamine lotion; antidiarrhea medicine containing chlorodyne. For mild pain, take one soluble aspirin dissolved in water after food.

Junior aspirin should be given only as directed. Do not give it to a child under five without consulting your doctor, and never longer than for two days. For bites, stings, or mild sunburn, calamine lotion is usually satisfactory.

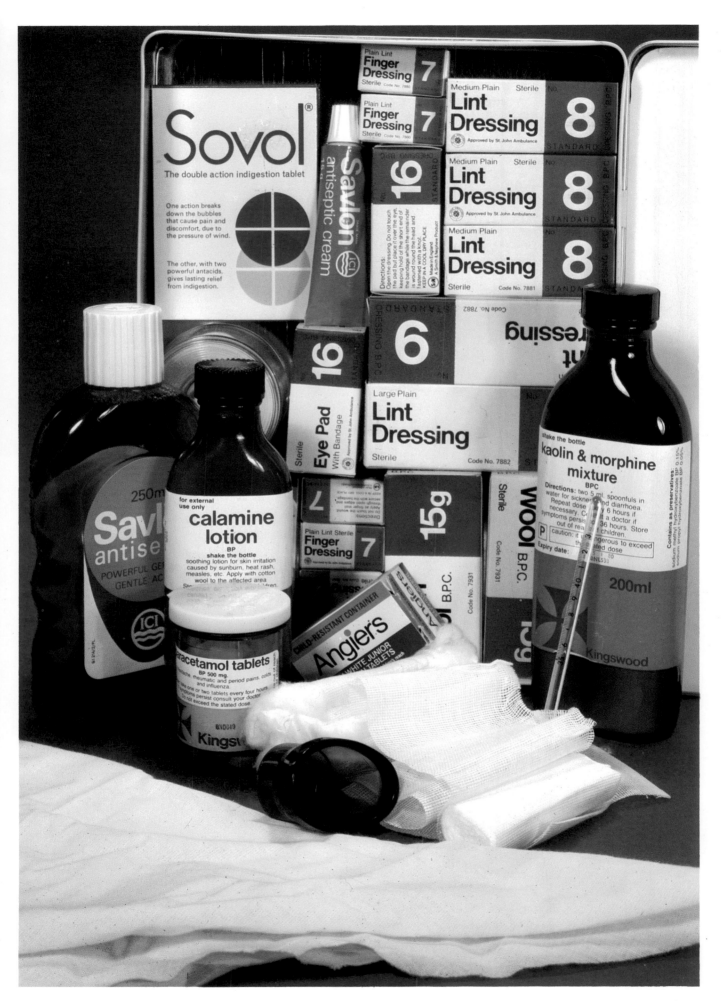

Safety in the Home

About 20 people die every day in the United Kingdom after an accident in the home or garden. Yet every one of these tragic accidents could almost certainly have been avoided. Above all it is important to be aware of the dangers that may lurk in and around your home. Such dangers are a threat to all the family, but each member, according to his age, capacity or activity in the home, may be more at risk from some hazards than from others.

More than half of all the accidents in the home are due to falls, and the majority of victims are aged 65 or more. Even minor falls can injure an old person whose bones have become frail. Usually the cause is falling down stairs. What can you do? First light all stairways and landings. In this respect two-way switches are most convenient. A handrail is a simple and important precaution. Loose or worn carpets should receive special attention and should be repaired if necessary. Many falls are due to people

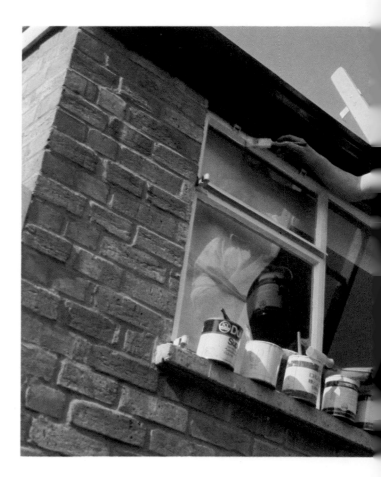

Are the electrical appliances in your home safe? Frayed protective cords should be repaired or replaced, otherwise live wires will be exposed. Unless you are sufficiently expert, have your appliances repaired professionally.

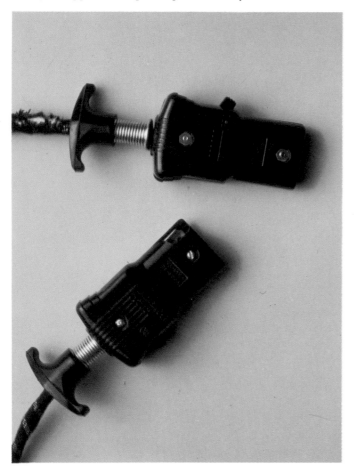

walking in stockinged feet. Wear nonslip shoes in the house at all times. Choose nonslip carpets and floor polishes. A vacuum cleaner, brushes or toys left on stairs are dangerous traps for the elderly. In winter you should beware of icy paths or broken exterior steps – these can be dangerous. Salt, ashes or sand are easy to obtain and should be sprinkled liberally as a precaution. Accidents in the bathroom can be prevented by placing a rubber mat in the tub or shower and installing hand rails by the bath and toilet.

Open windows present dangerous possibilities for children if they can be reached by a young explorer. It is therefore better to close all windows if you have to leave a young child unsupervized. Never leave a baby or small child in a cot unless the side rails are secure. To make sure a young child does not fall downstairs, safety gates should be fitted at the top and bottom of stairs.

One of the worst hazards in the home is fire. Use paraffin heaters with the greatest care, and do not move them while they are alight. If the electrical wiring in the house is old, have it inspected and renewed if it is necessary; look at the leads on appliances, particularly irons, and renew them at first signs of fraying. And see that all open fires are properly guarded.

Poisoning is a big risk for elderly people, who may get muddled over the number of sleeping tablets they have taken, misread directions on bottles or packets, or switch them from bottle to bottle. Keep them safe by labeling drugs in big, easy-to-read letters, or putting out a single dose of medicine before

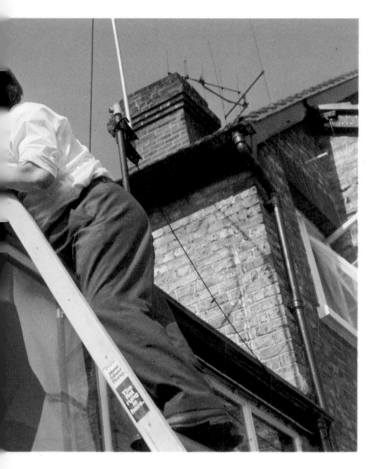

going to bed and locking the rest away. Remember, too, that all medicines should be disposed of once treatment is over.

Surprisingly, many more men than women are killed by accidents in their own homes. Such accidents as electrocution, falls off a ladder, and burns, are obviously bound to happen to men as they usually tackle any dangerous or difficult home maintenance jobs. You should always be careful if you are trying to fix an iron, to repair an oil burner, paint the ceiling, or heave an old piece of furniture down into the basement. All too often, people do these jobs in a hurry, or when they are tired or irritated at the end of a long day. This invariably results in carelessness and an inevitable accident. Many of these accidents are just unnecessary. Make sure that the ladder is safe, before you use it. If it is rickety with age, it is worth buying a new one. The same applies to broken plugs or frayed cords. Check on the safety of stairs, steps, and railings while you are cleaning the house.

It is better to get a professional to do a job for you if you feel you are not able to accomplish a necessary – or dangerous – repair in your home. Above all, it is not wise to fix something when you are tired. You have probably noticed how "accident prone" you are when you are tired or cross.

Above: many men feel pressurized to do household repairs in order to save money. However, their equipment may be old and unsafe, and they themselves may not be up to the job physically, especially at the end of the working day. It is not surprising therefore that many more men than women get killed by accidents in the home.

Below: most accidents that occur in the home are the result of fire. Keep all open fires guarded, especially when there are children around. Do not leave heated irons, connected soldering irons or open greasepans unattended. Keep matches away from children. Rubbish lying about, wooden shingles, cleaning fluids, and oil-stained rags are also fire hazards.

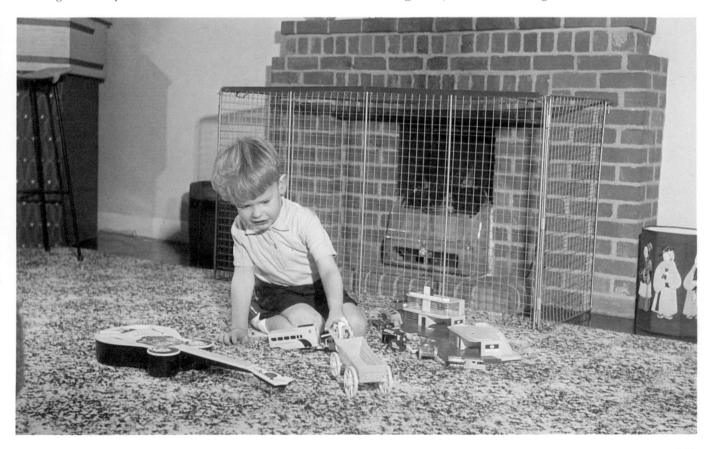

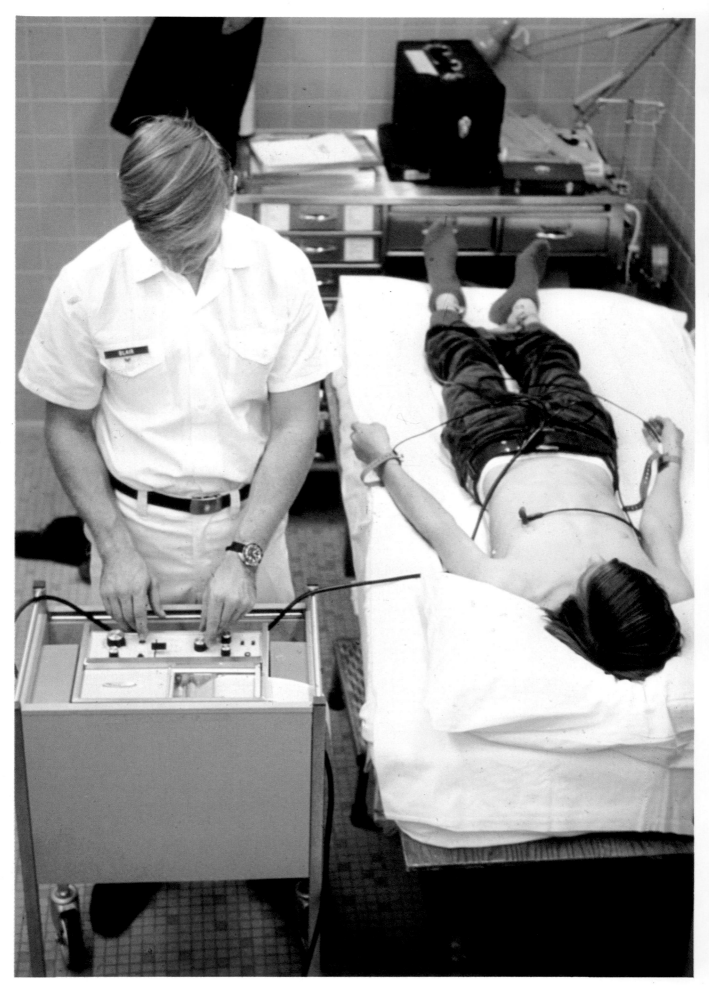

Index

Opposite: the wave pattern and frequency of the electrocardiogram will indicate abnormalities such as coronary thrombosis, cardiac muscle thickening, heart block or anatomical displacement.

References in *italics* are to captions.

A

ADH (antidiuretic hormone), 26, 29
ATP (adenine triphosphate), *14*
abdomen
  cross sectional X-ray, *250*
  palpation, 240, *240*
abortion, avoidance of, 137
accidents
  as result of carelessness, 319
  avoidance in the home, 318-19
  to young children, 158
achondroplasia, 179
acne, 185, *185*
acromegaly, 179
actin, *30, 33*
active transport, *14, 15*
adenine triphosphate (ATP), *14*
adolescence
  commitment phase, 175
  conflicts over discipline, *175*
  diet, 184, *185*
  drug addiction, 182-3
  emotional problems, 174-5
  health problems, 184-5
  incidence of anorexia nervosa, 181, *181*
  need for discussion of problems, *174*
  need for parental care, 174
  phases of development, 174-5
  physical changes, 174
  problems, 173
  variations in growth rate, *177*
adrenal medulla, 28, *29*
adrenaline, 28, *29*
afferent fibers, *31*
aging
  decreasing function of organs, *229*
  deteriorating faculties, *228*
  factors affecting, 228
  process, 228-9
  sexual activity, 126-7
  unnecessary deterioration, 220
  see also old people
aggression
  effect of regular exercise on, 211
  effect of upbringing, 191
  in children, 170
  induced by amphetamines, 183
  male trait, 202
  positive aspects, 203
  within family, 202-3
air
  intake (volume), 24
  warmed before reaching lungs, 24
albinism, 18
alcohol
  adopting sensible approach to, 183, *183*

avoidance by ulcer sufferers, 51
dangers of excess, 198
effect of excess on unborn babies, 136
effect on life expectancy, 229
factors affecting intoxication, *199*
for release from problems, *220*
intake by diabetics, 253
medical effects, 198, *198*
reduction before surgery, 266
stimulating old people's appetite, 236
symptoms of poisoning, 315
Alcoholics Anonymous, 199
alcoholism, 198-9
  treatment, 199
aldosterone, 26
alimentary canal, 22, *22*
  pinocytosis and phagocytosis, 15
  see also digestive system
alveoli, 24, *24*
amblyopia, 61
ambulances, 307
American Heart Association, blood
  pressure screening, *278*
amino acids, 10
  formation of proteins, *10, 11*
ammonia, as waste product, 26
amniocentesis, *139*
  to discover fetal abnormalities, 195, *195*
amoeba, 15, *15*
amphetamines, 183
amputation, in Middle Ages, *264*
analgesics, *290*
androgens, 116
anesthetics
  influence on surgical techniques, 264
  operating theater equipment, *270*
  "pre-med" injections, 267, 270
angina pectoris, 93
  prognosis, 103
animal foods, diet constituent, 20
anisometropia, 61
anorexia nervosa, 45, 181
antacids, 50
antibiotics, 103
antibodies, 36, 97
antidiuretic hormone (ADH), 26, 29
antigens, 36, 97
  conferring blood groupings, 97
antihistamines, sleep-inducing effect, 215
antiseptics, 264
anxiety
  "irritable colon syndrome," 53
  symptoms, 294
  treatment, 299
aphasia, 281
apoplexy *see* stroke
appendectomy, 263
appendicitis, 163, 262-3, *263*
  acute, 45
appetite, stimulation in old people, 236
art therapy, *296*

arterial circulation, 98
  of lower leg and foot, *99*
  see also blood: circulation
arteries
  development of atheroma, *103*
  effect of hypertension, *279*
  hardening, through lack of exercise, 210
  pressure points, 246
  section through, *99*
  state indicated by pulse, 247
  subject to stress, 102
  thrombus formation, *280*
arterioles, 26, 98
arteriosclerosis, 35, 102
  risk factors, 104
arthritis, 300
  maintaining independence, 303
  physical treatment, 303
  surgery, 303
  treatment, 302-3
arthrodesis, 303
arthroplasty, 303
artificial insemination, 124-5
  by donor, 125, *125*
  in cases of infertility, 122, *122*
  judging right time, 125
artificial respiration *see* resuscitation
aspirin, 316
  poisoning, 315
asthma, effect on lung capacity, 249
astigmatism, 65
atheroma, *103*
athletes, *9*
  enlarged hearts, 210, *211*
autoimmune diseases, 97
axons, *31*

B

babies
  acceptance by other children, *157*
  bathing, 148-9, *148*
  bedding, 149
  bottle feeding, 150, *150, 153*
  dangers of overfeeding, 150
  early needs, 148, *148*
  emotional needs, 156
  father's role in care, 152
  feeding requirements, 150
  influenced by parents' attitudes, 148
  learning to handle, 148, *149*
  postnatal checks, *151*
  reasons for crying, 156
  "soft spot" on skull, 157
  variety of development patterns, 157
  weight gains, 150-1
  see also children; pregnancy
backache, *292*
balance, 69, 76

326

gastric ulcers, 48-9, *49*
  bed rest useful, 51
  symptoms, 49
gastrin, 29, 48
gastritis, 44
gastrocamera, *251*
gastrointestinal tract, 22
gastroscopes, 250
genes, 10
  arrangement on chromosomes, *10*
genetic code, 10, 11
genetic counselling, 195
genetic research, 11
genetics, 12, 194-5
  effect on skin and hair condition, *218*
  Mendelian inheritance, *194*
geriatrics, 236
German measles
  dangers during pregnancy, 146
  producing congenital defects, 194
  vaccination, 167
Gesell, Arnold, 171
gigantism, 178
glands, 28
  enlargement in neck, 162
  examination, 240
  in alimentary canal, 23
  secretions to mucosa, 17
  specialized epithelia, 17
glandular fever, 162
glasses, 64
glaucoma, 59, *59*
  surgical treatment, 67
glomerulus, 26, *26*
glucose
  effect of insulin deficiency, *255*
  formation, 20
  mechanism of entry into cell, 252
glycosuria, 252
goblet cells, *53*
goiter, 194
gold salts, therapy for rheumatoid
  arthritis, 302
gonococci bacteria, *128*
gonorrhea, 128
gooseflesh, *39*
  vestigial process, 18
Gorer, Geoffrey, 189
gout, 194
granulocytes, 97
Gross, Leonard, 222
group behavior, 190
group practices, 277
growth rate
  controlled by pituitary gland,
    178-9
  in adolescence, 178
  increasing height of adults, 178
  of fetus, 178
guide dogs, 62, *63*
gums, infection, 89

H

hair, 219
  follicles, 18
  graying, 219
  keratin constituent, 18
  on the body, function, 18
Hales, Stephen, 278
hallucinations, from lack of sleep, 215
hallucinogens, 183
haustra, *52*
head
  change of shape during childhood, 178
  see also skull injuries
hearing, 55
hearing aids, 69, *75*
  for old people, 236
  types, 75
hearing defects, 70-1
  associated with other abnormalities, 72
heart
  abnormal valves, 103
  congenital malformation, 146
  defects
    associated with Down's syndrome, *197*
    encouraged by smoking, 213
  disease, 100-1
    avoidance, 104-5
    causes, 102-3
    changes in incidence pattern, 104
    deaths, 102, *102*
    surgical treatment, 111
    symptoms, 100-1
  double pumping system, 94
  examinations, 244-5
  failure due to insufficient blood flow,
    244
  increasing efficiency, 210
  length of survival without oxygen, 310
  murmurs, 245
  of heavy smoker, *105*
  pacemakers, 265
  pains associated with, 101, *101*
  posterior and anterior views, *92*
  restarting beat, 311-12
  routine investigation, 240
  section, *93*
  surgery, 270
  transplant surgery, 11, 264
  valve sounds, 245
  see also coronary thrombosis
heartbeats, 95
heart-lung machines, 265
heat
  distribution in body, *39*
  see also temperature control
hebephrenics, 296-7
height
  genetic effect, 178
  of certain tribes, *178*

see also growth rates
Heimlich manouver, 310
Hemery, David, *211*
hemiplegia
  characteristic gait, 77
  result of stroke, 280
hemoglobin, 21, 94
  effect of smoking, 212
  influence of exercise, 210
  role as oxygen transporter, 96
hemolytic jaundice, 194
hemophilia, 11, 147
Henle, loops of, *27*
hepatitis
  induced by drug injection, 183
  viral, 45
hereditary diseases, 10
  see also congenital defects: hereditary
heroin, 183
heterozygosity, 12
hobbies, *208*, 209
Hodgkin's disease, chemotherapy, 289
home, 193
homeostasis *see* osmoregulation;
  temperature control
homosexuality, changes in attitude, 130
homozygosity, 12
hormones
  effect on growth, 178-9
  female sex, 117
  function, 28
  in infertility treatment, 122
  influencing kidneys, 26
  influencing secondary sexual
    characteristics, 176
  male sex, 116
  production and excretion, 29
  production by placenta, 13
  secretions from endocrine glands, 28
  tests during pregnancy, *139*
hospitalization, patients' fears, *276*
Hughes, Robert, 180
human relationships, 190
  see also family
Huntington's chorea, 294
  progress of disease, *295*
hymen, 117
hypermetropia, 59, *59*
hypertension, 103, 278
  biofeedback technique of reducing, *279*
  causes, 279
  screening program, *278*
  treatment, 279
    following heart attack, 111
hypnosis, to induce sleep, 215
hypoglycemic coma, 253
hypotension, 279
hypothalamus
  monitoring blood constituents, 26
  role in childbirth, 28
  role in temperature control, 34

R

racial characteristics, *12*
  of skin, 18
radiation therapy, *284*
radioactive substances
  use in diagnosis, 258
radioactivity, cancer link, *286*
radiotherapy for cancer, 288
Ranvier, nodes of, 30
"reading" machines, *63*
receptors
  in the eye, 56, 57
  indicating pain, 290
rectum, 23
referred pain, 291
reflexes, *240*, 241
relaxation, *137*
  aided by exercise, 207
  as aid to fitness, 107
renal artery, 26
renal vein, 26
respiration, 24
  by embryo, 13
  routine investigation, 240
  see also breathing
respiratory infections, 160
rest
  during illness, 168
  during pregnancy, 136
  influencing health, 206
  see also bed rest
resuscitation, 306-7, 310-12
  equipment, *272*
  in cases of unconsciousness, 314
  in drug overdose cases, 316
  mouth-to-mouth, 310-11
  priorities, 310
reticuloblastoma, 59
retina, 56, *57*
  detachment, 67, *67*
retirement, 230-1
  benefits and problems, *230, 231*
  economic factors, 230-1
  individual response, 231
  influence on lifestyle, 231
  preparation, 231
rheumatic fever, 103
rheumatism, 300
  incidence, 300
rheumatoid arthritis, 300, *300*
  New York City study, 200
rhodopsin, 57
rhythm method of contraception, 121
ribonucleic acid (RNA), *11*
ribosomes, 10, *11*
rickets, 21, 194
ringworm, 160
Rinné's test, *74*
road accidents among children, 160

prevalence among teenagers, 184
Royal Canadian Air Force exercise
  program, 107
rubella *see* German measles
Ruffini, organs of, *35*

S

safety at home, 318-19
saliva
  to break down food, 42
salivary glands, 23, 47, *47*
salmonella infection, 52
salt
  body's requirements, 21
  concentration controlled by kidneys, 26
scabies, 19
scalds, 313
scanners, *275*
  use in diagnosis, 242, 258-9, *259*
  use in tumor diagnosis, *285*
schizophrenia, 296
  treatment, 299
school age children
  development of speech disorders, 78, *79*
  liability to infections, 160
  problems of adjustment, *171*
scratches, first aid treatment, 309
scrotum, 116
scurvy, 21
sea-sickness pills, sleep-inducing effect, 215
sebacious glands
  at puberty, 18
  on scalp, 219
secretory cells, 16
semen, 116
  following vasectomy, 122
  nocturnal emissions, 177
  preservation for artificial
    insemination, *124*
semicircular canals, 69
  role in balance, 76
Semmelweis, Ignaz, 264
senile gait, 77
sex
  capacity retained in later life, *126-7*
  changes in attitudes, 130
  commercial exploitation, 130
  compatability, *112*
  during pregnancy, 137
  education, *176*
  female sexuality, 114-15, *115*
  inducing sleep, 215
  in later life, 126-7
  influence of physical fitness, 209
  operations to change, 116-17
  phases of lovemaking, 118-19
  possible basis of anorexia, 181, *181*
  relief of stress, 109

role expectations, *190*
secondary characteristics, development
  of, 176, 177
taboos, 118
teenage sexuality, *173*
see also venereal disease
sex chromosomes, 12
sex-linked defects, 195
sex of offspring, determination, 12
sex organs
  female, 117
  male, 118
sexual response, 118-19
Sexual Revolution, 130
shivering, 35
shock
  first aid treatment, 309
  following blood loss, 308
  following burns or scalds, 313
  need for urgent medical care, 309
sight, 55
  see also eyes
skeletal muscle, 16
skeletal pain, 291
skeleton, 32-3
  function, 32
  protecting organ, 36
skin, 17, 18-19
  abnormalities, link with deafness, 71
  barrier against infection, 19, 36
  disorders, 19
    in children, 160
  effects of diet, 218
  excessive exposure to sun, 219, *219*
  factors affecting texture, 218
functions, 18
  pores, *35*
  premature aging, 218
  psychological aspects of harm, 18
  receptors, *35*
  sensations, routine testing, 241
  structure, 18, *19*
  teenage problems, *184, 185*
  variations with age and sex, 18, *18*
skull injuries, 312
sleep, 214-15
  differing requirements of children, 170
  purposes, 214-15
  varying requirements for adults, 215
sleep treatment, 299
sleeping pills, 215, *215*
  before surgery, 267
  problems for old people, 237
slimming diets, 180
small intestine, inflammation, 52
  see also intestines
smallpox, 167
smell, related to taste, 42
"smoker's cough," 213
smoking *see* cigarette smoking
social behavior, 190

Picture Credits

Key to picture positions: (T) top; (C) center;
(B) bottom; and in combinations, e.g. (TR)
top right; (BL) bottom left, etc.

Endpapers   Henry Grant, A.I.I.P.,
            London.
8   Colorsport
10(L)   Biophoto Associates
10(R)   Gene Cox
11(T)   Fratelli Fabbri Editori
11(B)   Brookhaven National
            Laboratory
12(T)   *Sunday Times* Colour
            Library
12(B)   C. James Webb
13(T)   David Cox © Aldus Books
13(B)   C. James Webb
14   Fratelli Fabbri Editori
15(L)   Biophoto Associates
15(R)   Photomicrograph Dr.
            Gordon F. Leedale, Leeds
            University
16(T)   C. James Webb
16(B)   Sidney W. Woods © Aldus
            Books
17(T)   Gene Cox
17(B)   Biophoto Associates
18   Patrick Thurston/*Daily
            Telegraph* Colour Library
19   Fratelli Fabbri Editori
20   © Aldus Books
21   Alan Hutchison Library
22(L)   David Cox © Aldus Books
22(R)   Sidney W. Woods © Aldus
            Books
23   Biophoto Associates
24   Gene Cox
25   Fratelli Fabbri Editori
26   Biophoto Associates
27   Fratelli Fabbri Editori
28   Jon Kenny © Aldus Books
29(T)   *Daily Telegraph* Colour
            Library
29(B)   C. James Webb
30(T)   Gene Cox
30(B)   Fratelli Fabbri Editori
31(T)   Camera Press
31(B)   Biophoto Associates
32   Fratelli Fabbri Editori
33(T)   © Aldus Books
33(B)   Biophoto Associates
34(T)   Ken Moreman
34(B)   Central Office of
            Information. British Crown
            Copyright
35(L)   Gene Cox
35(R)   Gene Cox
36-37(B)   Fratelli Fabbri Editori
37(T)   Gene Cox
38   © Aldus Books
39(T)   Z.E.F.A.
39(B)   Natural History
            Photographic Agency
40   Pictor International
43(T)   Dr. Gordon F. Leedale,
            Leeds University
43(B)   Fratelli Fabbri Editori
44   Sidney W. Woods © Aldus
            Books

45(T)   C. James Webb
45(B)   Gene Cox
46, 47(T)   © Aldus Books
47(B)   Biophoto Associates
48   Mike Busselle © Aldus
            Books
49(T)   Biophoto Associates
49(B)   Ken Moreman
50   Mike Busselle and Richard
            Hatswell © Aldus Books
51(T)   Ken Moreman
51(B)   Olympus Optical
            Company Ltd.
52(L)   Sidney W. Woods © Aldus
            Books
52(R), 53   Biophoto Associates
54   Picturepoint, London
56   Sidney W. Woods © Aldus
            Books
57(L)   Gene Cox
57(R), 58(T) Fratelli Fabbri Editori
58(B), 59(T) Institute of Ophthalmology
59(B)   Fratelli Fabbri Editori
60(T)   Sidney W. Woods © Aldus
            Books
60(B)   Central Office of
            Information. British Crown
            Copyright
62   Royal National Institute for
            the Blind
63(T)   Camera Press
63(B)   Keystone
64   Central Office of
            Information. British Crown
            Copyright
65(T)   Camera Press
65(B)   Central Office of
            Information. British Crown
            Copyright
66, 67(T)   Institute of Ophthalmology
67(B)   B.B.C. © photograph
68   Fratelli Fabbri Editori
69   Gene Cox
70   Mr. N. Shah
71(T)   © Aldus Books
71(B)   after Leo L. Beranek, *Noise*.
            © December, 1966 by
            Scientific American, Inc.
            All rights reserved
72   C. James Webb
73(T)   Sidney W. Woods © Aldus
            Books
73(B), 74   Mr. N. Shah
75(T)   Robert Bosch GmbH
75(B)   Central Office of
            Information. British Crown
            Copyright
76(L)   Biophoto Associates
76(R)   Jon Kenny © Aldus Books
77   Biophoto Associates
78   Syndication International
79(T)   *Sunday Telegraph*
79(B)   Henry Grant, A.I.I.P.,
            London
80   Syndication International
82(T)   Fratelli Fabbri Editori
82(B), 83(T) Royal Dental Hospital,
            courtesy of Dr. Graham

            Roberts
83(B)   Fratelli Fabbri Editori
84-85   Royal Dental Hospital
86(T)   Picturepoint, London
86(B), 87   Gibbs Oral Hygiene Service
88(T)   Biophoto Associates
88(B)   Fratelli Fabbri Editori
89   Royal Dental Hospital
90   Pictor International
92, 93(T)   Fratelli Fabbri Editori
93(B)   Central Office of
            Information. British Crown
            Copyright
94(L)   Sidney W. Woods © Aldus
            Books, after *Scientific
            American*, May, 1957
94(R)   Biophoto Associates
95(L)   Sidney W. Woods © Aldus
            Books, after *Scientific
            American*, May, 1957
95(R)   © Aldus Books
96   C. James Webb
97   Biophoto Associates
98(T)   C. James Webb
98(B)   Fratelli Fabbri Editori
99(T)   Gene Cox
99(B)   Ken Moreman
100-101   Mary Tomlin © Aldus
            Books, after *Reader's Digest*,
            November, 1973. © 1973
            by The Reader's Digest
            Assoc., Inc.
102   © Aldus Books
103   Biophoto Associates
104   Ken Moreman
105(T)   Lennart Nilsson. *Life*,
            1968 © Time Inc.
105(B)   © Aldus Books
106(T)   Mike Busselle © Aldus
            Books
106(B), 107 Health Education Council
108(T)   Mike Busselle © Aldus
            Books
108(B)   Mike Busselle and Richard
            Hatswell © Aldus Books
109   Hallinan/FPG
110   Central Office of
            Information. British Crown
            Copyright
111(L)   World Health Organization,
            courtesy C. James Webb
111(R)   John Moss/Colorific!
112   Pictor International
114   Camera Press
115(L)   Monty Coles © Marshall
            Cavendish Ltd.
115(R)   Robert McFarlane ©
            Marshall Cavendish Ltd.
116-117   Alan Holingbery © Aldus
            Books
118   Mike Busselle © Aldus
            Books
119(T)   © Aldus Books
119(B), 120(B) Mike Busselle © Aldus
            Books
122   C. James Webb
123   Alan Holingbery © Aldus
            Books

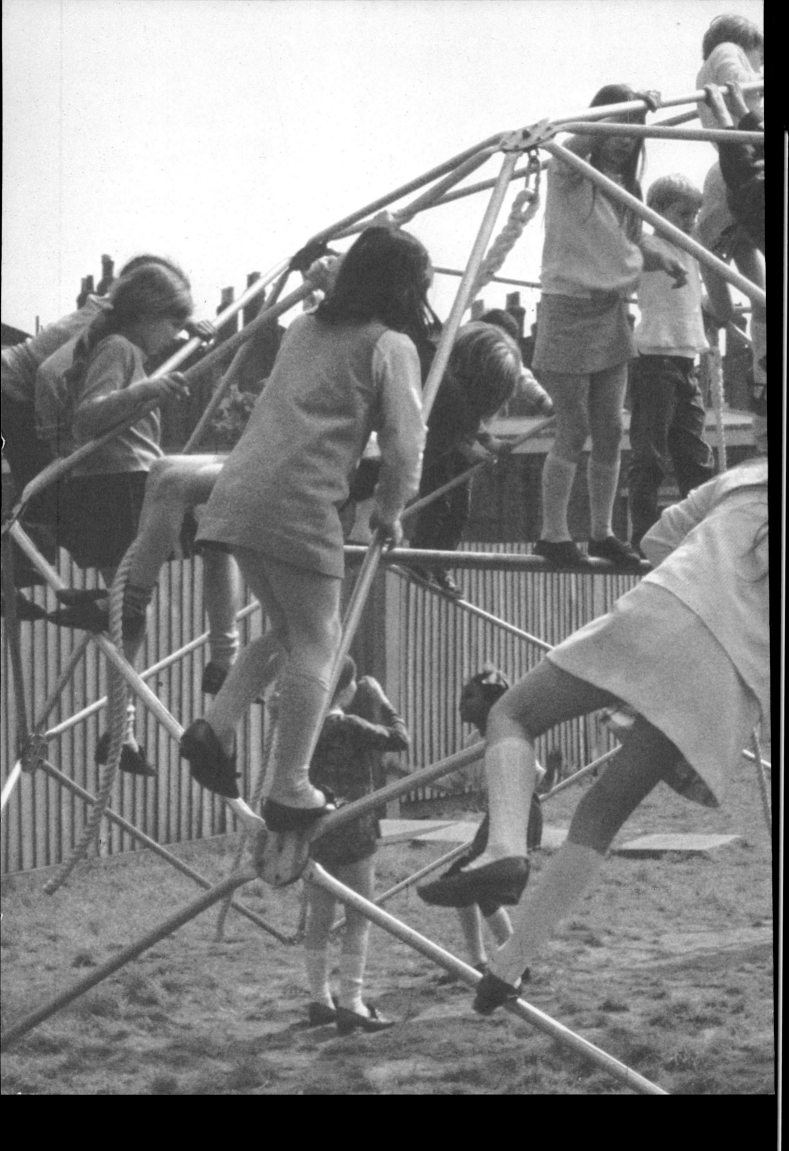